Second Edition

Radiographic Pathology

Second Edition

Radiographic Pathology

TerriAnn Linn-Watson, M.Ed., ARRT (R, M), CRT (R, M, F), MTRT

Professor, Radiologic Technology Program
Montana State University, Billings
City College
Billings, Montana

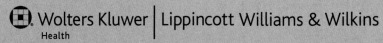
Wolters Kluwer | Lippincott Williams & Wilkins
Health
Philadelphia • Baltimore • New York • London
Buenos Aires • Hong Kong • Sydney • Tokyo

Publisher: Angus McDonald
Acquisitions Editor: Michael Nobel
Senior Product Manager: Amy Millholen
Production Product Manager: Priscilla Crater
Design Coordinator: Stephen Druding
Marketing Manager: Shauna Kelley
Compositor: Integra Software Services Pvt. Ltd
Printer: RR Donnelley Asia

Second Edition

351 West Camden Street   Two Commerce Square
Baltimore, MD 21201   2001 Market Street
                           Philadelphia, PA 19103

Printed in China

Library of Congress Cataloging-in-Publication Data
Linn-Watson, TerriAnn, author.
  Radiographic pathology / TerriAnn Linn-Watson. — Second edition.
     p. ; cm.
  Includes bibliographical references and index.
  ISBN 978-1-4511-1214-6
  I. Title.
  [DNLM: 1. Radiography—methods.   2. Pathology—methods. WN 200]
  RC78
  616.07'57—dc23

                                                        2013028819

DISCLAIMER
Care has been taken to confirm the accuracy of the information present and to describe generally accepted practices. However, the authors, editors, and publisher are not responsible for errors or omissions or for any consequences from application of the information in this book and make no warranty, expressed or implied, with respect to the currency, completeness, or accuracy of the contents of the publication. Application of this information in a particular situation remains the professional responsibility of the practitioner; the clinical treatments described and recommended may not be considered absolute and universal recommendations.

The publishers have made every effort to trace the copyright holders for borrowed material. If they have inadvertently overlooked any, they will be pleased to make the necessary arrangements at the first opportunity.

To purchase additional copies of this book, call our customer service department at (800) 638-3030 or fax orders to (301) 223-2320. International customers should call (301) 223-2300.
Visit Lippincott Williams & Wilkins on the Internet:
http://www.lww.com. Lippincott Williams & Wilkins customer service representatives are available from 8:30 am to 5:00 pm, EST.

10 9 8 7 6 5 4 3 2 1

RRS1310

This book is dedicated to the people who have made such a positive difference in my life this past year:

Kendrick, Kelly, Thomas, Christopher, and J.J. Watson
Kamden Watson
Jack Ryan
Tom And Carolyn Flaherty
Father Denis Keane
Dr. Allen and Jeanette Hill
Karla Uledalen

A special dedication to my mother Christen W. Linn
In memory of my father, Leslie L. Linn

A course that presents the most commonly seen pathologies that radiographers will be imaging should be an integral part of the core curriculum of every student radiographer's education. Understanding how the pathology occurs and recognizing the appearance on the diagnostic image will allow the technologist to aid the physician by adjusting images or patient positioning to best demonstrate the disease process. This ability makes the technologist invaluable to the diagnostic team.

Hallmarks of the Second Edition

As quickly as one edition of a textbook in this field is completely rewritten and published, the ARRT and ASRT revise and expand the curriculum for the profession. In an effort to impress upon the student of radiologic technology the importance of lifelong learning and professionalism and in an effort to ease the time constraints on the educator, this second edition has been largely expanded to be in line with the newest curriculum guidelines.

The chapters have been reordered to flow more in line with a semester as it advances from the basic to the more complex pathology. More radiographic images have been added to enhance the student's understanding of his or her role in providing quality images with which to help the radiologist make a diagnosis. Images of both normal and abnormal processes have been presented when the pathology is more subtle to the untrained eye. Modality images have been included to increase the awareness of the complementary roles that all modalities present with each other. Questions at the end of appropriate chapters are useful for guiding discussion to help the student critically think about the pathologies presented. The bulleted chapter summary, "Recap," is an extremely student-friendly format for reviewing the important and salient points presented in the chapter. Finally, the "Tech Tip" feature highlights something that the student should remember as important to either the obtaining of a diagnostic radiograph or things to look for on a radiographic image to help determine the next step in the process. Only the pathologies that should be recognized by the technologist are presented, making the material easier and more interesting to study.

I am very excited to bring this long-awaited second edition to radiologic technology students and instructors. The publishers and I feel that the improvements will significantly enhance the learning curve of the student and turn the question "Why do I have to learn pathology?" into "Wow, I know what that is and I am only a student! How cool is that?!"

TerriAnn Linn-Watson, M.Ed., ARRT (R, M),
CRT (R, M, F), MTRT

User's Guide

This User's Guide shows you how to the put the features of *Radiographic Pathology, Second Edition*, to work for you.

Goals and Objectives

Each chapter begins with Goals and Objectives that clearly outline the types of information students should expect to learn while reading and completing the activities of the chapter.

● Goals

1. To review the basic terminology related to general principles of pathology

    OBJECTIVE: Define the basic terms related to pathology

2. To learn the difference between structural and functional diseases

    OBJECTIVE: Define functional disease and give examples

    OBJECTIVE: Define structural disease and explain its formation

Key Terms

Following the Goals and Objectives, there is a list of Key Terms for the chapter. Key Terms are also bold at first mention in the chapter and defined in the Glossary.

● Key Terms

Abscess
Altered tissue growth
Anoxia
Atrophy
Benign neoplasm
Congenital
Congestion

Case Studies

Case Studies provide real-life applicability to obtaining and evaluating images of pathologic conditions.

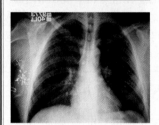

Congenital Anomalies

Case Study

This 21-year-old patient was brought into the emergency department approximately 1 AM. A chest radiograph was ordered. The technologist marked the image with his initials, the date, the fact that it was an upright image and a 40L next to the upright arrow. The radiologist read this out as a gun shot wound (GSW) to the right axillary area. It was discovered the following morning that the report was incorrect. The patient had been shot on the left side. Yet that is the opposite side of the heart's apex. Looking closely at the heart and the diaphragm it can be seen that there is air in the stomach below the heart. If the patient was truly shot on the left side (as was confirmed by visual inspection of the patient in the operating suite) then this patient has the condition known as situs inversus.

Congenital heart disease is a broad term and includes a wide range of diseases and conditions. These diseases can affect the formation of the heart muscle or its chamber or valves. Some congenital heart defects may be apparent right at the time of birth, while others may not be detected until later in life. Only the most common congenital defects are described here. Although the radiographer should be familiar with the various conditions that can be seen on a chest radiograph, it is not the intent here to cover areas that are rarely seen, or that only a physician can determine from advanced years of study.

Coarctation of the aorta is severe narrowing of the aorta (Fig. 8-8) that causes the left ventricle of the heart to suffer an increase in workload in order to push blood through a narrow passageway. The seriousness of the defect depends on the location of the constriction. If the narrowing is severe enough or complete, anastomotic vessels develop in an attempt to compensate

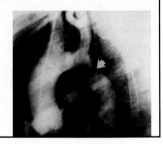

Tech Tips

Throughout the chapters, Tech Tips highlight important information related to obtaining a diagnostic radiograph and things to look for on a radiographic image to help determine the next step in the process.

TECH TIP

Assess the patient and the radiographic order. If the process reduces body or organ mass, decrease the kVp; if the process adds to the body tissue be sure to increase the kVp. Changing the mAs is not correct and changes the patient dose delivered. The kVp changes the penetration of tissue.

Recap

A bulleted summary provides a quick review of important chapter content.

RECAP

Anatomy
- Circulatory system
  - Heart has two atria (base) and two ventricles (apex)
  - Four valves that are important
    - Mitral valve is the left arterioventricular, also called bicuspid
    - Tricuspid valve is the right arterioventricular
    - Aortic semilunar valve is between the aorta and left ventricle
    - Pulmonary valve is between the pulmonary trunk and right ventricle
  - Vessels
    - Aorta is the major artery
    - Inferior vena cava is the major vein
    - Arteries become arterioles, then capillaries, then venules, and finally veins
- Lymphatic system
  - The major organs are the spleen, thymus, and tonsils and adenoids
  - Lymph vessels begin as lymph capillaries and are known as lymphatics
  - Lymphatics are the collecting vessels
  - Lymph nodes are found in the path of the lymphatics and are the filters

- Blood picks up oxygen from capillaries around alveoli and returns to the left atrium via the pulmonary veins
  - Systemic circulation
    - Blood flow is from left atrium through the mitral valve into the left ventricle
    - From left ventricle through the aortic valve and into the aorta to the body
    - Three branches off of the aortic arch send blood to upper body, while the rest goes to lower body
    - Blood gives off oxygen when in the capillaries of the tissues
  - Portal circulation
    - Blood of the abdominal digestive organs go through the portal circulation to be detoxified
    - After portal circulation, the blood goes to the right atrium for pulmonary circulation
- Lymphatic system
  - Plays a major role in immunity by
    - Producing lymphocytes and antibodies
    - Initiating phagocytosis
    - Producing blood when other ways are compromised

Critical Thinking Discussion Questions

Each chapter concludes with Critical Thinking Discussion Questions to guide discussion and help students think critically about the pathologies presented in the chapter.

 CRITICAL THINKING DISCUSSION QUESTIONS

1. Describe blood flow in the pulmonary circulation. Describe blood flow in the systemic circulation.

2. Explain "rib-notching." What causes it and when does it occur?

3. What are left-to-right shunts? How do the lungs become overloaded with blood in a shunt? What is the shunt flow from left to right? Explain fully the three major types of left-to-right shunts. Be sure to include their names, where they occur, where the blood flows, what the shunt causes, and what the radiographic appearance is.

4. Describe tetralogy of Fallot. What must exist for this condition to occur? What does this combination of defects cause? What type of shunt is produced with this condition? This condition is the most common cause of "blue baby." Why?

5. List and describe the appearance of the three types of aneurysms. What is the danger of an aneurysm?

6. What is congestive heart failure (CHF)? What causes it? What happens to the heart in left-sided heart failure? What happens to the heart in right-sided heart failure? What is the radiographic appearance of each?

7. What is pericardial effusion? What causes it? When should this condition be suspected? What modality is best suited for pericardial effusion? Why is it the best?

8. How is hypertension related to atherosclerosis?

9. What are the complications of one or more episodes of rheumatic fever?

10. What causes subacute bacterial endocarditis? What is a predisposing factor?

Clinical and Radiographic Characteristics of Common Pathologies Table

Found in each of the systems chapters, this table lists common pathologic conditions, along with the causal factors, manifestations, and radiographic appearance.

Bonus Ancillary Materials on **the**Point

Student Resources include Chapter Outlines, Student PowerPoints, and Image Bank.

Instructor Resources include PowerPoints, Lesson Plans, Test Generator, Key Terms and Concepts, Image Bank, Answers to Text Questions, and Answers to Workbook.

CLINICAL AND RADIOGRAPHIC CHARACTERISTICS OF COMMON PATHOLOGIES

Pathologic Condition	Causal Factors to Include Age, if Relevant	Manifestations	Radiographic Appearance
Atherosclerosis	As early as the 20s High cholesterol	Narrowing of vessel	A slight increase in opacity but not due to calcium
Arteriosclerosis	Elderly Latter stages of atherosclerosis	Hardening of vessel wall	Calcification of the vessel wall
Coarctation of aorta	Congenital Narrowing of aorta	Hypertension or hypotension	Rib-notching
Atrial septal defect	Congenital	Frequent pulmonary infections	Enlarged right atrium and ventricle
Ventricular septal defect	Congenital	Heart murmur	Enlarged left atrium and ventricle
Patent arterial duct	Congenital	Asymptomatic	Enlarged left atrium and ventricle
Tetralogy of Fallot	Congenital	Cyanosis	Coeur en sabot
Aneurysms Saccular Fusiform Dissecting	Any age Weakened vessel wall Tear in vessel wall	Usually asymptomatic	Localized ballooning Uniform dilation Diffuse enlargement
Arteriosclerotic heart disease	Hypertension	Dyspnea	Calcification, cardiomegaly
Congestive heart failure (CHF)	Any age (elderly) Hypertension	Easy fatigue	Cephalization, cardiomegaly
Pericardial effusion	Any age Tuberculosis Virus infection	Usually asymptomatic	Rapid increase in heart size
Rheumatic heart disease	Unknown	Endocarditis	Calcified mitral valve, Kerley B lines

Reviewers

Steve Forshier, M.Ed., RT(R)

Clinical Director
Pima Medical Institute
Tucson, Arizona

Michael Giovanniello, Ph.D.

Program Manager
Broward College
Davie, Florida

Robyn J. Potter, MS, RT (R)(M)

Program Director of Radiology
Bluegrass Community and Technical College
Lexington, Kentucky

Deena Slockett, MBA, RT(R)(M)

Associate Professor
Florida Hospital College of Health Sciences
Orlando, Florida

Angie Wilson, M.Ed.

Assistant Professor
St. Phillip's College
San Antonio, Texas

Acknowledgments

My greatest thanks go to Amy Millholen, Senior Product Manager, for helping me get through this very long endeavor and keeping me on track. You gave me much encouragement. Also, Jonathan Dimes, the artist, worked wonders and made excellent suggestions for the artwork and radiographic images used in the text. To the two of you, thank you!

I also wish to thank the reviewers for their input and suggestions to improve the text and student and instructor ancillaries.

Finally, the 2011 graduates from the Radiologic Technology Program at Chaffey College in Alta Loma, California, are to be thanked for their encouragement and submission of images of pathology for me to use as images in this text.

Table of Contents

The Pathologic Process

● Goals

1. To review the basic terminology related to general principles of pathology

   OBJECTIVE: Define the basic terms related to pathology

2. To learn the difference between structural and functional diseases

   OBJECTIVE: Define functional disease and give examples

   OBJECTIVE: Define structural disease and explain its formation

3. To learn the causes of diseases

   OBJECTIVE: List and define the causes of disease

4. To become familiar with the different types of injury and inflammation

   OBJECTIVE: Describe acute and chronic injury

5. To recognize the different types of growth disturbances

   OBJECTIVE: Explain growth disturbances and give examples of benign and malignant types

6. To review the types of tissue

   OBJECTIVE: List the different types of fundamental tissues and give examples

7. To learn the process of repair and healing

   OBJECTIVE: Explain the various aspects of inflammation and how inflammation aids in repair

● Key Terms

Abscess
Altered tissue growth
Anoxia
Atrophy
Benign neoplasm
Congenital
Congestion
Degeneration
Diagnosis
Differentiation
Disease
Embolus
Endogenous
Etiology
Exogenous
Exudate
Frequency
Functional disease
Grading
Growth disturbance
Hereditary
Hyperplasia
Hypertrophy
Hypoxia
Iatrogenic

● Goals *continued*

OBJECTIVE: Identify complications connected with the repair and replacement of tissue

8. To understand the different types of malignancies and how they are spread

   OBJECTIVE: Name the different types of cancer and what it affects

   OBJECTIVE: Describe how metastasis occurs

9. To determine how the pathology might affect the radiographic image

   OBJECTIVE: Describe the relevance of pathologic conditions to radiologic procedures

● Key Terms *continued*

Idiopathic
Incidence
Infarct
Infections
Inflammation
Invasion
Ischemia
Lesions
Malignant neoplasm
Manifestations
Metaplasia
Metastasis
Morbidity rate
Mortality rate
Necrosis
Neoplasia
Nosocomial
Pathogenesis
Pathology
Phagocytosis
Prevalence
Procedures
Prognosis
Purulent
Signs
Staging
Structural disease
Sublethal cell injury
Suppurative inflammation
Symptoms
Tests
Thrombus
Transudate
Trauma

An understanding of basic principles of pathology and an awareness of the radiographic appearances of specific diseases are essential goals in the training of a radiologic technologist. A technologist is aided in the selection of proper technical factors and in determining the need for a repeat radiograph when the disease process is fully understood. Many types of diseases exist, and many conditions can be demonstrated radiographically. The role of the radiologic technologist is to display visually the changes in normal anatomy and tissue density that are caused by disease.

Before the various components of disease processes and healing mechanisms can be fully understood, a review of basic terminology is required. A good foundation in medical terminology will be most helpful in digesting the somewhat difficult information presented in this and following chapters.

Definitions and Terminology

Pathology is, in the broadest sense, the study of disease processes. What then is **disease**? Disease is any abnormal change in the function or structure within the body. It is a morbid process, usually having specific characteristic symptoms and, in some cases, physical signs. A disease can primarily affect one or more organs, or it can target one organ and affect another one secondarily.

Pathology is also concerned with the sequence of events that leads from the cause of a disease to abnormalities and finally to the manifestations. This sequence of events that makes a disease apparent is called **pathogenesis**. **Etiology** is the study of the cause of a disease and is often misused as a synonym for the actual cause of a disease. Diseases that have no known cause are said to be **idiopathic**.

When the pathogenesis of a disease allows one to determine the actual disease, a **diagnosis** occurs. Once a diagnosis is made and the condition is fully assessed, the physician is now able to make a **prognosis**, that is, a prediction of the course of the disease and the prospects for the patient's recovery. In order to make a diagnosis and prognosis, a number of factors are considered. Clinical **manifestations** may point to a specific diagnosis. **Signs** are objective manifestations that are physically observed by a health-care professional. A mass, rash, or abnormal pulse rate is an example of a sign. **Symptoms** are the patient's perception of the disease, such as headache and abdominal pain. Symptoms are subjective, and only the patient can identify them.

If clinical manifestations are not adequate to make a diagnosis, the patient is evaluated by various **procedures**, such as a barium enema or a gall bladder ultrasound. An analysis of specimens taken from the patient, such as blood and excrement, can also help determine the disease process. These are known as **tests**.

All disease processes are measured as statistical data to help in the etiology of a disease and to help the Center for Disease Control map patterns of the occurrence of diseases. These measurements are frequency, incidence, and prevalence. **Frequency** is the rate of occurrence of a pathologic process that is measured over a given period of time, normally 1 year. **Incidence** is the number of newly diagnosed cases of a disease in 1 year. **Prevalence** is the number of people who have any given disease at any given point in time. Two other measurements are used: **morbidity rate** refers to the ratio of sick to well persons in a given area, and **mortality rate** is the ratio of actual deaths to expected deaths.

Radiographically, it is important to understand the disease process and its impact on the surrounding body tissues. Alterations in body tissue will most definitely alter the technical aspect of the normal radiograph and should not present a challenge to the technologist who understands that impact. If the disease process adds more tissues (tumors, masses, and edema), then the process is considered *additive* and the technical factors must be increased to penetrate the extra tissue. However, if the disease destroys tissue, such as osteoporosis and emphysema, it is considered to be a *destructive* process and the technical factors must be adjusted for less penetration. A sound understanding of these two types of processes will greatly alleviate a technologist's frustration when multiple images are necessary to adequately demonstrate a pathological condition.

Consideration for the patient's needs and comfort is much easier when the technologist has an understanding of the disease process that the patient is experiencing. A patient in end-stage renal failure will be experiencing multiple symptoms that a technologist might not be able to actually see. However, if the technologist is aware of the complications and impact of end-stage renal disease, the patient becomes more than just the next procedure that has to be completed before the end of the shift.

TECH TIP

Assess the patient and the radiographic order. If the process reduces body or organ mass, decrease the kVp; if the process adds to the body tissue be sure to increase the kVp. Changing the mAs is not correct and changes the patient dose delivered. The kVp changes the penetration of tissue.

Classification of Diseases

All diseases of the body are produced by an alteration either in structure or in function of an organ or system. Since disease is an abnormal change within the body, the two classifications of diseases are structural and functional.

Structural disease, also known as **organic** disease, involves physical and biochemical changes within the cell. These changes are known as **lesions**. For a disease to be considered of a structural nature, the organ involved must be altered in some way as to present a pathologic entity. Three broad categories classify most structural disease, although some diseases fall into more than one category and some are difficult to classify.

Genetic and *developmental* diseases are caused by abnormalities in the genetic makeup of the individual or abnormalities due to changes in utero. The range of abnormalities in this category is very broad, extending from deformities present at birth, known as **congenital** abnormalities, to changes caused by genes but influenced by the environment so that they are not manifested until later in life. **Hereditary** diseases result from developmental disorders genetically transmitted

from either parent to the child and are derived from ancestors.

Acquired injuries and *inflammatory diseases* are diseases caused by internal or external agents that destroy cells or cause the body to injure itself by means of inflammatory processes. External agents of injury include physical and chemical substances and microbes. The major internal mechanisms of injury are vascular insufficiency, immunologic reactions, and metabolic disturbances. **Necrosis** occurs when the direct effects of an injury kill the cells in the injured area. Any injury to a cell that does not cause the cell to die is known as a **sublethal cell injury**. Also known as **degeneration**, this is the initial cell response following injury. An **inflammatory** disease results from the body's reaction to a localized injurious agent. Types of inflammatory diseases include infective diseases, toxic diseases, and allergic diseases.

Hyperplasia and *neoplasia* are categories used to describe diseases characterized by increases in cell populations. **Hyperplasia** is a proliferative reaction to a prolonged external stimulus and usually regresses when the stimulus is removed. **Neoplasia** is presumed to result from a genetic change that produces a single population of new cells, which can proliferate beyond the degree that is considered normal. Both hyperplasia and neoplasia are discussed later in the chapter.

Functional diseases are those diseases in which the function of the organ may be impaired, but its structural elements are unchanged. The basic change is a physiologic or functional one and is referred to as a pathophysiologic change. The onset begins without the presence of any lesions, such as those diseases triggered by psychic or psycho-physiologic factors. Many mental illnesses are considered functional disorders. The most common functional disorders are tension headache and functional bowel syndrome, disorders that are caused by unconscious stimulation of the autonomic nervous system.

Causes of Diseases

Diseases are initiated by injury, which may be external or internal in origin. Causative agents that are external in nature are called **exogenous** agents, while those agents that are internal in nature are called **endogenous** agents.

External causes of diseases are divided into mechanical (also known as physical), chemical, and microbiologic.

Direct *physical* injury by an object is called **trauma**. This is a type of mechanical injury, such as an actual blow to the head. Other physical agents causing disease include extreme heat and cold, electricity, atmospheric pressure, and radiation. *Chemical* injuries are generally categorized by the manner of injury into poisoning and drug reactions. *Microbiologic* injuries are usually classified by the type of organism (such as bacteria and fungi) and are termed **infections**. These are common in a hospital environment, particularly when treatment involves the placement of a urinary catheter. Known as a **nosocomial** infection, patients contract a urinary tract infection (UTI) when catheters are not inserted with sterile technique. Infections resulting from treatment by a health professional produce **iatrogenic** diseases.

Internal causes of disease fall into three large categories: vascular, immunologic, and metabolic diseases. *Vascular diseases* may involve obstruction of the blood supply to an organ or tissue, bleeding, or altered blood flow such as that occurs with heart failure. Vascular insufficiency is the leading internal cause of structural disease and results in tissue necrosis due to **anoxia**. Without sufficient oxygen to feed the tissue, the muscle dies. Deficiency of oxygen and nutrient-laden blood in the muscle is termed **ischemia**, and an area of necrotic muscle tissue is called an **infarct**. Ischemic infarct occurring in the heart is known as myocardial infarct and is the leading cause of death from vascular insufficiency.

Immunologic diseases are those caused by aberrations of the immune system and affect the body's ability to fight disease. If the body produces agents that actually attack it, the process is known as autoimmune disease. Overreaction or unwanted reactions of the immune system cause allergic diseases. *Metabolic diseases* encompass a wide variety of biochemical disorders. These are the functional activities of cells that result in growth, repair, energy release, use of food, and secretions.

Injury

There are two types of injury: acute and chronic. Acute injury has a sudden onset and is severe although short-lived. Acute injury can involve a reduction in oxygen (**hypoxia**) or even anoxia. Such injuries can lead to

necrosis. When an acute injury occurs, a **thrombus** may accompany it. Thrombi can narrow the vessel, causing vascular insufficiency. If the thrombus dislodges and moves through the blood stream, it is called an **embolus**. Any particulate matter that moves through a vessel is an embolus. Fat or bone marrow in a major blood vessel following a severe fracture of a long bone is an example of an embolus. Emboli and thrombi are dangerous and should be treated promptly.

An injury that occurs several times is known as a chronic injury such as a shoulder that dislocates repeatedly. With chronic injury, atrophy is usually involved. **Atrophy** is an acquired process that is regressive. It results from a decrease in cell size or cell number or both. It is actually a progressive wasting away of any part of the body, causing impairment or loss of function. There are four types of atrophy as discussed below:

Senile: This type of atrophy occurs with age and involves shrinkage of the brain tissue. Memory is impaired. Senile atrophy is *not* Alzheimer's disease.

Disuse: When a body part is not used, it will atrophy. An example is a casted leg in which the muscle tissue shrinks considerably in 6 to 8 weeks of disuse.

Pressure: Atrophy as a result of steady pressure on tissue is not uncommon. Bedsores are an example of pressure atrophy.

Endocrine: This type of atrophy is caused by decreased hormonal production. For example, when a woman goes through menopause, estrogen and progesterone are no longer produced. The lack of these hormones causes the uterus and ovaries to shrink.

Inflammation

As with injury, there are acute and chronic inflammations. When an injury occurs, the body responds by becoming inflamed at the site of injury. Inflammation is what actually allows the healing process to begin. The inflammatory response serves a protective and defensive purpose by attempting to neutralize and destroy injurious agents. Leukocytes attack the cellular debris and clean the site, a process known as **phagocytosis**.

Acute inflammation has four clinical cardinal symptoms as mentioned below:

Red skin (rubor)

Swelling (edema)

Heat at the site (calor)

Pain (dolor)

A fifth symptom may be loss of function; however, this depends on the site and the extent of injury. Loss of function is not usually considered a "cardinal" symptom because of its variable occurrence. Both heat and redness of the skin are caused by increased vascularity at the site of injury. The blood vessels become dilated and there is increased permeability of the capillary walls. Vasodilatation allows an increase in blood supply to be delivered to the injured area, resulting in **congestion**. Congestion manifests itself by heat and redness of skin and becomes apparent within minutes after an injury. Swelling and pain occur as a result of exudates increasing interstitial fluid, which then presses on nerve endings. Inflammation will often lead to fluids being secreted by the body. As capillaries dilate and become permeable, passage of fluid from one side of the vessel wall to the other becomes possible. A **transudate** is a collection of fluid in tissue or in a body space caused by increased hydrostatic or decreased osmotic pressure in the vasculature system without loss of protein into the tissue. Transudates are clear, watery fluids with low protein content. When there is increased osmotic pressure in the tissue because of high protein content and there is inflammation of the lymphatic flow, **exudates** will most likely result. Exudates tend to be more localized than transudates because most inflammations are localized, whereas the effects of increased hydrostatic pressure or depleted serum proteins are usually generalized.

Purulent exudates (pus) are loaded with live and dead leukocytes. An inflammatory reaction with a lot of purulent exudates is called **suppurative inflammation**. A localized collection of pus is an **abscess**.

Chronic inflammation lasts for extended periods of time and is often associated with sublethal cellular degeneration. Tissue necrosis is uncommon. Examples of chronic inflammation are asthma, hay fever, and other allergies. Many are environmental.

Repair

Regardless of the cause or the type of inflammation, the sequence of events that occurs during repair is as follows:

Alteration in vascularity

Capillary permeability

Spread of white blood cells (leukocytes) to the site of inflammation

Phagocytosis

When the body attempts to heal itself and return to its normal status, repair is being accomplished. The repair process of wounds is separated into primary union and secondary union, depending on whether the wound edges are placed together or left separated. The best example of repair by *primary union* is that which follows a clean surgical incision of the skin in which there is minimal tissue damage, and tape or sutures closely approximate the edges of the wound. There is *regeneration* of normal parenchyma cells that are identical to the original cells. If the organization of the tissue is not altered, then the cells will go through mitosis and the damaged tissue is replaced. Since regeneration allows the original structure and function to be duplicated and restored, this is the most desired form of repair.

Repair by *secondary union* utilizes the same basic process as primary union, except there is greater injury, with consequent greater tissue damage and more inflammation to resolve. To fill the void left by tissue damage, there is a tremendous proliferation of capillaries and fibroblasts creating *granulation tissue*. This is a long process that leaves scars in the form of fibrous connective tissue. The original structure and function of the tissue is not restored.

Scar formation can create some complications. Because the function is not restored, there will be loss of function. Scar tissue in the digestive area can unite areas that are normally separate (adhesions) and these may cause obstructions. Because scar tissue tends to shrink over time, a stenosis (narrowing of the organ) is a distinct possibility.

Healing is not guaranteed in a specific time frame. When wound damage covers a large or deep area, there may be prolonged healing time resulting in large amounts of granulation tissue formation. Healing can be delayed in the elderly patient due to poor circulation and reduced mitosis. Complications can arise if the patient is too mobile and causes the wound to bleed or form a hematoma. If the wound is not clean or becomes disturbed in some manner, it is possible that bacteria can enter in and cause an infection.

Fundamental Tissue

The cells of the body are derived from one cell, the fertilized ovum. The cells of the developed organism can be divided into *germ cells* (normally confined to the gonads) and *somatic cells*. Somatic cells are classified into four major categories: epithelial cells, connective tissue cells, muscle tissue cells, and nervous tissue cells.

Epithelial cells are generally those that arise from the embryonic ectoderm and endoderm. Different forms of epithelial cells have different functions. Some create tissue to form the lining of body spaces (such as in the gastrointestinal tract), while others become a protective layer and cover surfaces of the various glands and organs (such as the skin). Most epithelial cells lack blood vessels and must depend on other cells for nourishment. Epithelial cells divide continuously making them extremely radiosensitive.

Connective tissue cells, which are mostly derived from mesoderm, are the most widespread in the body and provide multiple functions. They lend support wherever the body needs it, such as tendons and ligaments. They connect and bind, such as muscle and bone. Another function is to produce blood cells and to protect against infection. The cells found in connective tissue are fibroblasts, macrophages, mast cells, and other types. Mast cells produce heparin and histamine. Macrophages are infection fighters and help in phagocytosis.

Muscle tissue cells are also derived from mesoderm but resemble epithelial cells in their close approximation to each other. Muscle tissue cells are long and slender and are called fibers. The fibers decrease in length and increase in thickness to cause contraction and provide movement. Muscle tissue plays a role in vital body functions. There are three types of muscle tissues: *voluntary* (striated), *involuntary* (smooth), and *cardiac* (involuntary, striated).

Nerve tissue cells are derived from ectoderm and include nerve cells (neurons) and their supporting cells (neuralgia). Nerve tissue is the most highly specialized tissue in the body, making them one of the most radio-resistant cells in the body. It activates and integrates the body as a whole. Neurons have very long processes, known as axons, which carry electrical impulses to the brain and spinal cord, causing all conductivity in the body.

Altered Tissue Growth

The tendency of cells to undergo a growth alteration is related to their involvement in physiologic replacement. The proliferative capacity of cells relates to the process of maturation from a nonspecific cell type to a specialized cell. There is a direct relationship between the reproductive capability of the cell and the occurrence of disease. Two cell types that undergo continuous replacement are epithelial and endothelial. As such, these cells are most susceptible to growth changes. Muscle tissue has limited ability to reproduce; therefore, growth alterations are uncommon. Alterations in growth are very rare in nerve tissue in that neurons and neuralgia are incapable of reproduction.

Altered tissue growth, also known as **growth disturbance**, can be defined as a departure from normal tissue growth caused by the multiplication of cells. Since hyperplasias and neoplasms are both characterized by proliferation of cells that increase tissue mass, these can be classified as the two categories of growth disturbances. Hyperplasias and neoplasms differ on the basis of cause and growth potential.

Hyperplasia is an exaggerated response to various stimuli in the form of an increase in the number of cells in the tissue. Hyperplasia may recede if the stimulus is removed, provided permanent structural changes have not occurred. Hyperplasia typically involves tissues that undergo physiologic replacement, but it may involve stable tissue. Hyperplasia may be caused by a wide variety of stimuli, such as a remote response to inflammation, hormone excess or hormone deficiency, chronic irritation, or unknown factors. Hypertrophy should be distinguished from hyperplasia; both frequently occur together. **Hypertrophy** refers to an increase in cell size, whereas hyperplasia refers to an increase in cell numbers. The term hypertrophy is best applied to muscles, as the muscle fiber (cell) enlarges as a response to increased workload rather than undergoing hyperplasia. **Metaplasia** occurs when a normal cell becomes abnormal. This is unlike hyperplasia in that metaplasia is an abnormality of growth in an individual cell. As such, it has not taken on tumor characteristics.

Neoplasm means new growth and occurs when cell division does not progress in the usual pattern. A neoplasm will result if the developmental pattern is interrupted by an abnormal and uncontrolled growth of cells. Neoplasms are presumed to arise by mutation or altered genetic control. These tumors behave as if they are independent parasitic organisms. A neoplasm continues to grow after the agent is removed.

Neoplasms can be classified as **benign** or **malignant**. Benign neoplasms are single masses of cells that remain localized at their site of origin and limited in their growth. Adenoma, angioma, cystadenoma, fibroma, lipoma, and myoma are examples of benign tumors. Cancer cells grow without regard for the control exhibited by normal cellular growth. Malignant neoplasms (cancerous tumors) are defined by their potential to invade and metastasize at some point. **Invasion** refers to direct extension of neoplastic cells into surrounding tissue without regard for tissue boundaries.

Malignant neoplasms disseminate to distant sites of the body through a process known as **metastasis**. Metastasis means transplantation of cells to a new site. There are three ways for metastasis to occur as described below:

Lymphatic: This is the most common way tumor cells are spread. The cells travel through the lymph system to other areas. When the cells reach a lymph node that is too small for the cells to pass through, the tumor cells will permeate the lymph vessel wall and plant at that site.

Seeding: This is a diffuse spread of tumor cells. The tumor invades a body cavity by penetration. An example is a gastrointestinal tumor in which cells penetrate the peritoneum and travel to the bladder.

Hematogenous: This occurs when cells penetrate blood vessels and are then sent into the circulatory system. When the large cells get trapped in the smaller vascular channels, they pass through the vessel wall and into the tissue, where they multiply.

Cancer is classified by the tissue or blood cells in which it is derived. Most cancers originate from epithelial tissue and are called carcinomas. If the tumor is from non-epithelial tissue, such as connective, muscle, and bone tissue, the term **sarcoma** is used. **Lymphoma** is cancer of the lymphatic system, and **leukemia** is malignancy of the blood and related organs.

TECH TIP

Cancers of epithelial tissue such as adenocarcinoma are additive in nature and require increased kVp. Many bone cancers, such as osteosarcoma, will deplete the bone cells and are considered destructive. These require a decrease in kVp.

A cell can transform from normal to cancerous, thus a tumor can closely reproduce the normal structure of the cells. The term **differentiation** is used to describe this process. The more highly differentiated the tumor, the *less* the degree of malignancy, because it is most closely like the normal cells. The process of determining the degree of differentiation, and thus the degree of malignancy, is expressed as **grading**. Grade 1 tumors are the most differentiated and least malignant. Grade 4 tumors are the most malignant and least differentiated. The size of tumors at the primary site and the presence of any metastasis are evaluated through a process known as **staging**. Staging is critical, as the choice of treatment relies on this assessment.

Currently, in the United States, the leading cause of death due to cancer in women is lung carcinoma. Breast and colorectal carcinoma follow closely. Heart disease is the number 1 overall cause of death in women. In males, heart disease and prostate cancer are the leading causes of death. Over the last several years, bronchogenic carcinoma has fallen to third place as a major cause of death in males.

Throughout the remaining chapters of this book, it will be helpful to refer to this chapter as well as to the glossary. The pathologic conditions that are about to be studied are not easily memorized. There are many "classic signs" seen on the radiograph that help the radiographer identify the disease process, but the reader is encouraged to take the time necessary to fully understand the process occurring and not simply memorize the disease itself.

RECAP

- Disease processes are either
  - Functional (pathophysiologic)
    - Alters only the function of the organ
    - Shows no lesion, or
  - Structural (organic)
    - Actual structure of the organ or cell is changed
    - Characterized by lesions
      - Three broad categories include genetic and developmental, acquired, and hyperplasia and neoplasms
- Disease processes are caused by
  - Exogenous (external)
    - Three broad categories are physical (trauma), chemical (drug reactions or poisoning), and microbiologic (infections), and
  - Endogenous (internal)
    - Three broad categories are vascular diseases (blockage to the circulatory system), immunologic disease (problems with the immune system), and metabolic diseases (biochemical disorders)
- Injury can be either
  - Acute
    - Associated with a thrombus or embolus, or
  - Chronic
    - Associated with one or more types of atrophy (usually pressure or disuse)
- Inflammation is also either
  - Acute
    - Associated with four cardinal signs
      - Red skin
      - Edema
      - Heat
      - Pain
    - Allows the healing process to begin, or
  - Chronic
    - These are mostly environmental inflammations such as hay fever and asthma

Healing Process

- Begins with inflammation
- Vessel walls dilate increasing the permeability
- Congestion brings leukocytes to begin phagocytosis
- Wound repair is either primary or secondary, depending on the amount of damage
  - Primary repair is regeneration, which is desirable
  - Secondary repair is granulation formation, which is scar tissue
- Complications include
  - Infection
  - Bleeding or hematoma
  - Delayed healing
  - Obstructions or stenosis
- Types of fundamental tissues are
  - Epithelial cells (linings), connective tissue cells (support mechanisms), muscle tissue cells (for movement), and nerve tissue cells (most specialized)
  - Disease processes have a direct relationship with the reproductive capability of tissue cell

Growth Disturbances

- Hyperplasia is an increase in cell number; may recede if stimuli is removed
- Neoplasia is a separate entity of new cell growth; it is either benign or malignant
- Malignant tumors are named according to the cells from which they arise
  - Adenocarcinoma from glandular tissue
  - Leukemia from leukocytes
  - Lymphoma from lymphatic tissue
  - Sarcoma from connective, muscle, and bone tissues

Types of Metastasis

- Seeding (diffuse spread)
- Lymphatic (most common)
- Hematogenous (in the circulatory system)

Determination of Malignancy

- Grading determines the amount of differentiation of the tumor's cellular structure
- Staging determines the size of the tumor and the occurrence of metastasis

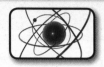 # CRITICAL THINKING DISCUSSION QUESTIONS

1. Describe how acute injury can be associated with vascular insufficiency.

2. Describe primary and secondary repair.

3. Why is regeneration the more desirable of the two types of repair?

4. Explain what "additive" pathology means and how it affects the radiographic exposure factors.

5. Explain what "destructive" pathology means and how it affects the radiographic exposure factors.

6. There are four clinical cardinal symptoms, but a fifth symptom may be present. Explain what it is and why it might occur.

7. Explain how secondary union occurs.

8. Describe the difference between carcinoma and sarcoma. What is lymphoma? How is lymphoma different from leukemia?

9. What are issues that the radiographer must be aware of when preparing to do a procedure on a patient with an infection?

The Skeletal System

● Goals

1. To review the anatomy and physiology of the skeletal system

   OBJECTIVE: Name the classifications of the skeleton and joints in the body

   OBJECTIVE: List and give examples of the five types of bones in the body

   OBJECTIVE: Describe the structure, physiology, and function of bones and joints

2. To learn the basic pathologic conditions of the skeletal system

   OBJECTIVE: Differentiate between osteogenesis imperfecta and osteopetrosis

   OBJECTIVE: Define transitional vertebrae and give examples

   OBJECTIVE: Explain how achondroplasia occurs

   OBJECTIVE: List the different types of osteochondritis dissecans

   OBJECTIVE: Describe the different types of osteopenia

   OBJECTIVE: Define chondromas and name its three types

   OBJECTIVE: Describe osteoclastomas

   OBJECTIVE: Differentiate between multiple myeloma and osteitis deformans

   OBJECTIVE: List three different types of arthritis

● Key Terms

Achondroplasia

Amphiarthrodial

Ankylosing spondylitis (rheumatoid spondylitis)

Appendicular

Arthritis

Axial

Bone cyst

Bursitis

Cancellous

Chondroma

Congenital dislocated hip

Cortical

Delayed union

Diarthrodial

Dislocation

Displacement

Distraction

Enchondroma

Endosteum

Exostosis

Fibrous dysplasia

Fracture

Legg-Calvé-Perth disease

Malunion

● Goals *continued*

OBJECTIVE: Define and describe different types of fractures and dislocations

3. To become familiar with how different imaging modalities serve to enhance and complement radiographic diagnosis of common pathologies of the skeletal system

OBJECTIVE: Describe how CT, MRI, and nuclear medicine are best to serve in the diagnosis of pathology of the skeletal system

● Key Terms *continued*

Medullary
Nonunion
Osgood-Schlatter
Ossification
Osteitis deformans
Osteoblast
Osteochondritis dissecans
Osteoclast
Osteoclastomas
Osteodystrophy
Osteogenesis imperfecta
Osteomalacia
Osteomyelitis (osteitis)
Osteopenia
Osteopetrosis
Osteoporosis
Periosteum
Scoliosis
Sequestrum
Spina bifida
Subluxation
Synarthrodial
Transitional vertebra

Bone radiography is the "bread and butter" of the radiologic technologist's work. As such, the technologist must not only memorize the many projections and positions for all the areas of the body but also be able to critically think outside the box when the patient is not in a condition that will allow a normal radiograph as taught in the classroom. In addition, the pathology that can occur will change the technical factors that are required to adequately expose the body part for a diagnostic radiograph. It is for this reason, it is so important to have a full understanding of anatomy, pathology, and the resulting impact on positioning and technique.

Anatomy

Classification and Structure of Bones

The skeletal system, composed of 206 bones, is commonly divided into the axial skeleton, which contains 80 bones of the skull, spine, ribs, and sternum; and the appendicular skeleton, which contains the remaining 126 bones of the extremities, pectoral and pelvic girdles. There are five types of bones:

1. Long bones, such as the femur
2. Short bones, such as those present in the carpal bones
3. Flat bones, such as the parietal bones found in the skull
4. Irregular bones, such as the vertebrae
5. Sesamoid bones, such as the patella

Bone is a type of connective tissue, but it differs from other connective tissue because of its calcified matrix. All bones, except articular surfaces that are covered with articular cartilage, are covered with two layers of periosteum. The outer layer is made up of dense, fibrous tissue and the inner layer is made up of cells called osteoblasts that are associated with the production of bone.

Beneath the inner layer of periosteum is a layer called cortical, or compact, bone. This is a dense,

closely knit bone. The cancellous, or spongy, bone is below the cortical layer. This is porous, loosely knit bone with a honeycomb appearance.

The medullary, or marrow cavity, is the open canal that runs down the center of the diaphysis (shaft) of long bones and contains the bone marrow. A layer of endosteum lines the marrow cavity. Figure 2-1 shows coronal and cross-sectional slices through a long bone, indicating the various structures within it.

Two types of tissue are found in the cavities of bones. Red bone marrow is found in the open areas of spongy bone and forms red blood cells. Yellow bone marrow contains predominantly fat and is found in the marrow cavity of long bones.

Classification and Structure of Joints

Joints are a part of the skeletal system and must be considered along with the bones. There are three types of joints:

1. **Synarthrodial** joints are immovable joints that have a layer of fibrous tissue between the bones. The sutures of the skull are an example of this tissue. Later in life, the tissue atrophies and disappears, and the bone ends become fused.
2. **Amphiarthrodial** joints are slightly movable joints with a layer of cartilage on the bone ends. Between the two bone ends of an amphiarthrodial joint is a disk made of cartilage and fibrous tissue. The intervertebral joint spaces are amphiarthrodial joints and the intervertebral disks are the fibrocartilaginous plates.
3. **Diarthrodial** joints are freely movable because there is a space between the ends of the bones. The bones are held together by a capsule that is filled with synovial fluid. This fluid acts as a lubricant and nourishes the hyaline cartilage that lines the articular surface of the joint. Nerve endings are located in the joint capsule to transmit to the brain the signal of movement of the joint. There are six types of synovial joints:

Gliding, or plane, joints have flat surfaces and they glide over each other, such as the vertebrae (Fig. 2-2).

Hinge joints allow angular motion in one direction, such as the elbow (Fig. 2-3).

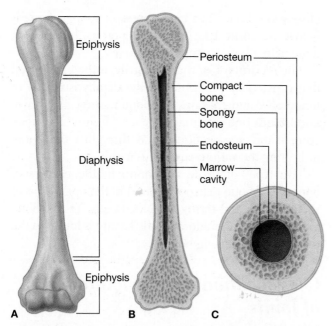

FIGURE 2-1   (A) The two major areas of a long bone. (B) Inside portions of a long bone including the marrow or medullary cavity. (C) A cross section of a long bone.

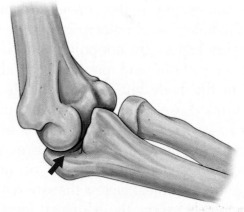

FIGURE 2-3   The humerus and the ulna meet to make a hinge joint.

Pivot joints allow rotation by being kept in place by a ring of cartilage or bone around the head of another bone. The joint of C1/C2 is a pivot joint (Fig. 2-5).

Ball-and-socket joints have a head-shaped bone end that fits into a cup-shaped socket, as in the hip (Fig. 2-6).

Condylar joints (also called ellipsoidal) have a head-shaped bone that fits into a concave surface that allows motion of flexion, extension, abduction, adduction, and circumduction. The wrist is an excellent example (Fig. 2-4).

Saddle joints are similar to condylar joints except that one bone end is convex while the other end is concave. The thumb is a saddle joint (see Fig. 2-4).

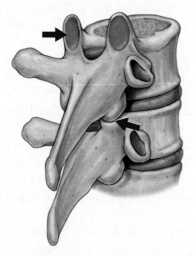

FIGURE 2-2   The superior and inferior articulating facets meet to form a gliding joint.

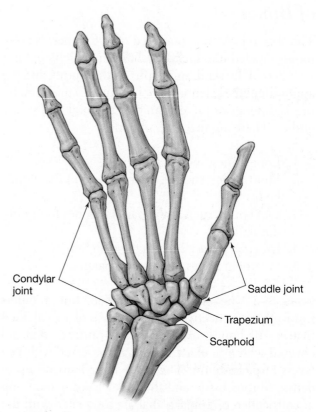

FIGURE 2-4   The first metacarpophalangeal joint and the carpometacarpal joints are examples of saddle joints. The wrist and metacarpophalangeal joints are condylar joints.

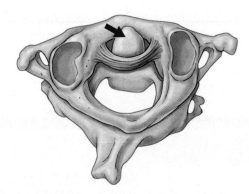

FIGURE 2-5   The ring of cartilage between the dens and C1 forms a pivot joint.

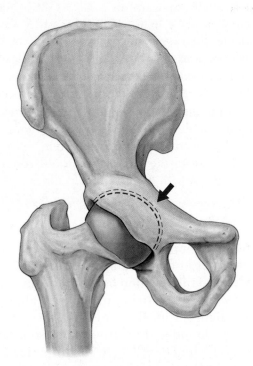

FIGURE 2-6   The head of the femur as it fits into the acetabulum is a ball-and-socket joint.

Physiology and Function

Although it is beyond the scope of this text to provide an in-depth description of the formation of bones, a general overview is needed in order to understand certain pathologic conditions.

While still an embryo, the skeleton is really a fibrous membrane or hyaline cartilage. Ossification is the process of bone replacing these membranes and begins with the appearance of osteoblasts, which are bone-forming cells. The osteoblasts form bone matrix, which is composed of large amounts of mucopolysaccharide substance accumulated around each osteoblast and embedded with bundles of collagenous fibers. As soon as bone matrix is formed, complex calcium salts are deposited that calcify the matrix, making it hard.

Bones grow longer as a result of cells multiplying in the epiphyseal cartilage. Ossification then occurs in this new cartilage. Bones grow in diameter by the action of two cells. Osteoclasts are cells associated with the absorption and removal of bone. They "eat away" the inside of the marrow cavity while the osteoblasts build up the outside of the bone.

Functions of the skeletal system are given below:

1. **Support:** The body and the surrounding tissue are supported by the body's skeleton.
2. **Protection:** The organs housed within the body are protected from trauma by the framework surrounding them.
3. **Movement:** The bones and joints are levers and the muscles are the applied force. When a muscle contracts, the bone moves.
4. **Production of blood cells:** The red bone marrow manufactures new blood cells.
5. **Storage:** Important mineral salts such as phosphorus and calcium are stored in the skeletal system.

Pathology

Congenital Anomalies

There are many congenital syndromes that are confusing as there is overlap in the radiographic abnormalities among them. There are some congenital anomalies that are so slight and nonharmful that they are considered nothing more than a variance of the normal skeleton. For example, a small sesamoid bone is sometimes found at the base of the fifth metacarpal. Others are more significant and demonstrate specific radiographic qualities. Only the more common congenital abnormalities are discussed in this text.

Scoliosis is the lateral deviation and rotation of the spine. There are various types of scoliosis: idiopathic, congenital, or acquired. Since congenital scoliosis creates the majority of varieties, it will be the only type discussed. Congenital scoliosis is commonly the result of vertebral abnormalities such as a hemivertebrae, wedge vertebrae, or neuromuscular development. The ribs will be affected with the rotation of the vertebrae and this will create chest abnormalities. There are associated anomalies of the urinary system with congenital scoliosis.

Wedged vertebra or hemivertebrae is a failure of formation of the vertebrae. Bars are failure of segmentation of the spine causing unbalanced growth. The thoracolumbar area is the most commonly affected. Figure 2-7 shows how a "wedge" shape of vertebrae fits into the normal vertebral column and affects the normal structure.

Imaging is the most definitive and important diagnostic tool for scoliosis. Radiographic evaluation must include excellent quality erect anterioposterior (AP) and lateral projections of the entire spine. Lateral-bending views may be required to determine fixation. In severe cases, chest radiographs may be requested to determine the anomalies of the lungs and heart.

Other imaging modalities include computed tomography (CT) and magnetic resonance imaging (MRI) which are helpful in detecting laminar fusion. Ultrasonography is only helpful prenatally. Nuclear medicine three-phase bone scans are used when the patient presents with pain.

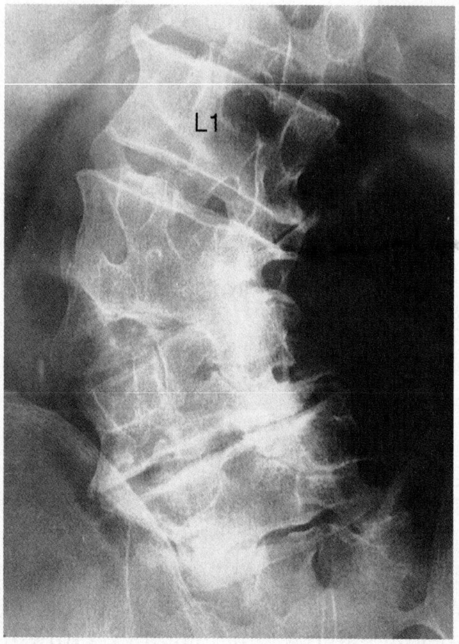

TECH TIP

The patient's shoes must be removed so the patient is imaged standing bare feet. If the equipment has the capability, the SID should be 84" and a single exposure on a 14" × 36" image receptor must be made. If this size of IR is not available, then separate exposures on 14" × 17" image receptors must be made. A high ratio grid is desirable to reduce scatter as a high kVp (approximately 125) is best. A 300 mA station is necessary to produce the optimum density. Gonadal shadow shielding is required on all patients. In the AP projection, lateral collimation must be used but not to the extent that would compromise anatomy with its curvatures.

FIGURE 2-7   L2, AP lumbar spine. Observe the fused hemivertebra at L2, with no separating intervertebral disk. There are only four lumbar-type vertebrae. The wedging of the hemivertebra has created a significant structural scoliosis. (Donald E. Freuden, DC, DABCO, Denver, CO.)

A **transitional vertebra** is one that takes on the characteristics of the vertebrae on either side of it. This occurs at the junction between the divisions of the spine. The L1 vertebra may have rudimentary ribs articulating with the transverse process, similar to those found at T12. Ribs may also be found at the C7/T1 junction. Cervical ribs project off of C7 (Fig. 2-8) and are of more concern than ribs found at L1, as they may exert pressure on nerves or arteries and require surgical removal. Ribs off of L1 are another incidental finding on abdominal radiographs (Fig. 2-9).

Another type of transitional vertebrae can occur at the L5/sacral junction. In this instance, L5 may have an enlarged transverse process that actually looks like the upper portion of the sacrum (Fig. 2-10). This condition may be unilateral or bilateral. In some cases, the enlarged process is actually fused to the sacrum. If this occurs, the process is known as sacralization (Fig. 2-11).

Congenital dislocated hip (CDH), also known as developmental dysplasia of the hip, occurs when the capsule of the hip joint relaxes and allows

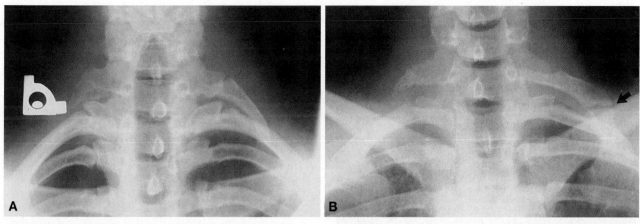

FIGURE 2-8   Cervical ribs. (A) AP lower cervical spine. Observe the complete cervical rib at C7 on the right side. An attenuated cervical rib is present at the same level on the left side. (B) AP lower cervical spine. Note the cervical rib with an accessory articulation (*arrow*). A small cervical rib is also noted on the opposite side. (Donald E. Freuden, DC, DABCO, Denver, CO.)

dislocation of the hip (Fig. 2-12A, B). This will occur more often in Caucasian females than in any other ethnicity. There seems to be relevance between breech deliveries and oligohydramnios as predisposing factors. Although the process is common in neonatal periods, 75% to 95% of the newborns showing clinical signs will revert to normal after 6 to 8 weeks of age. Radiographs of the hips

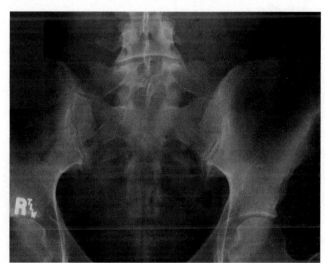

FIGURE 2-10   The fifth lumbar vertebra (L5) demonstrates a transitional transverse process on the patient's left side that is in contact but not fused with the sacrum.

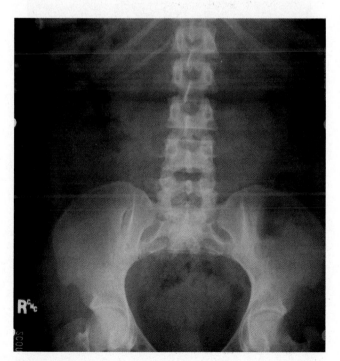

FIGURE 2-9   Lumbar ribs. AP lumbar spine demonstrates ribs coming off L1.

performed prior to 6 weeks of age have a high false-negative rate. However, these radiographic images can rule out other possibilities of one leg being shorter than the other. Since radiography cannot demonstrate cartilaginous margins of the acetabulum, ultrasound is a much better tool to assess the condition immediately following birth and up to 2 months of age.

If CDH has not been diagnosed and treatment is not put into place, there are a few complications that may occur. Avascular necrosis is a risk that can be reduced by traction. There is the possibility that a pseudoacetabulae may develop from pressure of

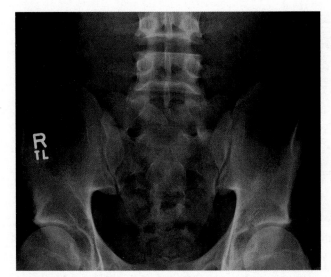

FIGURE 2-11   In this case, the transverse process is completely fused to the sacrum, causing a process called sacralization.

a displaced femoral head in the iliac wing that will produce mechanical problems later in life. Finally, secondary osteoarthritis will occur later in life in the 50s or 60s.

TECH TIP

When the technologist is presented with an infant patient for bilateral hips to rule out CDH, it is imperative that the legs are perfectly straight and even. The pelvis must be straight and flat on the table. Without perfect positioning, the possibility of falsely diagnosing CDH is high. The technologist must obtain as much help as necessary to hold the patient perfectly still.

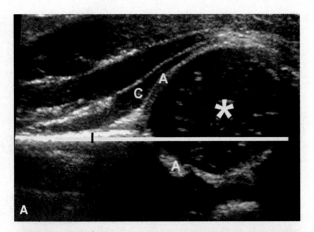
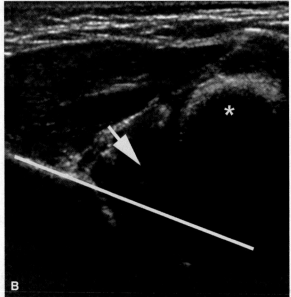

FIGURE 2-12   Congenital hip dysplasia. (A) Ultrasound examination shows lateral subluxation of femoral head (*) with application of pressure. Normally, an extension of a line drawn along the ischium (I) should pass through the center of the femoral head. (B) Dislocation of femoral head. With pressure, the femoral head echoes disappear (*arrow*) and the echoes of the femoral neck now can be seen (*). A, acetabulum; C, cartilaginous portion of acetabular roof. (Courtesy of Leonard E. Swischuk, MD, University of Texas at Galveston.)

Spina bifida is the failure of fusion of one or more vertebral arches. There are types of spina bifida that are based upon the degree and pattern of deformity. *Spina bifida occulta* (SBO) occurs when the two halves of the posterior arch fail to unite. The first sacral vertebra is the most common location. SBO can also occur at T12 but this is much less common. In SBO, there is no protrusion of the spinal cord or its membrane, however if neural elements project though the defect

without any meninge covering, a myelocele is present (Fig. 2-13A). When a cerebrospinal fluid (CSF)-filled sac is covered with the meninges of the cord, it is called a meningocele (Fig. 2-13B). There is a wide bony defect in the posterior arch of the lumbar vertebrae in *spina bifida aperta*. This leaves room for a protrusion of the spinal cord contents beyond the spinal canal. A sac containing CSF and some of the neural elements of the cord protruding is called a myelomeningocele

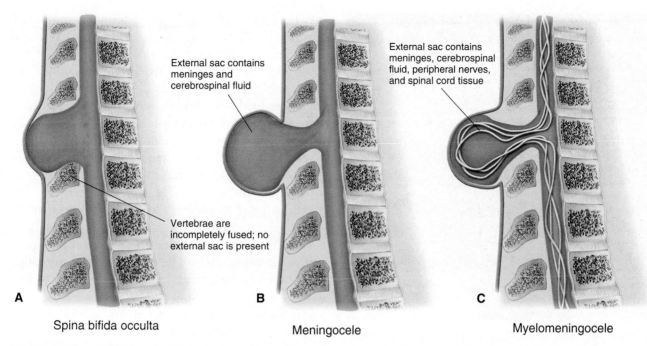

External sac contains
meninges and
cerebrospinal fluid

Vertebrae are
incompletely fused; no
external sac is present

External sac contains
meninges, cerebrospinal
fluid, peripheral nerves,
and spinal cord tissue

A

B

C

Spina bifida occulta

Meningocele

Myelomeningocele

FIGURE 2-13   (A) Myelocele; (B) meningocele; and (C) myelomeningocele. (Asset provided by Anatomical Chart Co.)

(Fig. 2-13C). These protrusions can be diagnosed through sonography as early as 12 weeks of gestational age. Plain radiographs will show the absence of the lamina and spinous processes, along with widening of the space between the thinning pedicles (Fig. 2-14). MRI is helpful in determining involvement of neural elements.

Osteogenesis imperfecta (OI) is called "brittle bone" disease because of the extreme vulnerability of bones to fracture. It is an inherited connective tissue disorder that affects multiple organs and not just the skeletal system. Blue sclera, osteoporosis, wormian bones in the skull, and multiple fractures are the most common abnormalities. There is a lack of osteoblastic activity and abnormal collagen formation so that the skeleton does not ossify properly. This leads to a form of congenital osteoporosis. It is estimated that OI affects between 20,000 and 50,000 people in the United States with 1 in every 20,000 births being afflicted.

Clinically, there are two types: congenital and tarda. The congenital form is the most severe with multiple fractures at birth. Infants with congenital OI are stillborn or die very early. The rare survivors develop other problems involving cystic formation. The long bones are short, thick, and bowed, resembling dwarfism (Fig. 2-15). The tarda form appears after puberty with multiple fractures and milder deformities of the long bones at varying times following birth.

The long bones are characterized by thin cortices, allowing for fracture with minimal trauma. Fractures can even occur in utero. Multiple fractures in the

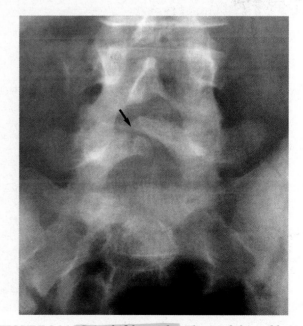

FIGURE 2-14   **Spina bifida occulta. There is failure of fusion of the laminae of L5, producing a cleft (*arrow*).** (Daffner RH. *Clinical Radiology: The Essentials.* 3rd ed. Philadelphia, PA: Lippincott Williams & Wilkins; 2007.)

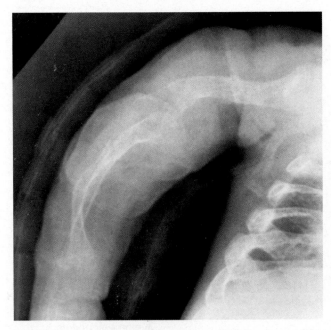

FIGURE 2-15   Osteogenesis imperfecta (OI). Pronounced osteoporosis and cortical thinning of all bones with evidence of previous fractures and resultant deformities. (Eisenberg RL. *Clinical Imaging: An Atlas of Differential Diagnosis.* 5th ed. Philadelphia, PA: Lippincott Williams & Wilkins; 2010.)

newborn can result in limb deformities and small stature (Fig. 2-16A, B). Often, deafness is associated with this disease since the small ossicles can easily fracture. The connective tissue that surrounds the ossicles may be abnormal as well. The abnormal collagen production leads to deformed, hypoplastic teeth. The condition of OI tarda becomes less severe with age, depending on the type of OI that has developed. Type I (OI tarda 1) is the most common and mildest form, while type IV is the most severe and it is not unusual for the patient to have experienced over 100 fractures prior to puberty. Multiple fractures in the lower extremities are the radiographic hallmark of OI. Subsequent healing leads to shortening, bowing deformities (Fig. 2-17). The excessive callus formation around the fracture areas (pseudo tumors) may be mistaken for osteosarcoma.

Dual-energy X-ray absorptiometry (DXA) is used in the initial diagnosis of OI. Children may receive annual DXA scans for assessment of skeletal development and future fracture predictions.

Radiographic features include diffuse osteoporosis with thin cortices. The extremities are short and thick

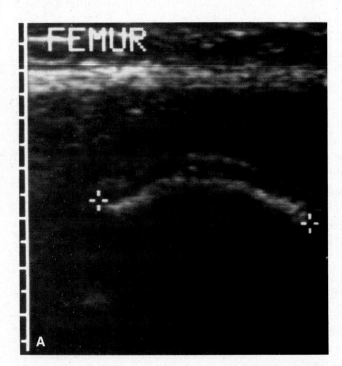

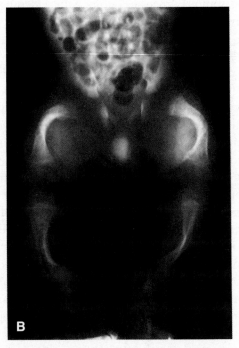

FIGURE 2-16   Osteogenesis imperfecta type III. **(A)** Longitudinal image of a fetal thigh at 38 weeks of gestation demonstrates a short, bowed femur (*cursors*). **(B)** Radiograph after delivery confirms the presence of short bowed femurs, tibia, and fibula bilaterally. (MacDonald MG, Seshia MMK, Mullett MD. *Avery's Neonatology Pathophysiology and Management of the Newborn.* 6th ed. Philadelphia, PA: Lippincott Williams & Wilkins; 2005.)

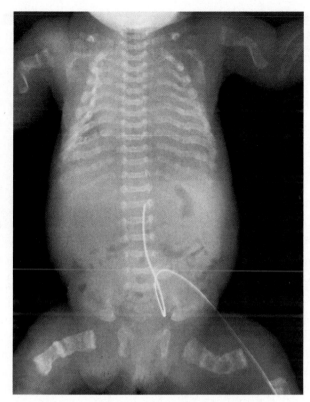

FIGURE 2-17   Osteogenesis imperfecta. Generalized flattening of vertebral bodies associated with fractures of multiple ribs and long bones in an infant. Note the femurs with multiple healed and healing fractures. (Eisenberg RL. *Clinical Imaging: An Atlas of Differential Diagnosis*. 5th ed. Philadelphia, PA: Lippincott Williams & Wilkins; 2010.)

(resembling dwarfism), while the pelvis is narrow. The fractures will be obvious as the healing process can be easily identified.

T E C H   T I P

The radiographer must understand the process of OI so as to be able to adjust the technique for quality radiographs. As will be discovered later in this chapter, fractures heal by producing more bone. This requires a need for a slight increase in kVp. Additionally, the radiographer must have excellent positioning skills, as routine positioning may not be possible owing to the deformities produced by the multiple fractures/healing processes.

A process that is basically the exact opposite of OI is **osteopetrosis**. There is a deficiency of osteoclasts and therefore, faulty bone absorption. There is no certain cause of this faulty bone absorption but it leads to a generalized increase in bone density (Fig. 2-18). The increase in density leads the disease to be called "marble bone" disease. The long bones are sclerotic (Fig. 2-19A, B) and fragile with frequent transverse fractures. As is true in other disease processes, there are several clinical forms of this condition. *Osteopetrosis infantile* frequently ends in blindness and deafness and then death by the age of 2 years. *Osteopetrosis tarda* remains asymptomatic with detection being made with anemia or pathologic fractures (Fig. 2-20A, B). *Osteopetrosis intermediate* falls somewhere in between the other two forms. In severe forms, there is obliteration of the marrow cavity and a deformed skull. Patients who suffer from osteopetrosis are prone to osteomyelitis.

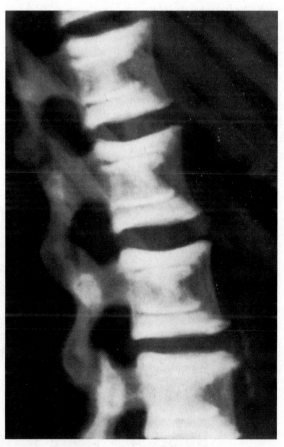

FIGURE 2-18   Osteopetrosis. A miniature inset is seen in each lumbar vertebral body, giving it a bone-within-a-bone appearance. There is also sclerosis at the end plates. (Eisenberg RL. *Clinical Imaging: An Atlas of Differential Diagnosis*. 5th ed. Philadelphia, PA: Lippincott Williams & Wilkins; 2010.)

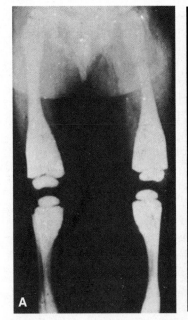
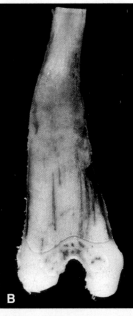

FIGURE 2-19   Osteopetrosis. (A) A radiograph of a child shows markedly misshapen and dense bones of the lower extremities, characteristic of marble bone disease. (B) A gross specimen of the femur shows obliteration of the marrow space by dense bone. (Rubin R, Strayer DS. *Rubin's Pathology: Clinicopathologic Foundations of Medicine.* 5th ed. Philadelphia, PA: Lippincott Williams & Wilkins; 2008.)

Radiography is the best diagnostic procedure and is supported by CT. The increased sclerosis creates increased density with little definition of the trabecula and obliteration of the marrow cavity. This creates a "bone-within-a-bone" appearance.

TECH TIP

With such a high increase in density of the bones, the technical factors will need to be increased. The kVp will need to be increased but not above 75 for extremities, as the scatter will be greater. Even though the bones are radiopaque, they are quite brittle and break easily. Therefore, care must taken when moving extremities, as a normal outward appearance of fracture may not be apparent.

Achondroplasia is the failure of the cartilage that becomes bone to form properly, thus not allowing ossification to proceed as it should. It is caused by an abnormal gene located on one of the chromosomes. In 80% of cases, achondroplasia is not inherited but results from a new mutation occurring in the egg or the sperm cell that forms the embryo. The parents are normal sized in these cases.

Achondroplasia is the most common cause of disproportionate short stature, occurring in 1 in 15,000 to 1 in 25,000 live births. It occurs in all races and in both sexes. Affected individuals have short extremities while the trunk and skull are of normal size. Often the arms are shorter than the lower extremities making the abnormality even more apparent at birth.

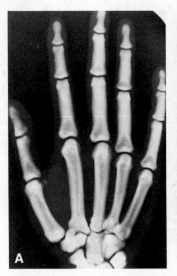
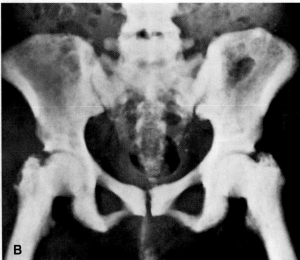

FIGURE 2-20   Osteopetrosis. (A) Striking sclerosis of the bones of the hand and wrist. (B) Generalized increased density of the lower spine, pelvis, and hips in a 74-year-old woman with the tarda form of the condition. (Eisenberg RL. *Clinical Imaging: An Atlas of Differential Diagnosis.* 5th ed. Philadelphia, PA: Lippincott Williams & Wilkins; 2010.)

Other malformations include lordosis of the lumbar spine, bowed legs, and a bulky forehead with a saddle-shaped nose. Nasal passages are narrowed contributing to ear infections. The jaw is small so that the teeth may be crowded and poorly aligned. It is important to remember that the intelligence of achondroplastic individuals is not impaired even though the cranium is deformed.

Because the cartilage is not ossified as it should, radiographs taken of infants with achondroplasia will not require the higher kVp settings that other infants would normally require. Since the foramen magnum is narrowed, CT or MRI is used to monitor for compression on the spinal cord from the foramen magnum.

Radiographically, the skull, spine, pelvis, and limbs will show abnormalities. Narrowing of the spinal canal is a classic radiographic sign. There is shortening of all long bones. The ulna will be shorter than the radius, and the tibia will be shorter than the fibula causing a splayed and cupped metaphyses (Fig. 2-21A). The ribs are short and would not extend around the thorax. Soft tissue is prominent in the abdomen and buttock area (Fig. 2-21B).

Nonneoplastic Bone Changes

Osteopenia is a nonspecific radiographic finding that indicates increased radiolucency of bone. There are two types: osteoporosis and osteomalacia.

When osteoblasts fail to lay down sufficient amount of bone matrix, an abnormal decrease in bone density called **osteoporosis** occurs. There is a lack of bone formation (osteoid), but calcium production is normal. The calcium that would normally go to the bone is drained from it and is excreted through urine. Because of this, kidney or bladder stones may be associated with osteoporosis. Age, gender, and race are prime factors associated with osteoporosis. It occurs more often in women and among Whites and Asians than in African Americans. It is believed that about 25 million Americans are affected, with 80% being women.

Osteoporosis may occur in a variety of clinical conditions. *Primary osteoporosis* is more common and is not associated with an underlying illness. *Secondary osteoporosis* occurs in less than 5% of the cases and is due to some other problem. An example of underlying conditions that cause secondary osteoporosis is disuse

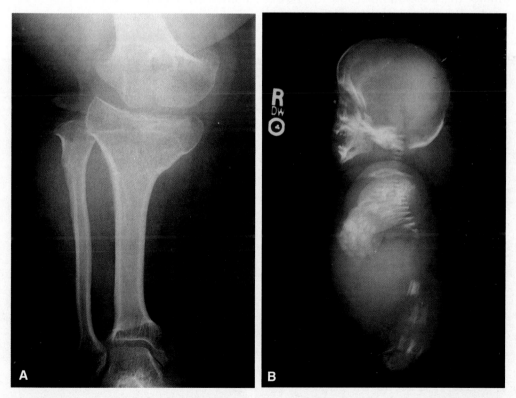

FIGURE 2-21   (A) Achondroplasia (lower limb). Observe the splayed and cupped metaphyses as well as the shortening of the leg. (B) Lateral view of a stillborn achondroplastic infant. Note the absence of the pelvis and the protruding abdomen. (A: Yochum TR, Rowe LJ. *Yochum and Rowe's Essentials of Skeletal Radiology*. 3rd ed. Philadelphia, PA: Lippincott Williams & Wilkins; 2004.)

atrophy, as seen in cases of paralysis, that causes the bone formation to be diminished and calcium to be drained away. People who are under prolonged administration of steroids or suffer from adrenocortical hormone hyperactivity, as in Cushing syndrome, are also more susceptible, as the hormone increases the body's ability to reabsorb bone. Postmenopausal women are more prone to osteoporosis because of a deficiency in the gonadal hormone level that leads to decreased bone formation (Fig. 2-22). Common locations for osteoporosis include the spine, pelvis, hips, femurs, distal radius/hand, and proximal humerus/shoulder.

Pathologic fractures are common in those who suffer from this disease, particularly compression fractures of the thoracic spine causing kyphosis from anterior wedging. Other common fractures include fractures of the hip. One-third of the women who live to 80 years of age will suffer from a hip fracture and 20% of those will die.

Radiographs show lack of density in the bones due to loss of calcium and thin cortices with fewer trabeculae. In known cases of osteoporosis, the technical factors (particularly kVp) should be decreased so as not to overexpose the image and cause a repeat radiograph. If osteoporosis is demonstrated on radiographic images, it can be determined that a minimum of 30% to 50% of the bone density has been lost. In the spine, the classic "empty box" syndrome is demonstrated when there is increased density at the endplates of the vertebrae and loss of density in the vertebral body (Fig. 2-23). High-resolution CT is better at making an early diagnosis but the best modality is the DXA, which measures bone density.

Osteomalacia also falls under the classification of osteopenia because it is an abnormal decrease in bone density caused by a lack of calcium and phosphorus. This defect of mineralization leads to softening of the bone in an adult, even though a normal amount of osteoid is present. This condition is the reverse of osteoporosis in which there is deficient bone formation but normal calcium production. Vitamin D deficiency is a cause of osteomalacia. Pregnancy is another cause, owing to the drain on the calcium in a woman's bones that occurs.

If osteomalacia occurs before the growth plate at the epiphysis closes in children, it is known as *rickets*. Rickets is often called infantile osteomalacia, since the bones lack hardening. In the infantile form, the osteoid tissue in growing bones is not calcified or hardened, and deformities of the skeleton result. Bowing of the lower legs is a common manifestation (Fig. 2-24). Radiographic signs are a generalized reduction in bone density due to decreased number of trabeculae seen in both osteomalacia and rickets. There may be

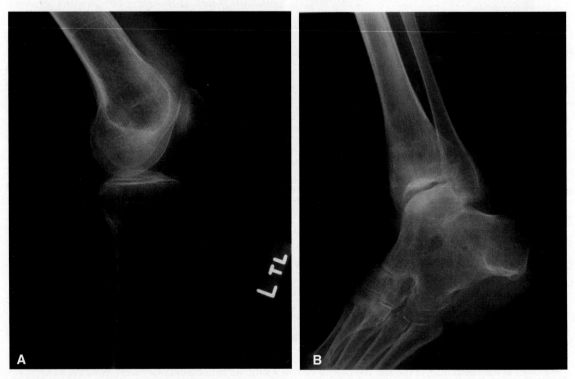

FIGURE 2-22   (A) Knee and (B) ankle of a 73-year-old woman with osteoporosis.

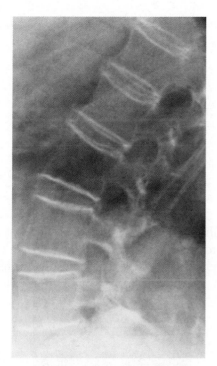

FIGURE 2-23　Osteoporosis of aging. Generalized demineralization of the spine in a postmenopausal woman. The cortex appears as a thin line that is relatively dense and prominent (empty box). (Eisenberg RL. *Clinical Imaging: An Atlas of Differential Diagnosis*. 5th ed. Philadelphia, PA: Lippincott Williams & Wilkins; 2010.)

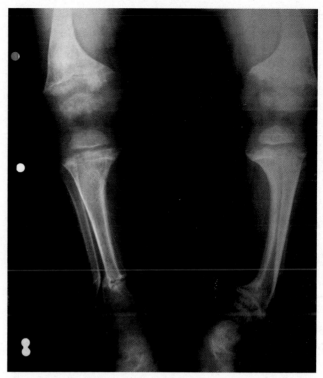

FIGURE 2-24　Osteomalacia in the form of rickets. Note the pseudofracture of the right tibia and fibula. There is bowing of the bones, a classic sign of rickets.

coarsened trabeculae due to osteoid deposition on remaining trabeculae without adequate mineralization seen in both processes.

Osteodystrophy is a disturbance in the growth of bone. Some disturbances are caused by lack of vitamins, as in osteomalacia, and others are a result of renal failure and are known as renal osteodystrophy.

Associated brown tumors are caused by large amounts of osteoclasts that "eat" away the inside of the bone, causing a lesion. Increased osteoclastic activity results in subperiosteal bone resorption. This results in a highly characteristic lace-like pattern of the outer cortex of the digits, femur, and humerus (Fig. 2-25). In addition to subperiosteal resorption, there is trabecula

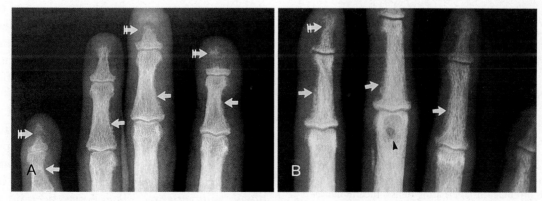

FIGURE 2-25　PA hands. Note the radial margins of the proximal and middle phalanges bilaterally are frayed, irregular, and lace like (*arrows*) owing to characteristic subperiosteal resorption. Also note the brown tumor (*arrowhead*) and osteolysis of the distal phalanges (*crossed arrows*). (Yochum TR, Rowe LJ. *Yochum and Rowe's Essentials of Skeletal Radiology*. 3rd ed. Philadelphia, PA: Lippincott Williams & Wilkins; 2004.)

bone resorption. This leads to a fuzzy, moth-eaten appearance of the skull known as the "salt and pepper" skull. When renal osteodystrophy occurs in the spine, it causes a "rugger jersey spine." The spine has spaced areas of osteosclerosis (light stripes from increased density of bone) and areas of osteolysis (dark stripes caused by increased radiolucency of the bone) giving it the appearance of a striped rugby jersey (Fig. 2-26).

Infection of the bone and bone marrow is termed **osteomyelitis**. **Osteitis** is infection of only the bone. The infection is most commonly caused by Staphylococci bacteria carried through the blood, but it can be caused directly if bacteria enter the bone from outside due to conditions such as a compound fracture. The usual site for development of osteomyelitis is the long bones of the lower limbs (Fig. 2-27).

In the acute stages, the inflammation causes a rise in pressure within the bone, but the periosteum constricts this buildup. This causes the vessels in the bone to become compressed. Within 24 to 48 hours the

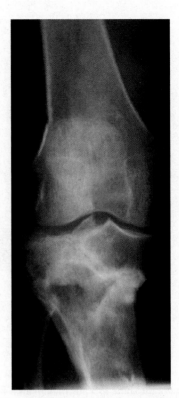

FIGURE 2-27   **Chronic osteomyelitis of proximal tibia after open fracture.** (Bucholz RW, Heckman JD. *Rockwood and Green's Fractures in Adults.* 5th ed. Philadelphia, PA: Lippincott Williams & Wilkins; 2001.)

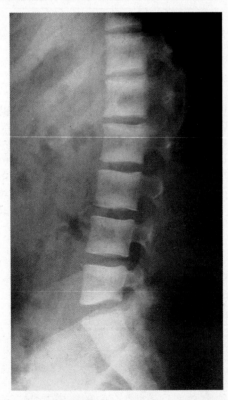

FIGURE 2-26   **Lateral lumbar spine. Note the prominent linear sub-endplate densities at multiple contiguous levels, which produce this alternating dense–lucent–dense appearance, simulating the transverse bands of a rugby jersey (*rugger jersey spine*).** (Yochum TR, Rowe LJ. *Yochum and Rowe's Essentials of Skeletal Radiology.* 3rd ed. Philadelphia, PA: Lippincott Williams & Wilkins; 2004.)

bone will die. This dead bone is called **sequestrum** and causes a linear opacity on a radiographic image. Unfortunately, radiography is not a very sensitive means of diagnosing this disease, since approximately 50% of the bone is destroyed before the changes are visible on a radiographic image. The first radiographic abnormality occurs in about 2 weeks and is poorly defined area of lucency at the site of infection. If sequestra are seen, it is highly suggestive of osteomyelitis as opposed to a neoplasm. A more reliable and faster means of demonstrating the bone destruction is a nuclear medicine bone scan. Areas of increased uptake or "hot spots" identify the infected site, allowing an early diagnosis (Fig. 2-28).

Osteitis deformans, or **Paget disease**, is overproduction of bone. It is an idiopathic disease but appears to be associated with an increased blood flow to the affected bones. This disease is more common in men over 55 years of age and occurs principally at the skull, tibias, and vertebrae. The bones become softened because of the over action of osteoclasts removing calcium. As the bones become sufficiently soft, they bow. This is particularly true of the tibias. After the

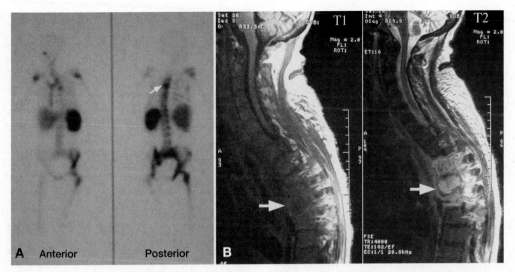

FIGURE 2-28 (A) Radionuclide bone scan shows retention of the tracer in a thoracic vertebra (*arrow*). Notice also the uptake in the pelvis and hip (also a result of osteomyelitis). The liver and spleen are routinely visualized with this technique. (B) MRI scan of the thoracic spine of the same patient. In the T1-weighted image (*left*), loss of bony structure in a vertebra is seen (*arrow*). In the T2-weighted image (*right*), the high signal intensity owing to water molecules shows edema and infiltrate in the same vertebra. (Engleberg NC, Dermody T, DiRita V. *Schaecter's Mechanisms of Microbial Disease*, 4th ed. Baltimore, MD: Lippincott Williams & Wilkins; 2007.)

period of softening, the bones become hard, causing the deformities to be permanent.

As the bone tries to repair itself, ossification takes place at the outside of the bone (recall the discussion of bone diameter growth). This constant destruction of the inside of the bone with simultaneous production at the outside of the bone, leading to enlargement is known as acromegaly (Fig. 2-29). Since the destruction and production are occurring simultaneously, radiographs demonstrate mixed areas of radiolucent osteolysis and radiopaque osteosclerosis known as the "cotton wool" appearance (Fig. 2-30A–C). Radionuclide scanning is always positive because of the increased metabolic activity.

Osteochondritis dissecans means bone dissected or separated from cartilage. Two forms that are important in radiography are Legg-Calvé-Perth disease and

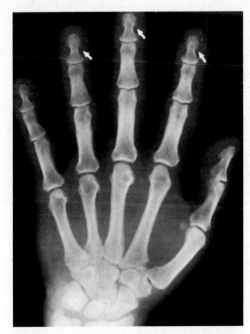

FIGURE 2-29 Acromegaly. Widening of the metacarpophalangeal joints, thickening of the soft tissues of the fingers, and overgrowth of the tufts of the distal phalanges (*arrows*). (Eisenberg RL. *Clinical Imaging: An Atlas of Differential Diagnosis*. 5th ed. Philadelphia, PA: Lippincott Williams & Wilkins; 2010.)

TECH TIP

This characteristic appearance of cotton wool is evident before any deformity is outwardly evident. Normal technical factors should be sufficient to demonstrate the extra thickness of the skull table on a lateral projection; however, an increase in kVp should be done when performing any anterior–posterior or axial projections.

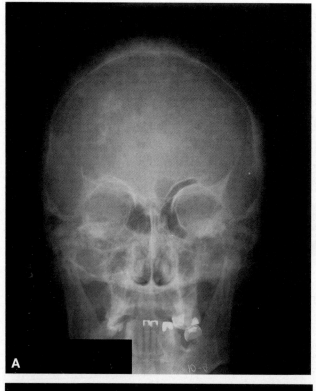

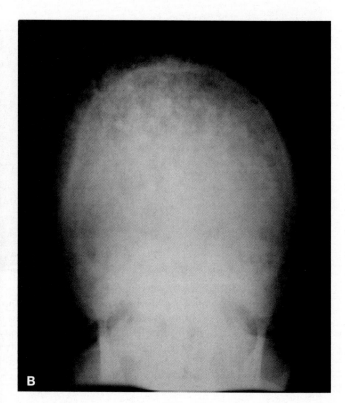

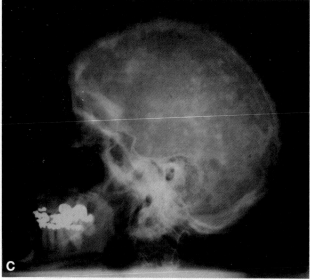

FIGURE 2-30   (A) Anteroposterior; (B) AP Axial; and
(C) lateral view skull images show the classic "cotton wool"
appearance of Paget disease.

Osgood-Schlatter disease. Legg-Calvé-Perth disease is
a common lesion of the head of the femur. It is most
often found in young boys around the age of 3 to 12
years; however, it can occur in females. This ischemic necrosis is usually unilateral but in about 15%
of the cases it is bilateral. The head of the femur at
the center of the epiphysis is fragmented. Because of
this, the femoral head becomes flattened and splayed
(Fig. 2-31). The hallmark of this disease is a flattened
femoral head that remains even after the lesion has

healed and the bone regains some of its structure. The
earliest clinical signs are pain and Trendelenburg gait,
a limp, but the radiograph will make the diagnosis
since early stages of tuberculosis can cause the same
clinical manifestations.

Anteroposterior and frog-leg oblique views show a
small joint space at the femoral head and acetabula.
There may be lucent or necrotic areas evident in the
epiphysis. MRI is useful for evaluation in the early
stages before the epiphysis has ossified.

Case Study

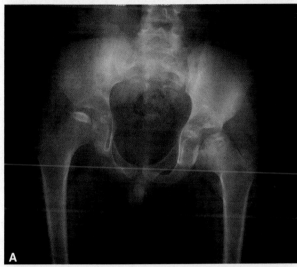

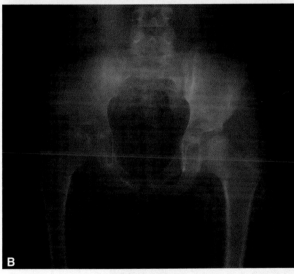

The above images show the progression of a male patient with Legg-Calvé-Perth process. Image A, taken a few months before the male patient's 8th birthday, shows involvement of the left femoral head. Image B was taken 2 weeks after the patient's 10th birthday, 2 years and 3 months from the last image. There is now clear destructive bone process bilaterally.

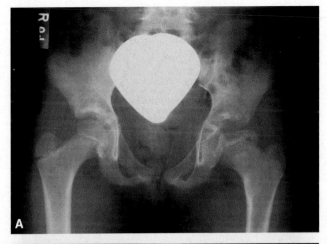

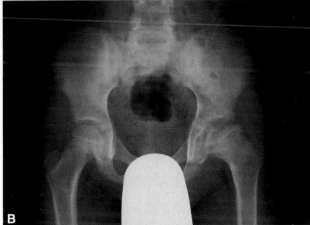

FIGURE 2-31   Legg-Calvé-Perth disease: (A) female and (B) male. Both have involvement of the left femoral head.

Osgood-Schlatter disease is characterized as a painful incomplete separation, avulsion, or strain of the epiphysis of the tibial tuberosity from the proximal anterior tibial shaft. There is bilateral involvement in 75% of the cases. It is more common in males between 10 and 15 years of age. It is thought to be traumatically induced avulsion due to repeated knee flexion against a tight quadriceps muscle. This causes soft tissue swelling and pain. Both of these symptoms should be present in addition to the avulsion to warrant a diagnosis of Osgood-Schlatter disease. Radiographic images show epiphyseal separation and fragmentation on the lateral knee image (Fig. 2-32).

Neoplastic Bone Changes

Benign

Fibrous dysplasia is the fibrous displacement of osseous tissue. Osteoblasts fail to undergo normal morphologic differentiation and maturation. The age of

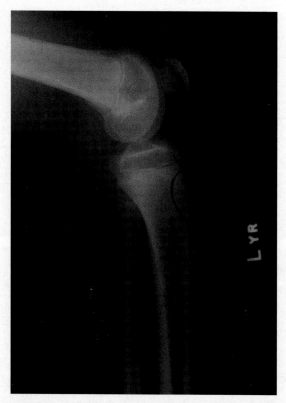

FIGURE 2-32   This lateral projection of the knee demonstrates Osgood-Schlatter disease with fragmentation of the tuberosity.

patients ranges from 10 to 70 years, but the process is seen more often in the 20s and 30s. The bones that are involved are the long bones, ribs, and facial bones. There may be solitary (monostotic) or multiple (polyostotic) lesions in one or more bones. Pathologic fractures are common because of expansion of the bone causing thin, eroded cortices. Angulation deformities result. The radiograph shows well-circumscribed lesions in the shaft of a long bone containing bands of sclerosis causing a multilocular effect (Fig. 2-33).

A bone cyst is a wall of fibrous tissue filled with clear fluid, occurring in the proximal humerus and knee of adolescents and young adults. Males outnumber females by a ratio of 3:1. A bone cyst develops beneath the epiphyseal plate but migrates down the shaft with growth (Fig. 2-34A). The cysts are not usually noted on a radiograph but are detected only when pain due to cyst growth or a pathologic fracture occurs (Fig. 2-34B). When they do appear radiographically, they show as a lucent focus with a thin cortex and sharp boundary. There may be septae to cause a loculated appearance. As can be seen in Figure 2-34C, there is a classic sign "fallen fragment sign," which occurs with pathologic fractures through a bone cyst. CT scans of a bone cyst show a fluid density within

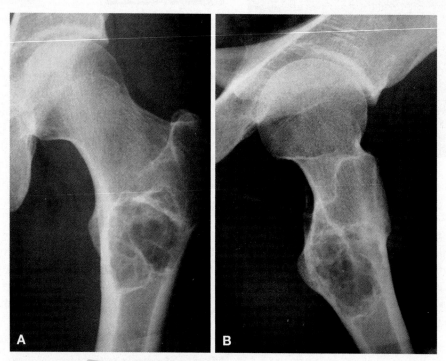

FIGURE 2-33   Fibrous dysplasia: (A) AP femur and (B) oblique femur. (Yochum TR, Rowe LJ. *Yochum and Rowe's Essentials of Skeletal Radiology*. 3rd ed. Philadelphia, PA: Lippincott Williams & Wilkins; 2004.)

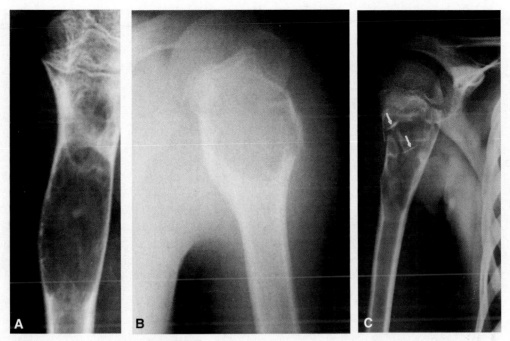

FIGURE 2-34   (A) Simple *bone cyst* in the proximal humerus. The cyst has an oval configuration, with its long axis parallel to that of the host bone. Note the thin septa that produce a multiloculated appearance. (B) Radiograph showing a 12-year-old boy sustained a pathologic fracture through a simple *bone cyst*. The fracture healed within 6 weeks. (C) A single box-like bone cyst in a humerus. The pathologic fracture through the cyst shows the "fallen fragment sign" (*arrows*). (A: Eisenberg RL. *Clinical Imaging: An Atlas of Differential Diagnosis*. 5th ed. Philadelphia, PA: Lippincott Williams & Wilkins; 2010. B: Bucholz RW, Heckman JD. *Rockwood and Green's Fractures in Adults*. 5th ed. Philadelphia, PA: Lippincott Williams & Wilkins; 2001. C: Berquist TH. *Musculoskeletal Imaging Companion*, 2nd ed. Baltimore, MD: Wolters Kluwer/Lippincott Williams & Wilkins; 2007.)

a well-defined lesion with bony septations within it. This will help differentiate it from fibrous dysplasia.

A **chondroma** is a cartilaginous tumor that is sharply delineated with a thin inner cortex, as seen on the radiographic image. The underlying bone is completely normal. The two benign types are as follows:

1. Exostosis
2. Endochondroma

The most common is **exostosis,** also called **osteochondroma**. It is the most common benign skeletal growth or tumor. It represents 50% of all benign bone tumors. More than 70% occur before the age of 20 years and has a male dominance of 2:1 over females. Most are asymptomatic unless surrounding nerves or blood vessels are disturbed. Occasionally, the stalk of bone will fracture causing pain at the site.

It arises from the cortex and grows parallel to the bone. The tumor points away from the adjacent joint and is capped by radiolucent cartilage. This cap may contain flake-like calcifications. Exostosis is caused by localized bone overgrowth at a joint, seen often at the knee (Fig. 2-35A). It enlarges during bone growth and then becomes static. Flat osteochondromas can occur in areas such as the pelvis and scapula.

An **enchondroma** arises in the medullary canal of the bone and is found most often in the bones of the hands and feet of adolescents and young adults. This benign tumor has little malignant potential when located in the hands or feet; however, the more centrally located the tumor, the greater the possibility of malignant transformation. Enchondromas are slow-growing tumors that are localized and small (Fig. 2-35B).

Osteoclastomas, or giant cell tumors, are benign tumors seen in young people in their early 20s. It is relatively common, representing about 15% of all primary tumors. The proportion of stromal cells to giant cells in the lesion will determine the tendency of the tumor to be benign or malignant. This, however, cannot be determined radiographically but must be done so clinically.

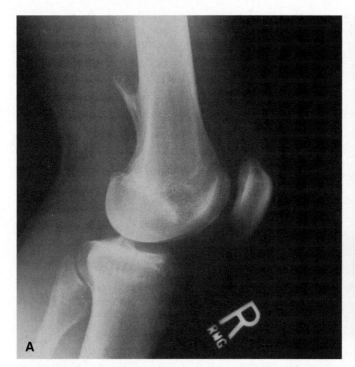

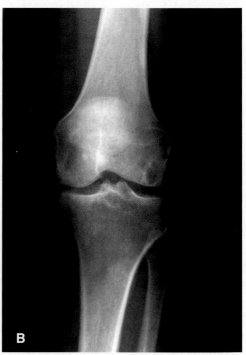

FIGURE 2-35   (A) Lateral knee demonstrating exostosis and (B) anteroposterior knee with an endochondroma.

The most common location is in the long bones arising from the epiphysis after closure (Fig. 2-36). The joint space is not involved. The tumor does extensive local damage to the bone, but does not metastasize. The cortex is thinned out as the lesion extends transversely across the end of the shaft of the long bone. It is seen on a radiograph as large lytic lesions separated by thin strips of bone. The lesions will expand the bone causing the characteristic "soap bubble" appearance on a radiographic image.

Surgical intervention is the only way to ensure removal of the tumor. Liquid nitrogen freezing, bone packing, and grafting are all planned with the surgery to minimize the likelihood of recurrence.

Malignant

The four chief primary malignant tumors of bone are chondrosarcoma, osteogenic sarcoma, Ewing sarcoma, and multiple myeloma. Because only multiple myeloma is easily identifiable on radiographic images, the other three will be covered briefly with more attention paid to multiple myeloma.

A **chondrosarcoma** is third most common malignant bone tumor. It occurs two times more often in men over the age 45 than in women. The pelvis and

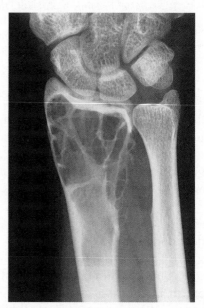

FIGURE 2-36   Giant cell tumor, soap bubble pattern (in distal radius). Note the subarticular, expansile, geographic lesion in the distal portion of the radius. This tumor has removed numerous trabeculae by its neoplastic growth, prompting reinforcement of the remaining trabeculae and rendering a classic soap bubble pattern. *Comment*: Giant cell tumors in the distal radius carry a higher incidence of malignancy than giant cell tumors at any other skeletal site. (Yochum TR, Rowe LJ. *Yochum and Rowe's Essentials of Skeletal Radiology.* 3rd ed. Philadelphia, PA: Lippincott Williams & Wilkins; 2004.)

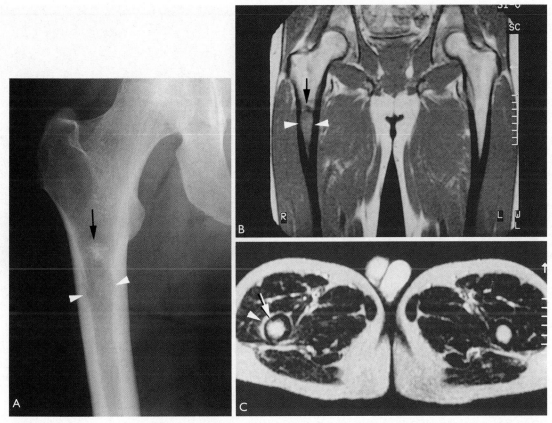

FIGURE 2-37   Chondrosarcoma (in femur). (A) AP spot hip. Note the intramedullary stippled calcification (*arrow*) in the right femoral diaphysis. There is a subtle radiolucency with early endosteal erosion of the femur (*arrowheads*). (B) T1-weighted MRI of coronal pelvis. Note the low signal intensity intramedullary calcification (*arrow*). The intermediate signal intensity tumor has replaced the normal marrow and expanded the medullary space (*arrowheads*). The left side is normal. (C) T2-weighted MRI of bilateral axial femur. Note that the tumor infiltration has caused endosteal erosion (*arrow*). The high signal intensity region along the cortical perimeter represents edema (*arrowhead*). No cortical fracture or soft tissue tumor invasion is identified. *Comment*: This 35-year-old male patient presented with a deep ache in his right hip. (Yochum TR, Rowe LJ. *Yochum and Rowe's Essentials of Skeletal Radiology*. 3rd ed. Philadelphia, PA: Lippincott Williams & Wilkins; 2004.)

long bones are the sites of a chondrosarcoma (Fig. 2-37). When the primary tumor is removed, there is often rapid growth or metastasis and prolonged recovery times. However, the outlook for a chondrosarcoma is better than that for other malignant sarcomas with a 5-year survival rate approaching 90% after removal.

Radiographic images reveal a large, radiolucent lesion with an oval or round shape. Scalloping of the endosteum is caused by the lobular outlines of the tumor. The cortex may be eroded which indicates an advanced stage.

Ewing sarcoma is the most common primary malignant bone tumor seen in a child of 5 to 15 years of age. It ranks as the fourth most common primary

malignancy overall. It occurs in the diaphysis of long bones. This tumor is often misdiagnosed as osteomyelitis because of the constant low-grade pain, fever, and leukocytosis that are present. This unique feature appears to be due to the tumor outgrowing its blood supply. This will cause extensive degeneration and necrosis. With healing, the bone has a stratified new bone formation, causing the "onion peel" appearance (Fig. 2-38). By the time the tumor is seen on a radiograph, the prognosis is poor. Nuclear medicine bone scan is the best imaging modality for this condition.

There is a 5-year survival rate in only about 5% of all Ewing sarcoma cases. Amputation is usually necessary if the lesion is in the knee joint to help prevent metastasis. If there is reoccurrence after resection of

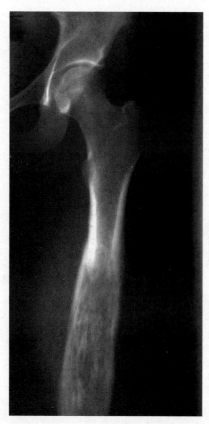

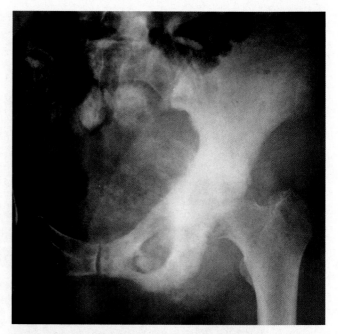

FIGURE 2-39   Osteosarcoma of the pelvis demonstrating osteoid matrix. Notice how dense the lesion is because of the osteoid matrix formation. (Daffner RH. *Clinical Radiology: The Essentials.* 3rd ed. Philadelphia, PA: Lippincott Williams & Wilkins; 2007.)

FIGURE 2-38   Ewing sarcoma. This image demonstrates expansile cortical destruction with poor circumscription and a delicate interrupted periosteal reaction. (Rubin R, Strayer DS. *Rubin's Pathology: Clinicopathologic Foundations of Medicine.* 5th ed. Philadelphia, PA: Lippincott Williams & Wilkins; 2008.)

the tumor, regardless of the location, the prognosis is usually fatal.

Osteogenic sarcoma, also known as **osteosarcoma** (Fig. 2-39), is a highly malignant primary tumor occurring at 10 to 30 years of age, with the peak incidence rate at 20 years of age. A second peak incidence rate is found at age 60, if Paget disease is already manifested. This common neoplasm occurs most often in the long bones, particularly at the lower ends of the femurs and upper ends of the humerus or radius. There is extensive destruction of bone and metastasis occurs to the lungs at an early stage. The periosteum is lifted from the bone by the tumor. Spicules of new bone are laid down, which radiate outward from the central mass. The patient presents with painful swelling at the site of the lesion. However, usually the tumor is found as an incidental finding while investigating recent trauma to the bone. This is known as traumatic determinism.

Radiographically, this presents as dense areas, radiolucent areas, or mixed areas to give it the characteristic "sunray" appearance. Osteogenic sarcoma carries a poor prognosis with a 5-year survival rate in about 20% of cases even if the patient is otherwise healthy. Amputation is the best treatment if the lesion is surgically accessible.

Of all the primary tumors of the bone, **multiple myeloma** is the most common. There may be only one tumor or, as the name suggests, multiple lesions in various areas of the body, particularly the flat bones. The disease is rare in persons younger than 40 years of age and is most often seen in persons over the age of 50 years. The tumor actually arises from the bone marrow plasma cells and occurs in bone marrow that is actively hemopoietic. Therefore, this is not a true osseous tumor.

The hallmark radiographic sign of multiple myeloma is punched-out osteolytic lesions, not unlike a "Swiss cheese" (Fig. 2-40) effect. The chance of pathologic fractures increases as the destruction of the bone continues. Also, the possibility of paraplegia increases as the bone marrow of the spinal column hypertrophies and exerts pressure on the spinal cord.

In patients with multiple myeloma, the overall prognosis is poor. Over 90% of the patients die within

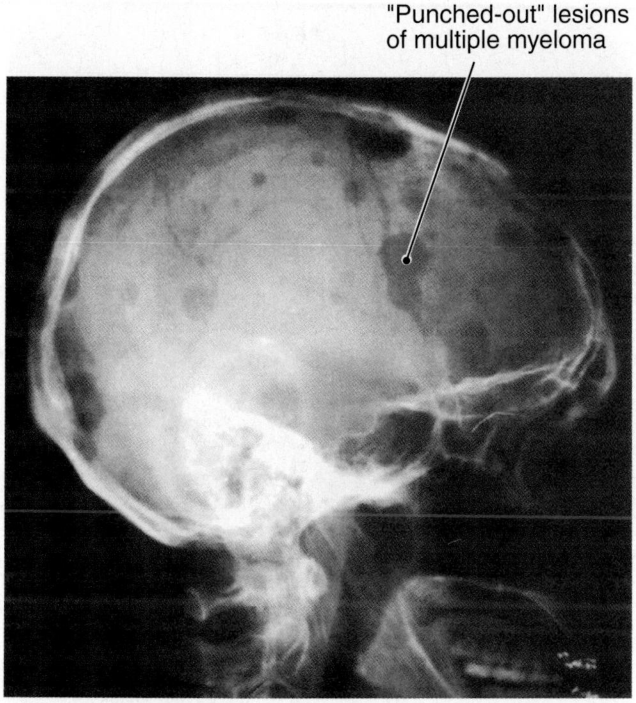

"Punched-out" lesions
of multiple myeloma

FIGURE 2-40   In this image of the skull showing multiple myeloma, the "punched-out" radiolucent lesions are the result of destruction by nodules of plasma cells. (Reprinted with permission from Rubin E. *Pathology.* 4th ed. Philadelphia, PA: Lippincott Williams and Wilkins; 2005.)

3 years of diagnosis. The average survival rate is 33 months. Treatment is mainly palliative with the aim for easing the patient's suffering.

Metastatic bone tumors are much more common than primary bone tumors. A metastatic tumor is the first sign that cancer is present somewhere else in the body; usually, the breast, lung, prostate, and kidney are the primary sites. Metastatic tumors reach the skeleton through the circulatory system or lymph system or by invasion. Pathologic fractures occur as a result of the tumor weakening the bone. The bones that contain red bone marrow are the first to be affected by metastasis, including the spine, skull, ribs, pelvis, and femurs.

Fractures and Dislocations

The most frequent injury to the skeletal system is a **fracture**. A fracture is a discontinuity of a bone caused by force applied either directly or indirectly to the bone. When a fracture occurs, there is a break in the endosteum and damage to soft tissue and surrounding vessels. Fracture of long bones can lead to shock because as much as one liter of blood can be lost in the surrounding tissue.

Bleeding is necessary for the healing of fractures, however. The blood loss leads to inflammation and the formation of fibrous tissue. Blood, lymph, and tissue form a fibrin clot at the fracture site. Fibroblasts are then embedded in this clot, forming a stabilizing type of tissue called granulation tissue. This tissue in turn becomes a temporary callus (a fibrocartilaginous mass) that knits the fracture. Calcium is later deposited by osteoblasts to complete the healing process.

Since complication of a fracture is possible, care must be taken to prevent this from occurring. Infection is likely with a compound fracture and delays union. Injuries to other organs, such as a lung punctured by a broken rib, with resulting pneumothorax, is another factor that must be watched for. There also may be ossification in surrounding muscles due to extensive soft-tissue damage or a fat embolism caused by the fat from the bone marrow entering the circulation.

Types of Fractures

Most fractures are named or classified by the direction of the fracture line, whether the overlying skin is intact, and the shape, position, and number of the fragments of the fractured bone.

A *complete* fracture is one that occurs through the entire cross section of the bone, while an *incomplete*, or *fissure*, fracture breaks only one cortex. If skin is not broken, the fracture is known as a *closed* fracture. In order to be classified as a *compound* (open) fracture, the skin or mucosal surface must be pierced by at least one end of the fracture bone.

Simple fractures divide the bone into two complete pieces. *Comminuted* fractures (Fig. 2-41) may be "shattered" but there must only be three or more fragments for the fracture to be termed comminuted.

Terms such as *transverse*, *spiral*, *oblique*, and *longitudinal* simply describe the direction of the fracture in relation to the long axis of the bone (Fig. 2-42). Radiographs seen in Figure 2-43 show these different types of fractures. A star-shaped fracture, particularly on the patella or the calvarium, is termed as *stellate*. If the cortical shaft is driven into the cancellous bone by some force, the bone becomes *impacted* and the fracture is termed as such (Fig. 2-44A, B).

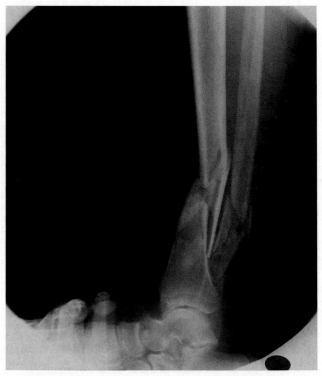

When a spiral fracture occurs in an adult ankle in the tibia, the force of the torque will almost always fracture the head of the fibula. If a knee radiograph or tib-fib radiograph has not been requested, it is incumbent on the technologist to alert the requesting physician or the radiologist to determine if this should be done at time the patient is in the department.

FIGURE 2-41   Comminuted fracture of the tibia and fibula.

The positioning of the fragments must be determined so that the fracture can be reduced (put back into place) prior to a cast being applied. **Displacement** refers to the lateral positioning of the fragments and **distraction** refers to the gap between the fragments.

When the tibia or fibula (or radius or ulna) is fractured, the other end of the paired bone should be checked for fractures. This is especially true in the case of spiral fractures, as the torquing force applied at one end of the bone is carried through to the other end and usually causes a second fracture (Fig. 2-45).

Not all bones fracture when they are involved in trauma. They may become **dislocated**, which means the bones that form a joint no longer articulate (Fig. 2-46). If there is **subluxation** of the joint, it is only partially dislocated (Fig. 2-47).

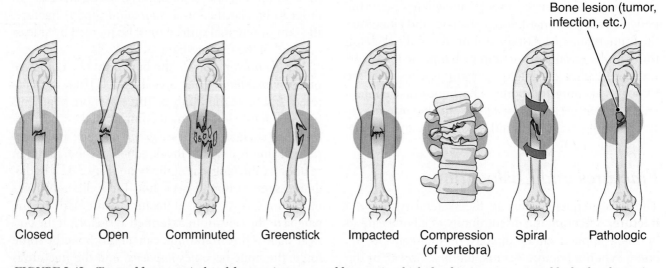

Bone lesion (tumor, infection, etc.)

Closed   Open   Comminuted   Greenstick   Impacted   Compression (of vertebra)   Spiral   Pathologic

FIGURE 2-42   Types of fractures. A closed fracture is any type of fracture in which the skin is not punctured by broken bone. An open fracture is one with protruding bone. Compression fractures are most common in vertebrae. (McConnell TH. *The Nature of Disease Pathology for the Health Professions*. Philadelphia, PA: Lippincott Williams & Wilkins; 2007.)

Case Study

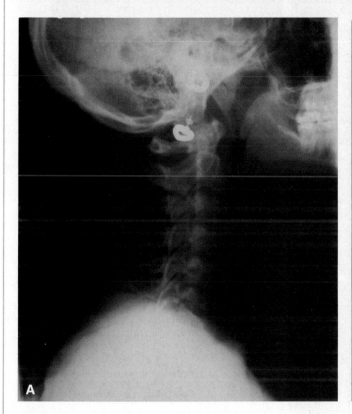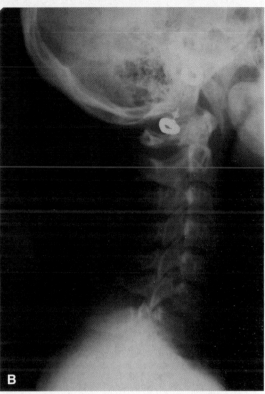

These two images demonstrate how important it is to demonstrate all seven cervical vertebrae. Image A demonstrates only six vertebrae, while image B shows the spine after the shoulders were pulled down. It can now be seen that C6 is subluxated over C7.

Finally, there can be problems with healing of the fracture. When healing does not occur in the normal time it is referred to as **delayed union**. **Malunion** occurs when the bone ends have not been properly reduced and are misaligned, which impairs normal function. It is possible for the bone ends to never join at all, particularly in certain pathologies. This is known as **nonunion**.

Common Fractures

All fractures can be broken down into general categories, such as those just described, or can be labeled by terminology that refers to a specific type of fracture. There are many types and classifications of fractures that can occur; however, only the most common

fractures that should be known by every radiographer will be discussed here.

Fractures that occur in children are usually not as serious as those that occur in adults because of the softness of children's bones. *Plastic* fractures occur when the soft young bone bends, but the cortex does not actually break (Fig. 2-48). A *greenstick* fracture (Fig. 2-49), on the other hand, is a break in the cortex but only on one side of the shaft. This is a type of fissure fracture. This angulated fracture produces a bowing of the bone. Another fracture that occurs in children is known as a *torus* fracture (Fig. 2-50A, B). This is a type of greenstick fracture in which a driving force pushes down the shaft of bone, causing the cortex to fold back onto itself. A final fracture that

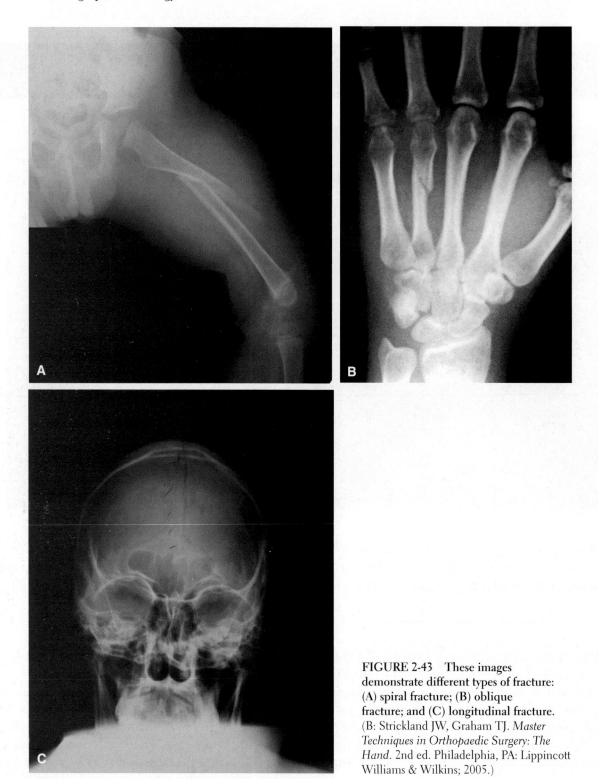

FIGURE 2-43   These images demonstrate different types of fracture: (A) spiral fracture; (B) oblique fracture; and (C) longitudinal fracture. (B: Strickland JW, Graham TJ. *Master Techniques in Orthopaedic Surgery: The Hand.* 2nd ed. Philadelphia, PA: Lippincott Williams & Wilkins; 2005.)

involves children is the *epiphyseal* fracture that occurs through un-united areas of epiphyses (Fig. 2-51). There is no displacement, as a comparison projection is needed. There are several classifications of epiphyseal fractures, but it is beyond the scope of an imaging radiographer to diagnose these types.

Fatigue (also known as a *march* fracture or a *stress* fracture) occurs at sites of maximum stress, usually the metatarsal bones. The fracture is the result of repeated, relatively trivial trauma to an otherwise normal bone. Its name derives from the fact that these fractures are most commonly found in persons unaccustomed to

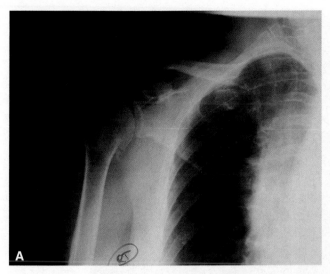

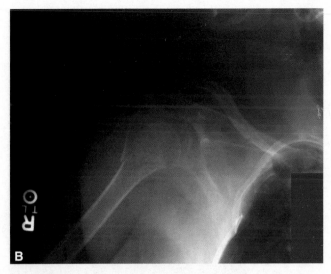

FIGURE 2-44   Both A and B show an impacted fracture of the right shoulder. The humeral shaft has been driven into the head of the humerus.

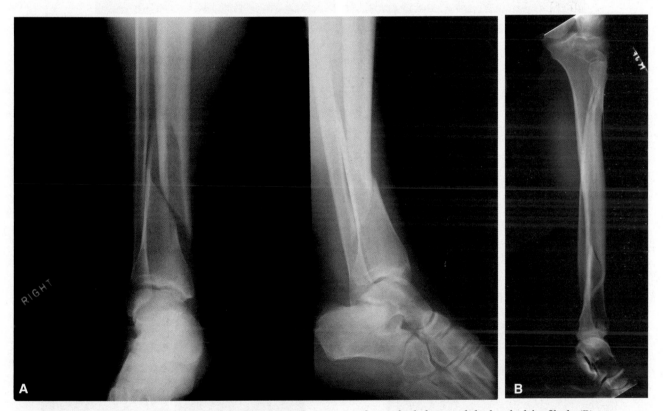

FIGURE 2-45   (A) This spiral fracture of the tibia created a torquing force which fractured the head of the fibula (B).

vigorous physical activity in the form of marching or hiking. Often the fracture is not seen on an initial radiographic image. It is usually seen after new bone formation has been completed. A fracture that occurs when normal stress is placed on diseased areas of bone is known as *pathologic* fracture (Fig. 2-52).

The disease must be treated for healing of the fracture to take place.

Fractures can easily occur around joint articulations. When a small chip of bone breaks away when a joint has dislocated, an *avulsion* fracture (Fig. 2-53) has occurred. Compressing forces applied to both sides of

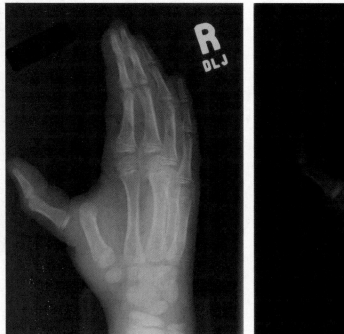

FIGURE 2-46   A dislocated right thumb.

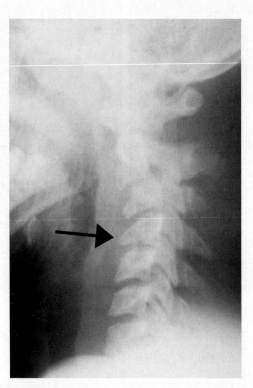

FIGURE 2-47   This adolescent swam with full speed into the pool wall. He has a crush injury of C4 and C2–C3 subluxation (*arrow*).

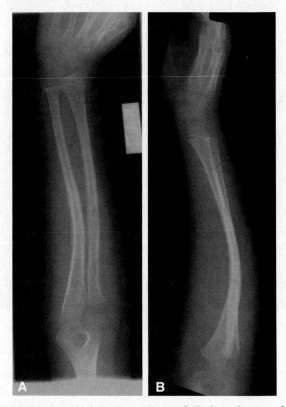

FIGURE 2-48   (A) Anteroposterior and (B) lateral views of the forearm of a young child showing bowing (plastic fracture) of bones but no actual fracture of the cortex.

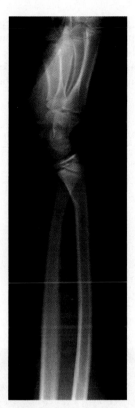

FIGURE 2-49   Greenstick fracture: the cortex is broken on one side, producing an angulated bowing of the bone.

the bone ends cause *compression* fractures (Fig. 2-54). These usually occur in the spine in postmenopausal women. As osteoporosis sets in, the bones become brittle. The spine, which normally holds the weight of the body upright, literally becomes bowed under the weight pushing down on the top of the vertebrae and the force of standing pushing up on the vertebrae. The anterior vertebral bodies collapse under the force.

Other fractures that will be encountered during the career of the radiographer have specific eponymic names to identify them. The *Galeazzi* fracture (Fig. 2-55A) is of the radial shaft at the junction of the middle and distal thirds. It is associated with dislocation of the distal ulna. The *Monteggia* fracture (Fig. 2-55B) involves the proximal third of the ulna with anterior dislocation of the radial head. Both fractures involve only one bone. It is essential in these instances to examine the elbow and wrist to determine whether any associated dislocations and possible avulsion fractures have taken place. The elbow itself may be fractured. A hallmark indication of a fracture here is the "sail" sign (Fig. 2-56). On lateral projections of a normal elbow, the anterior fat pad lies close to the distal end of the humerus and the posterior fat pad

is not visible. When trauma occurs at this site, fluid effusion, either synovial or hemorrhagic in nature, displaces both fat pads. The anterior one separates from the bone surface. The normally hidden posterior fat pad becomes displaced posteriorly and shows up as a crescent-shaped lucency. Since this fat pad is normally not seen, its presence is an excellent indicator of effusion present within the joint. The most common fracture associated with a fat-pad sign is a radial head or neck fracture. The posterior fat pad is a more reliable indicator of fracture because the anterior fat pad may be poorly visualized or present in normal patients.

Both *Colles* and *Smith* fractures occur at the wrist. A Colles fracture occurs when the distal radius fractures with the fragment being displaced posteriorly (Fig. 2-57A). Conversely, a Smith fracture can be identified by the anterior displacement of the fragments (Fig. 2-57B). Either of these fractures can be accompanied by an avulsion fracture of the ulnar styloid process. Fractures of the hand seen most often are the *Bennett* fracture, which is at the base of the first metacarpal (thumb) with proximal displacement (Fig. 2-58A), and the *boxer's* fracture, which occurs at the neck of the fifth metacarpal (Fig. 2-58B–D). A boxer's fracture is so named because it usually occurs when the person hits a solid object with a tightly closed fist, causing the metacarpal of the little finger to snap.

The last fractures to be identified are of the ankle. A *bimalleolar* fracture (Fig. 2-59A) is of the lateral and medial malleoli, and a *trimalleolar* fracture (Fig. 2-59B, C) is of the lateral, medial, and posterior malleoli of the ankle. These serious fractures require surgery to screw the fragments into place. A less drastic fracture of the ankle is the *Pott* fracture that involves injury to the distal tibial articulation. This was originally described as a fracture of the fibula with dislocation of the tibia. Today, a Pott fracture refers to a bimalleolar fracture with an avulsion fracture of the medial malleolus caused by abduction and external rotation of the ankle.

Common Dislocations

Radiographers must be aware of the direction of dislocations of the shoulder and hip to avoid further injury to a patient. The shoulder dislocates anteriorly, with the head slipping into the subglenoid fossa (Fig. 2-60A). A chip fracture is common with a shoulder dislocation. The hip dislocates posteriorly against the sciatic notch (Fig. 2-60B).

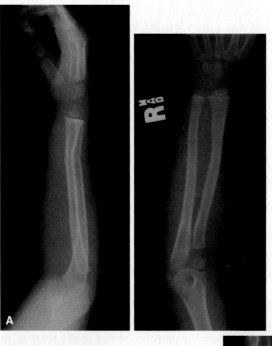

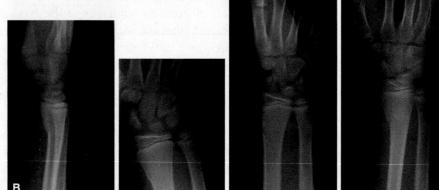

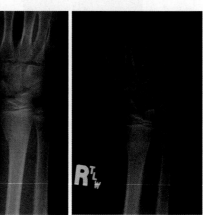

FIGURE 2-50   Torus fracture. (A) This lateral and AP radiograph shows that a torus fracture can sometimes only be seen on the lateral view. (B) This radiographic image shows five positions taken for a wrist examination. The torus fracture can be seen in all five images.

TECH TIP

Both dislocations are easily detected simply by observing the patient. A patient whose shoulder is dislocated will carry the affected arm across the chest or abdomen while the shoulder droops noticeably below the ipsilateral shoulder. A patient with a dislocated hip will usually have the knee of the affected side bent while the lower extremity is rotated outwardly, similar to a fractured hip. The patient is most comfortable if the knee is supported slightly. The alert radiographer will avoid further injury to a patient if the situation is assessed prior to any movement of the body part.

Joint Pathology

Arthritis is the most common joint disease. It is an inflammation of the joint, but there can be degenerative changes without infection. Following are descriptions of several types of arthritis that are important radiographically.

Osteoarthritis, also known as *degenerative joint disease* (DJD), is the most common of all types of arthritis and occurs in older patients who have put a lot of "wear and tear" on the large weight-bearing joints of the body, such as the knees, or in obese patients who have extra weight that the joints have to carry. Joint changes in this disease are found to some degree in all persons older than 50 years of age. Approximately 80% of all Americans are affected.

Osteoarthritis is a noninflammatory deterioration of the articular cartilage with new bone forming at the

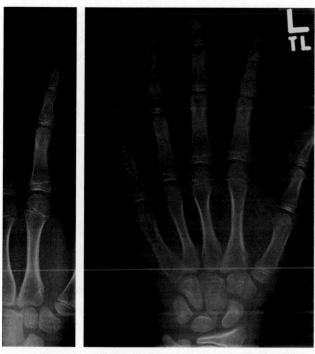

FIGURE 2-51   Epiphyseal fracture of the second digit. The actual fracture is located on the proximal epiphyseal plate of the middle phalanx.

surface of the joint. Radiographic images of the joint show the hallmark sign of "spurring" (Fig. 2-61A, B), or in severe cases, mild subluxation or loose bodies within the joint space (Fig. 2-61C). Narrow joint spaces and some erosion may occur. The smaller joints that are affected, such as the hands, will show nodules and increased size at the interphalangeal joint spaces.

Rheumatoid arthritis (RA) affects the small joints of the hands and feet. RA affects women in their 30s and 40s three times more often than males. It is an autoimmune disease characterized by chronic and progressive inflammatory involvement of the joints and atrophy of the muscles. The cause of RA is not known.

Widespread inflammation in the synovial membrane takes place, causing pain, stiffness, and thickening of the tissue. This thickened tissue grows inward and damages the cartilage. Later, the tissue becomes fibrous, which prevents motion of the joint (fibrous ankylosis). As the disease progresses, the fibrous tissue becomes calcified and becomes osseous tissue (bony ankylosis).

In the early stage of the disease, the radiograph shows soft-tissue swelling around the joints. Later, the films show a decrease in the joint space, with eroded bone ends and subluxation (Fig. 2-62). This leads to the gross deformities often encountered with RA.

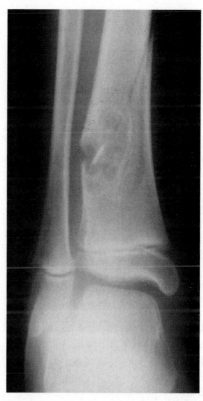

FIGURE 2-52   Anteroposterior radiograph of the distal tibia of a 10-year-old boy. The well-developed reactive rim of bone around the eccentric, metaphyseal, radiolucent lesion is virtually diagnostic of a nonossifying fibroma (NOF). The patient had no symptoms until he slid into second base and caught his foot, twisting his lower leg. He heard a crack and had acute pain immediately. The fracture was treated in a cast and healed, but the NOF took another 2 years to fill in with bone. (Bucholz RW, Heckman JD. *Rockwood and Green's Fractures in Adults.* 5th ed. Philadelphia, PA: Lippincott Williams & Wilkins; 2001.)

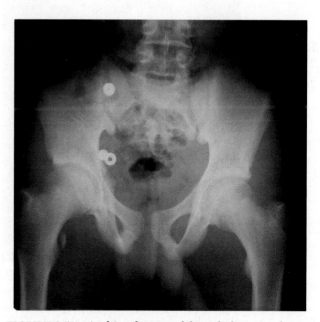

FIGURE 2-53   Avulsion fracture of the right lesser trochanter.

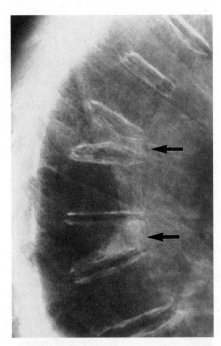

FIGURE 2-54   Lateral thoracic spine showing compression fractures. Two levels of compression fracture are evident in the midthoracic spine (*arrows*). (Yochum TR, Rowe LJ. *Yochum and Rowe's Essentials of Skeletal Radiology*. 3rd ed. Philadelphia, PA: Lippincott Williams & Wilkins; 2004.)

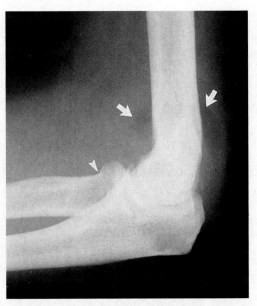

FIGURE 2-56   Fat-pad sign: Subtle radial neck fracture (lateral elbow). Note two triangular areas of radiolucency projecting away from the distal humeral shaft at the anterior and posterior aspects (*arrows*). A subtle fracture of the radial neck is also identified (*arrowhead*). *Comment*: Whenever both the anterior and posterior fat pads are visible in this projection, a careful search must be performed to rule out a subtle intra-articular fracture. (Yochum TR, Rowe LJ. *Yochum and Rowe's Essentials of Skeletal Radiology*. 3rd ed. Philadelphia, PA: Lippincott Williams & Wilkins; 2004.)

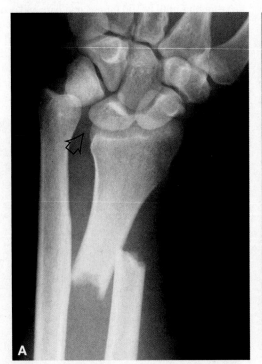

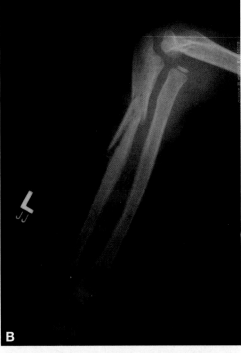

FIGURE 2-55   (A) Severely displaced Galeazzi fracture. The distal radioulnar dislocation (*open arrow*) is secondary to the marked shortening of the radius caused by the severe ulnar displacement and dorsal angulation of the distal radial fragment. (B) Monteggia fracture shows classic displacement of the radial head. (A: From Harris JH Jr, Harris WH. *The Radiology of Emergency Medicine*, 3rd ed. Philadelphia, PA: Lippincott-Raven; 2000:390, with permission.)

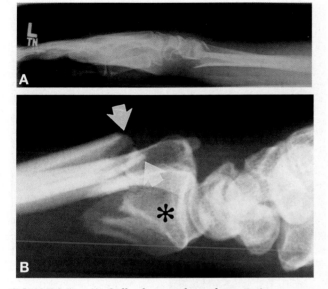

FIGURE 2-57 **(A) Colles fracture shows the posterior displacement of the radius and ulna. (B) This Smith fracture is characterized by a transverse fracture (*arrows*) of the distal radius with displacement of the distal radial fragment (*).** (B: Harris JH Jr, Harris WH. *The Radiology of Emergency Medicine*, 3rd ed. Philadelphia, PA: Lippincott-Raven; 2000:386.)

Ulnar deviation of the wrist with either "boutonniere deformity" (flexion) or "swan neck deformity" (hyperextension) of the proximal interphalangeal joint occurs (Fig. 2-63). The distal interphalangeal joint is rarely affected.

Ankylosing spondylitis, or **rheumatoid spondylitis**, is a chronic inflammatory disorder that predominantly affects the sacral iliac joints and lumbar spine. It is a common cause of chronic low back pain. The age of onset is between 15 and 35 years with an average age of approximately 26 years. Ninety percent of the patients who have ankylosing spondylitis are male.

Ankylosing spondylitis starts in the lumbar spine and progresses upward. As it reaches the thoracic area, kyphosis develops and breathing becomes difficult due to limited chest expansion. It causes extensive calcifications of the anterior longitudinal ligament. This creates the characteristic "bamboo-spine" appearance on a radiograph (Fig. 2-64). Bone density is normal until the ankylosis becomes debilitating and disuse osteoporosis occurs.

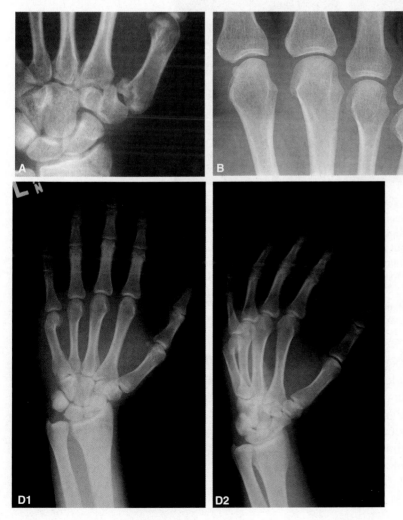

FIGURE 2-58 **(A) Bennett's fracture in the first metacarpal base. (B) Boxer's fracture in the head of fifth metacarpal. Note that a transverse fracture is seen at the junction of the fifth metacarpal head and shaft (*arrow*). Some slight radial displacement of the head is also present. (C) PA oblique hand. Note that this view reveals the significant anterior displacement of the metacarpal head, common in these injuries. These metacarpal head fractures are common after a direct blow to the metacarpal phalangeal joints, particularly on the ulnar side of the hand. (D1), (D2) These two projections show the head of the fifth metacarpal fractured with slight displacement which is better seen on the oblique projection.** (A: Bucholz RW, Heckman JD. *Rockwood and Green's Fractures in Adults*. 5th ed. Philadelphia, PA: Lippincott Williams & Wilkins; 2001. B and C: Yochum TR, Rowe LJ. *Yochum and Rowe's Essentials of Skeletal Radiology*. 3rd ed. Philadelphia, PA: Lippincott Williams & Wilkins; 2004.)

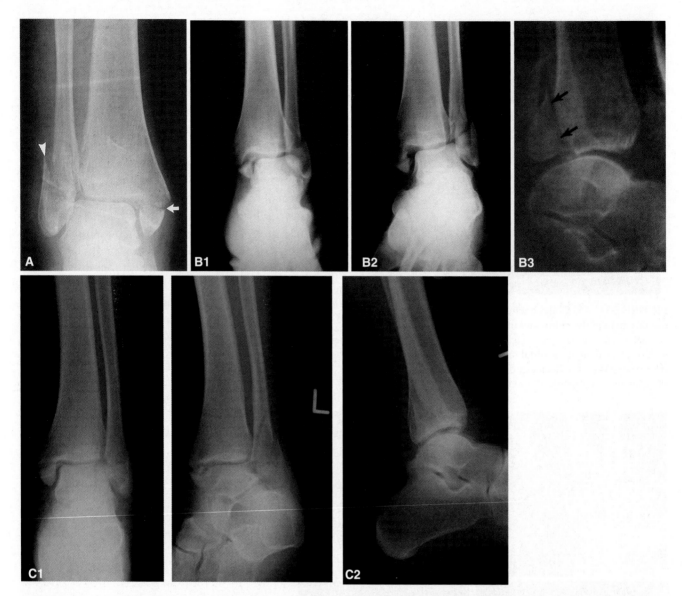

FIGURE 2-59   (A) Bimalleolar fracture (AP ankle). Note the characteristic transverse fracture through the medial malleolus (*arrow*), along with a spiral fracture of the lateral malleolus (*arrowhead*). (B1–B3) Trimalleolar fracture. These AP (B1), mortise (B2), and lateral (B3) projections demonstrate how important it is to show the part in two projections at 90° to each other. The posterior fractures could have been missed without the lateral projection. (C1) The AP and oblique projections show only the medial and lateral malleoli fractures. (C2) This lateral image shows that the posterior malleoli is also fractured making this a trimalleolar fracture. (A: Yochum TR, Rowe LJ. *Yochum and Rowe's Essentials of Skeletal Radiology.* 3rd ed. Philadelphia, PA: Lippincott Williams & Wilkins; 2004. B1, B2 and C: Koval KJ, Zuckerman JD. *Atlas of Orthopaedic Surgery: A Multimeidal Reference.* Philadelphia, PA: Lippincott Williams & Wilkins; 2004; B3: Bucholz RW, Heckman JD. *Rockwood and Green's Fractures in Adults.* 5th ed. Philadelphia, PA: Lippincott Williams & Wilkins; 2001.)

Not all joint diseases are arthritis. Many other types of disease processes, as well as trauma or infection, can destroy a joint. Probably the most common non-arthritic ailment of joints is **bursitis**. This is an inflammation of the synovial bursa caused by excess stress on the joint. Bursitis is generally found in the shoulder, and the radiographs may show calcified deposits in the tendon above the greater tuberosity of the humerus (Fig. 2-65).

TECH TIP

To see any calcification that might be present, the technologist should lower down the technical factors when he/she sees a diagnosis of bursitis on a radiographic imaging request.

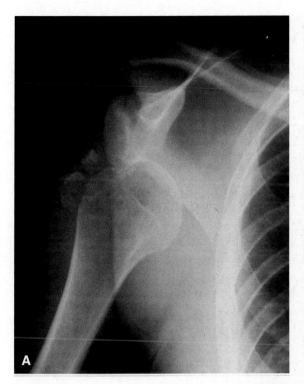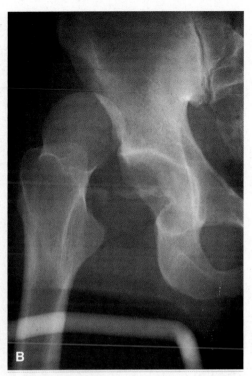

FIGURE 2-60   (A) A patient in his 40s sustained this fracture dislocation of the shoulder with evidence of rotator cuff disruption. (B) A 53-year-old woman with a posterior hip dislocation demonstrating fragments in the joint prior to hip reduction and an inferior femoral head fracture. (Bucholz RW, Heckman JD. *Rockwood and Green's Fractures in Adults*. 5th ed. Philadelphia, PA: Lippincott Williams & Wilkins; 2001.)

Low back pain is the most common complaint of radiologic technologists. This is usually caused by improper body postures when moving heavy objects. Diseases of the kidneys, prostate area, or disk problems may be the cause of the pain in patients.

Spondylolisthesis is the forward displacement of one vertebra on top of another, usually occurring at the L5/S1 junction (Fig. 2-66A). However, spondylolisthesis will occur anywhere that a vertebral body will slide forward over the vertebrae below it. A less common type is seen between L4 and L5 (Fig. 2-66B–E). This is usually caused by some kind of defect of the pedicle. **Spondylitis** is inflammation of the spinal vertebrae, and **spondylosis** is a condition of the spine characterized by fixation and stiffness.

Disk herniations are common in the lumbar spine area. The fibrous ring of the disk degenerates to the point that the pulpy nucleus is forced out of the disk. Posterior herniation results in pressure on the spinal cord and nerve roots. This can cause neurologic symptoms. Radiographs show narrowing of the disk. CT and MRI demonstrate the extent of the damage (Fig. 2-67A, C). Myelography was a procedure that was done prior to the advent of CT and MRI. The utilization of contrast media injected into the spinal canal would show the filling defect as the herniation pushes in on the cord (Fig. 2-67B).

Imaging Strategies

TECH TIP

Excellent quality conventional radiography of the skeletal system is usually all that is necessary to adequately demonstrate bone lesions and most fractures. It is extremely important, though, that the technologist honestly provides the best quality images possible. For long bone radiography, both joints must be demonstrated. All parts of the body must be imaged at the very minimum of 90° to each other (such as anterior posterior and lateral). Bone radiography must utilize contrast so the kVp will be in the lower ranges with the mAs increased to compensate.

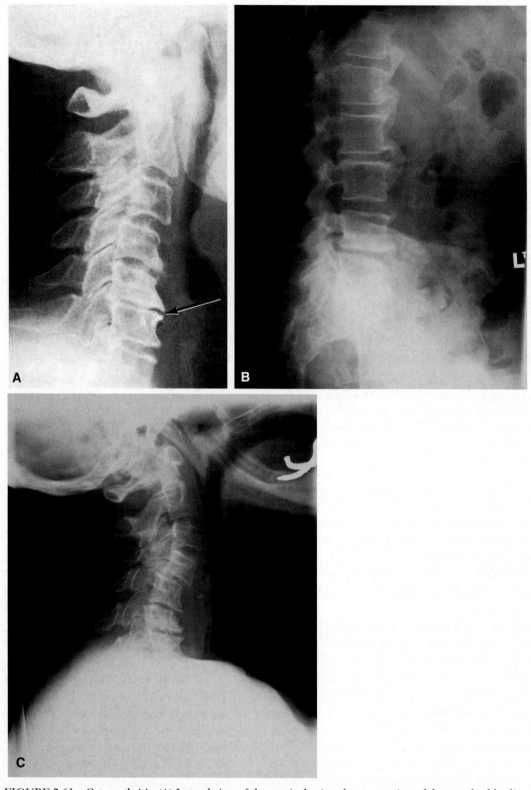

FIGURE 2-61   Osteoarthritis. (A) Lateral view of the cervical spine shows spurring of the vertebral bodies.
(B) Note the blurring of the vertebrae as well as the lipping along the anterior borders of the lumbar
vertebrae. (C) Lateral view of the cervical spine demonstrating subluxation and erosion. (A: Koopman
WJ, Moreland LW. *Arthritis and Allied Conditions: A Textbook of Rheumatology.* 15th ed. Philadelphia, PA:
Lippincott Williams & Wilkins; 2005.)

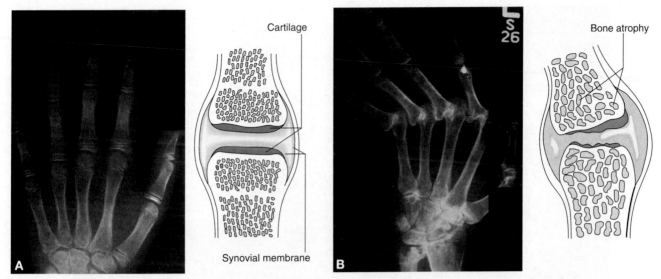

FIGURE 2-62   Joints of the hand affected by rheumatoid arthritis (RA). (A) Radiographic image of normal hand.
(B) Radiographic image of hand with RA. (Harris JH, Harris WH, Novelline RA. *The Radiology of Emergency Medicine*, 3rd ed.
Baltimore, MD: Williams & Wilkins; 1995:440, 467.)

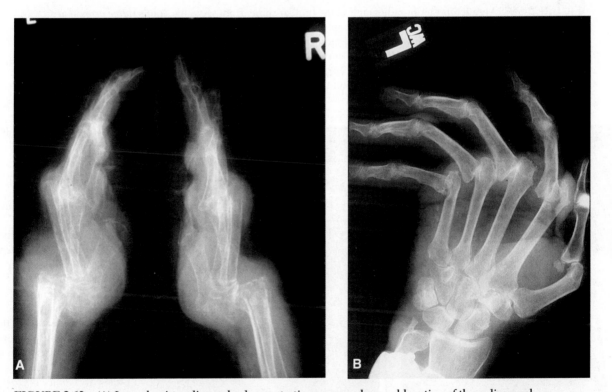

FIGURE 2-63   (A) Lateral wrist radiographs demonstrating severe palmar subluxation of the radiocarpal
joint. Metacarpophalangeal joint subluxation also is seen in this patient. (B) Severe metacarpophalangeal joint
subluxations in the volar and ulnar directions. There is rotation of the carpals on the distal radius causing "zigzag"
deformity. Erosion of the ulnar styloid and metacarpal heads is evident. (Koopman WJ, Moreland LW. *Arthritis and
Allied Conditions: A Textbook of Rheumatology*. 15th ed. Philadelphia, PA: Lippincott Williams & Wilkins; 2005.)

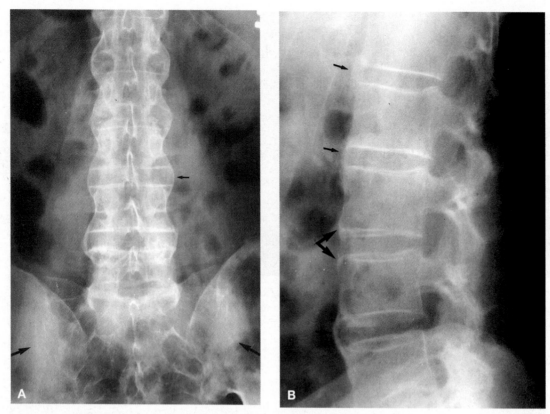

FIGURE 2-64   (A) Anteroposterior radiograph of the lumbar spine. Both sacroiliac joints (*large arrows*) are fused and there are bilateral, symmetric syndesmophytes (*small arrow*), resulting in the typical "bamboo" appearance of ankylosing spondylitis. (B) Lateral radiograph of the lumbar spine in ankylosing spondylitis with marginal erosions of vertebral bodies (*large arrows*) and typical marginal sclerosis (*small arrows*) on the anterior margins of the disks. (Koopman WJ, Moreland LW. *Arthritis and Allied Conditions: A Textbook of Rheumatology*. 15th ed. Philadelphia, PA: Lippincott Williams & Wilkins; 2005.)

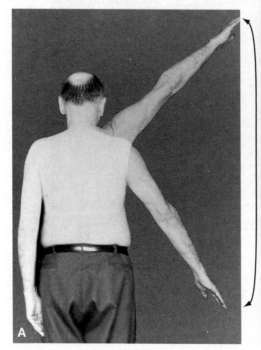

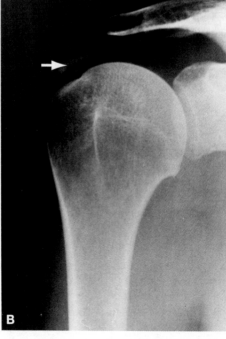

FIGURE 2-65   (A) Double-exposure photograph of a middle-aged man demonstrating the painful arc syndrome associated with calcific supraspinatus tendinitis in the right shoulder. Abduction of the shoulder joint (*two-headed arrow*) causes severe pain because of subacromial bursitis. (B) Calcium (*arrow*) deposits in the supraspinatus tendon of the musculotendinous rotator cuff, close to its insertion into the humerus. (Moore KL, Dalley AF. *Clinically Oriented Anatomy*. 4th ed. Baltimore, MD: Lippincott Williams & Wilkins; 1999.)

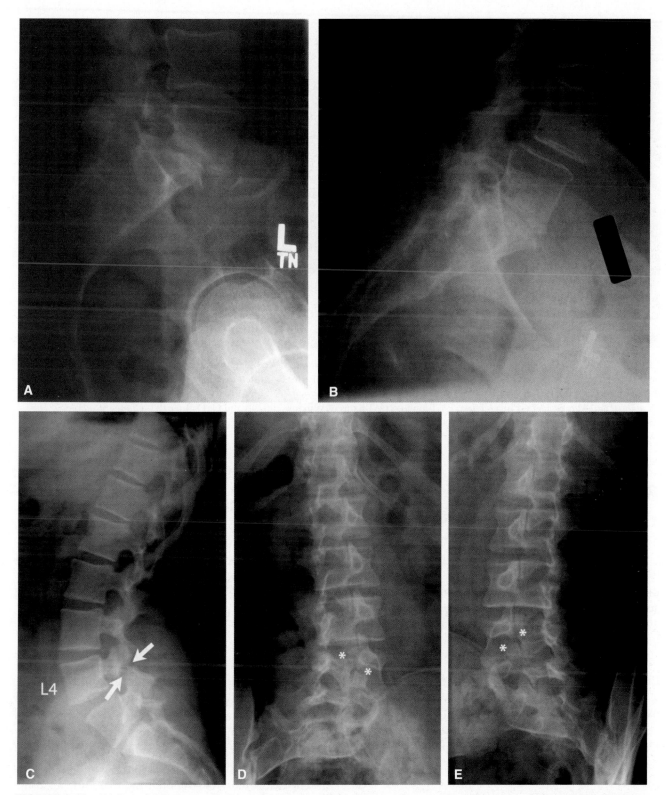

FIGURE 2-66   (A) Spondylolisthesis of L5 over the sacrum. (B) In this case, there is spondylolisthesis of L4 over L5, which is not as common as shown in (A). Lumbar radiographs, including lateral (C) and bilateral obliques (D and E), nicely demonstrate the bony break (*arrows* in C) within the region of the bilateral L4 pars interarticularis, with the infraction seen in the region of the so-called Scotty dog (* in D and E).

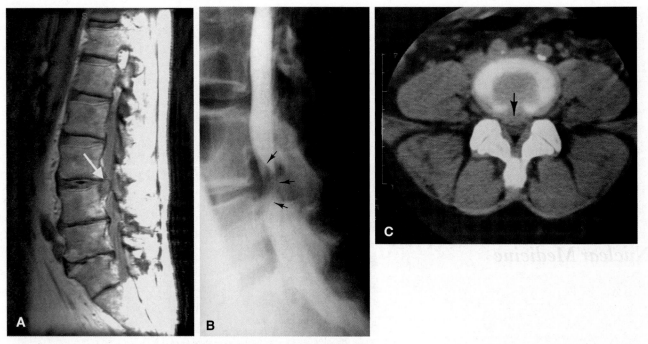

FIGURE 2-67   (A) This patient had a left-sided extruded L3–L4 *herniated disk* as seen on the sagittal T1-weighted images (*white arrow*). (B) Myelogram shows compression of the subarachnoid space by the *herniated disk* material (*arrows*). (C) Computed tomography (CT) scan in the same patient shows the *herniated disk* (*arrow*). (A: Schwartz ED, Flander AE. *Spinal Trauma: Imaging, Diagnosis, and Management*. Philadelphia, PA: Lippincott Williams & Wilkins; 2007. B and C: Daffner RH. *Clinical Radiology: The Essentials*. 3rd ed. Philadelphia, PA: Lippincott Williams & Wilkins; 2007.)

Bone Density Test

A bone mineral density (BMD) scan uses the energy of X-ray to pass through bone. Since bones will absorb the radiation, the scanner will count the amount of radiation that exits the patient. As demonstrated in regular X-ray, the greater the density of the bone, the greater the attenuation of the radiation and the less energy that is detected. This is what is desired. The bone mineral content that is being measured is the amount of calcium and other minerals that are contained in bones. The higher the mineral content, the denser the bones are and the stronger they are. Bones with decreased density, as occurs in osteoporosis, are more susceptible for fracture.

Bone density is measured through a scanning technique that requires the patient to be placed on a scanner and remain motionless until the scan is completed. Do not be confused by the use of the term "scan." Bone scans are reserved for those procedures performed by nuclear medicine.

DXA measures the spine, hip, or total body for mineral content. It is the most widely used technique today because radiation levels are low, the scan time is short (usually 5-15 minutes to complete) and it is relatively

non-invasive. Another significant advantage is its sensitivity. Remembering that bone loss must be approximately 30% to 50% for conventional radiography to detect the radiolucency, DXA scanning is much more sensitive and does not need such a high percentage of bone loss to detect pathology. Single-energy X-ray absorptiometry (SXA) measures only the wrist or heel and is not as reliable as the DXA equipment.

Computed Tomography

CT is used to help diagnose muscle and bone disorders, such as bone tumors and fractures, localize infection or blood clots, act as guidance for biopsy or surgery, and detect internal injuries and internal bleeding. Quantitative CT (QCT) scans can provide detailed, three-dimensional images and takes into account the effect of aging and diseases other than osteoporosis on bones. CT using three-dimensional capabilities is phenomenal in visualizing the anatomy of the facial bones to see small fractures that may have occurred there (Fig. 2-68). QCT is also another excellent method to measure BMD; however, there is a significant increase in radiation exposure. At the peripheral sites, it is up to 98% accurate.

Magnetic Resonance Imaging

In this procedure, radio waves and a magnetic field provide images of organs and tissues. Any joint can be seen well on MRI. Because of the structures near and around bones, it is usually the best choice for examination of the body's major joints, the spine for disk disease, and soft tissues of the extremities. MRI is widely used to diagnose sports-related injuries, as well as work-related disorders caused by repeated strain, vibration, or forceful impact. In addition, MRI allows visualization of degenerative disorders, deterioration of joint surfaces or a herniated disk (Fig. 2-67A).

Nuclear Medicine

Isotope uptakes of the skeletal system utilize technetium-labeled bone-seeking pharmaceuticals (technetium 99m) that provide high-resolution images. A three-phase bone scan (bone scintigraphy) is probably the initial imaging modality used when the clinician suspects bone disorders. Nuclear medicine is more sensitive than X-rays in diagnosing infections, tumors, and fractures. Boney destruction must be about 30% to 50% for a diagnostic radiography to detect some of the conditions, while nuclear medicine can detect bone destruction with only a 10% loss. A nuclear medicine bone scan can be used to detect arthritis, infection, tumors, and evidence of prior trauma such as an old sports injury.

Nuclear medicine will remain clinically and diagnostically useful despite the advancements made in CT and MRI, as the bone scan provides earlier diagnosis and demonstrates more lesions than other imaging modalities (Fig. 2-69).

Interventional Radiography

Angiography determines the vascularity of a bone tumor and the extent of the lesion. However, with the advent of MRI and CT, angiography is no longer indicated as a diagnostic tool. Nuclear medicine is as capable of identifying increased vascularity in a lesion.

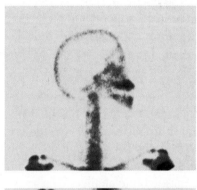
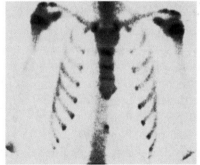
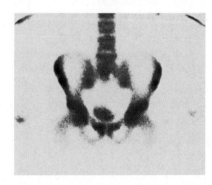

FIGURE 2-69   **Bone scans of the head and neck, thorax, and pelvis. The images can be viewed as a whole or in cross section.** (Moore KL, Dalley AF. *Clinically Oriented Anatomy*. 4th ed. Baltimore, MD: Lippincott Williams & Wilkins; 1999.)

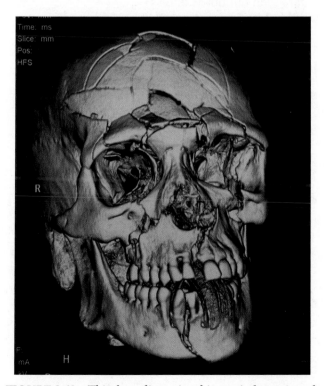

FIGURE 2-68   **This three-dimensional image is dramatic and shows the fractures quite easily.**

RECAP

Anatomy, Physiology, and Function of the Skeleton and Joints

- Two types of skeleton are axial and appendicular
- Five types of bones are long, short, flat, irregular, and sesamoid
- Three types of joints are synarthrodial, amphiarthrodial, and diarthrodial
- The six types of synovial joints are gliding, hinge, condylar, saddle, pivot, and ball-and-socket
- Ossification is the process of bone replacing the cartilage through osteoblastic and osteoclastic activity
- Skeleton provides support and protection, produces RBC, and stores minerals. Joints provide movement

Pathology

- Congenital bone pathology includes transitional vertebrae such as cervical or lumbar ribs; osteogenesis imperfecta (OI) (brittle bone disease); osteopetrosis; and achondroplasia. Achondroplasia is the most common cause of short stature
- Nonneoplastic bone changes
  - Osteopenia (umbrella term for osteoporosis and osteomalacia)
  - Osteodystrophy is disturbance in bone growth and has associated brown tumors leading to salt and pepper skull or rugger jersey spine
  - Osteomyelitis or osteitis is an infection that can cause sequestrum within 48 hours due to constriction of blood vessels
  - Osteitis deformans (Paget disease) causes cotton wool sign. Because of the overproduction of bone from osteoblasts, acromegaly can be associated with this condition
  - Osteochondritis dissecans includes Osgood-Schlatter disease (separation of the tibial tuberosity from the tibia) and Legg-Calvé-Perth disease that is the flattened head of one or both femurs in young males
- Neoplastic bone changes
  - Benign
    - Fibrous dysplasia and cysts have similar radiographic appearances: that of well-circumscribed lesions
    - Most notable chondroma seen on a radiograph is the exostosis. Classic appearance is a thin shaft of bone seen growing away from a joint space and parallel to the long bone
    - Osteoclastoma has a classic appearance of "soap bubble" because it is a hemorrhagic mass
  - Malignant
    - Three types are not as important radiographically as multiple myeloma: chondrosarcoma, Ewing sarcoma (seen in children aged 5 to 15 years and is sometimes misdiagnosed for osteomyelitis), and osteogenic sarcoma (poor outlook—seen in 10- to 30-year-olds)
    - Multiple myeloma is most common primary bone tumor. It involves the bone marrow plasma cells. Shows as "Swiss cheese" skull
    - Metastasis is more common than the three aforementioned primary tumors

Fractures and Dislocations

- The most common fractures seen that must be recognized by the technologists are the boxer's, Colles, and greenstick fractures. All other fractures are seen but not as often
- Shoulders dislocate anteriorly and hips dislocate posteriorly

Joint Pathology

- Osteoarthritis is the most common joint pathology. Degeneration of the joint spaces causes pain and stiffness. It is also called degenerative joint disease (DJD). Rheumatoid arthritis (RA) is an autoimmune disorder that will affect young women in their small joints of the hands and feet
- Bursitis is inflammation of the bursa (synovial sac) usually in the shoulder. Calcifications may be present, so kVp should be lowered
- Spondylolisthesis is the forward displacement of a vertebra over the one below it. Usually seen at L5/S1 junction
- Disk herniation is common in lumbar region. Center of fibrous disk protrudes and pushes on the spinal cord causing pain

Special Imaging Modalities

- Bone density tests are done to see the amount of density left in bones to rule out osteoporosis

- Computed tomography (CT) is useful in diagnosing tumors, fractures, infection, and other injuries. Quantitative CT is three-dimensional and provides stunning visualization of the skeleton
- Magnetic resonance imaging (MRI) is usually the best choice to visualize the joint spaces and the spine for disk disease

- Nuclear medicine bone scan is the true form of "bone scans." It is used to see arthritis, fractures, sports injuries, and is the first modality to demonstrate infection and tumors
- Interventional radiography in the form of angiography was used to determine the blood supply to tumors growing in the bones. Now it is no longer warranted

TABLE 2-1　CLINICAL AND RADIOGRAPHIC CHARACTERISTICS OF COMMON PATHOLOGIES

Pathologic Condition	Age (if known) Causal Factors	Manifestations	Radiographic Appearance
Osteogenesis imperfecta	Congenital, autosomal dominant gene	Hypoplastic teeth, limb deformities	Multiple fractures, both old and new
Osteopetrosis	Congenital, deficiency of osteoclasts	Obliteration of marrow cavity, osteomyelitis, deformed skull	Extreme density of bones
Achondroplasia	Congenital, autosomal dominant gene	Failure of bone growth, dwarfism, bowed legs, bulky forehead, saddle nose	Scalloped posterior margins of lumbar vertebra
Osteoporosis	Adulthood, aging, disuse of bone, hormonal changes, Cushing syndrome, prolonged steroid use	Back pain, fractures, normal calcium, lack of osteoid, kidney stones	Thin cortices and radiolucent bones due to decrease in density
Osteomalacia	Lack of calcium, vitamin deficiency, pregnancy	Normal osteoid, lack of calcium and phosphorus, skeletal deformities, bowing of lower limbs	Loss of density
Renal osteodystrophy	Renal failure	Brown tumor, heightened subperiosteal bone resorption, trabecula bone resorption	Salt and pepper skull, rugger jersey spine, lace-like pattern of digits, femur, and humerus
Osteomyelitis	Bacterial infection (Staphylococcus), idiopathic	Inflammation, Brodie abscess	Poorly defined radiolucency
Osteitis deformans	Idiopathic	Overproduction of bone, soft, bowed tibias, acromegaly	"Cotton wool" mixed areas of radiolucent and radiopaque densities
Legg-Calvé-Perth	Males, 3–12 y Ischemic necrosis, osteochondritis	Femoral head fragments, limp, muscle spasm, muscle atrophy of thigh	Flattened femoral head
Osgood-Schlatter	Males, 3:1 age 10–15 y Due to repeated knee flexion such as sports	Pain and swelling	Lateral knee shows avulsed tibial tuberosity with possible fragmentation
Osteochondroma	Localized bone overgrowth at joint	Benign cortical tumor capped by radiolucent cartilage which may contain calcifications	Growth parallel to bone pointing away from joint
Osteoclastoma	20–40 y, after epiphyseal closure	Extensive local bone damage, joint space not involved	"Soap bubble," large radiolucencies separated by thin strips of bone

(continued)

TABLE 2-1 CLINICAL AND RADIOGRAPHIC CHARACTERISTICS OF COMMON PATHOLOGIES *(continued)*

Pathologic Condition	Age (if known) Causal Factors	Manifestations	Radiographic Appearance
Ewing sarcoma	5–15 y	Low-grade fever, leukocytosis, misdiagnosed as osteomyelitis, located in diaphysis of long bone	"Onion peel" lesion, shows stratified layers of new bone formation
Multiple myeloma	40–60 y, idiopathic	Possible paraplegia, pathologic fractures, multiple lesions	"Swiss cheese," punched-out osteolytic lesions
Osteosarcoma	10–25 y, after 60 if Paget disease is present, idiopathic	Mass in bone, pathologic fractures	"Sunray," radiolucent areas mixed with dense areas
Osteoarthritis	Late adulthood, wear/tear on joints, obesity	Pain, decreased mobility, enlarged joints, knees and hips involved	"Spurring" at joint space, mild subluxation
Rheumatoid arthritis	Adulthood, possibly auto–allergic	Pain, stiffness, deformity, soft tissue swelling	Decreased joint space, swan neck and boutonniere deformities
Rheumatoid spondylitis	Late teens, early adulthood	Fused sacroiliac joints, kyphosis, difficult breathing	"Bamboo spine" squared off vertebrae

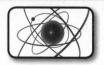 **CRITICAL THINKING DISCUSSION QUESTIONS**

1. Which two conditions fall under the umbrella disease of osteochondritis dissecans? Where does each of these occur? What are the radiographic appearances of each? Who is more prone to have these conditions?

2. What is the condition of bursitis? Where is it usually located? What do the radiographic images show? What technical factors should a radiographer use to demonstrate bursitis?

3. What is a bone mineral density test? How is it performed and what pathology can be proven with this test?

4. Why is nuclear medicine bone scan much better for diagnosing bone lesions than regular X-ray? What are the different conditions that can be seen on nuclear medicine bone scan? Why is angiography no longer performed?

5. How do CT and MRI work in conjunction with each other to demonstrate the entire aspect of the skeletal system? Which modality is best for which parts of the body and for which conditions?

6. Define arthritis. How does osteoarthritis differ from rheumatoid arthritis? What are the appearances of each on radiographs? What patient manifestations occur with rheumatoid arthritis?

7. What two diseases fall under the umbrella disease of osteopenia? How are they different from each other? What technical requirements must be considered to avoid repeat radiographic exposure?

8. Explain how two projections taken at 90° to each other will demonstrate the relationship of bone fragments to each other in a spiral fracture.

9. Explain the appearance of Legg-Calvé-Perth disease on a radiograph. What two projections should be taken to demonstrate this pathology? What happens to the femoral head in this disease?

10. What will osteomyelitis show on the radiograph prior to new bone formation? After the healing process has begun, how should the technical factors be adjusted to accommodate the new bone formation?

The Respiratory System

● Goals

1. To review the basic anatomy and physiology of the respiratory system

   OBJECTIVE: Identify anatomic structures on both diagrams and radiographs of the respiratory system

   OBJECTIVE: Describe the physiology of the respiratory system

2. To become acquainted with the pathophysiology of the respiratory system

   OBJECTIVE: Explain how pathologies of the respiratory system affect the patient throughout life

3. To describe the various pathologic conditions affecting the respiratory system

   OBJECTIVE: Describe the various pathologic conditions affecting the respiratory system and the radiographic manifestations

4. To learn how respiratory pathology affects technical factors in X-ray

   OBJECTIVE: Explain how a specific pathologic process will affect the technical factors that the radiographer must consider

5. To learn about different imaging modalities of the respiratory system

   OBJECTIVE: Explain how the various imaging modalities used in the diagnosis of pathology of the respiratory system help in diagnosis

● Key Terms

Alveoli
Asthma
Atelectasis
Bronchiectasis
Bronchitis
Bronchogenic carcinoma
Chronic obstructive pulmonary disease
Croup
Cystic fibrosis
Emphysema
Hamartoma
Perfusion
Pleural cavity
Pleural effusion
Pneumoconiosis
Pneumonia
Pneumothorax
Pulmonary edema
Pulmonary emboli
Respiratory distress syndrome (RDS) (ARDS, adult RDS)
Respiratory syncytial virus (RSV)
Tuberculosis (TB)
Ventilation

The respiratory system consists of the nose, pharynx, larynx, trachea, bronchi, and two lungs. For a detailed anatomic description of the nasal cavity and its related paranasal sinuses, refer to an anatomy and positioning book for radiographers. Anatomy and physiology books give a description of this area, but without the relationship to radiography. The pharynx, larynx, trachea, and bronchi are described in this chapter only briefly. The lungs and mediastinum are more important radiographically and are dealt with in detail.

Anatomy

The pharynx extends from the skull to the esophagus. Both air and food pass through this tube. The larynx is located between the pharynx and the trachea. The thyroid cartilage makes up a portion of the box-like structure of the larynx, and the epiglottis is the lid to this box.

The trachea is anterior to the esophagus and extends from the larynx to the level of T5, which corresponds with the level of the sternal angle. The trachea divides here into the right and left main bronchi. The area of bifurcation is known as the carina. Unlike the esophagus, the trachea is not collapsible because of the rings of cartilage that make its walls. The trachea is flattened on its posterior wall, allowing for the expandable esophagus to press into it if needed during swallowing.

The right bronchus is shorter, wider, and more vertical than the left bronchus. Each bronchus enters the lung medially at the hilum. The right hilum should always be lower than the left, as the heart displaces the left hilum upward. The presence of pathology should be considered if this is not the case.

As soon as the main bronchi enter the lungs, they divide into bronchi that go to each lobe of the lung. These lobar bronchi in turn branch into the bronchi that go to each segment of the lobe. The segmental bronchi continue branching until bronchioles (little bronchi) are formed. From these, the alveolar sacs (**alveoli**) are formed, which are the functional units for gas exchange. Figure 3-1 shows the anatomy of the lungs, pleural cavity with an inset image of the alveoli.

The lungs are cone-shaped organs that fill the pleural spaces of the thoracic cavity. Each lung is located in its respective hemithorax. The lungs are separated by the mediastinum. Both lungs should extend from the diaphragm, which is the base of the lung, to just slightly above the clavicle, which is the apex of the lung.

Each lung is divided into lobes by fissures. The right lung has three lobes and two fissures. The right horizontal (minor) fissure separates the upper (superior) lobe from the middle lobe. The right oblique (major) fissure separates the middle lobe from the lower (inferior) lobe. The left oblique (major) fissure divides the upper (superior) lobe and the lower (inferior) lobe. The lower part of the upper lobe of the left lung is called the lingula, and, in some cases, a horizontal fissure can be found between the upper lobe proper and the lingula.

Each lobe of each lung is divided into segments that are the structural units of the lung. The number of segments varies from lobe to lobe. The right lung contains a total of 10 segments, and the left lung contains either 8 or 9 segments. The number of segments in the lower lobe of the left lung can vary from individual to individual. This accounts for the discrepancy often found between authors as to the total number of segments in the left lung. For radiologic technologists' purposes, segments are not as important as the lobes.

The lungs are encased in a double-walled, serous membrane sac called the pleura. The inner layer is called the visceral, or pulmonary, pleura and actually covers each lung except the hilum. The outer layer is called the parietal pleura and lines the chest cavity. The pleura secrete a thin watery fluid that prevents friction between the visceral and the parietal pleurae. The space between the two pleural walls is the **pleural cavity**. The thoracic wall and diaphragm meet at the costophrenic angle, also known as the sulcus. This creates a space called the costophrenic sinus. The heart and the diaphragm meet at the cardiophrenic angle.

Another portion of the thoracic cavity is the mediastinum. It is a compartment separating the two lungs from top to bottom and from front to back. Boundaries of the mediastinum are the sternum, thoracic spine, pharynx, and the diaphragm.

Four divisions of the mediastinum are used when defining pathology. These are the superior, anterior, middle, and posterior sections. Of these four, only the superior mediastinum is not used in radiography. Located within the mediastinum are the heart and

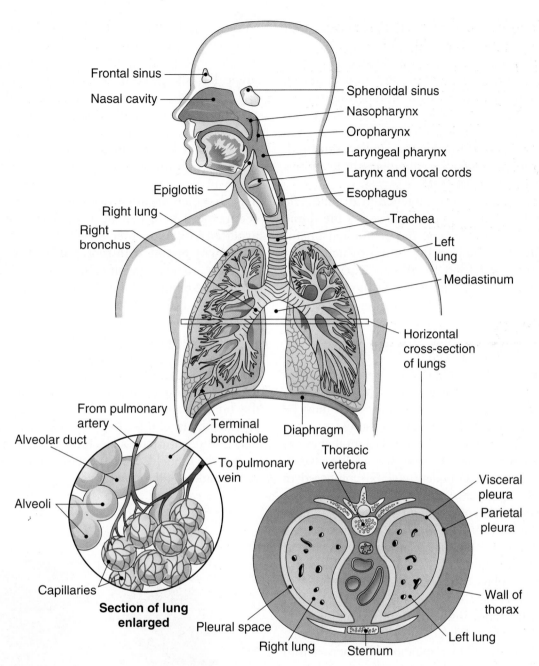

FIGURE 3-1   **The lungs, bronchi, pleural cavity, and alveoli.** (Cohen BJ, Wood DL. *Memmler's the Human Body in Health and Disease.* 9th ed. Philadelphia, PA: Lippincott Williams & Wilkins; 2000.)

aortic arch, the great blood vessels, the trachea, the esophagus, lymph tissue, the thymus gland, nerves such as the vagus and phrenic nerves, and the main bronchi.

Physiology and Function

The pharynx, larynx, trachea, and bronchi each have a limited function, but are indispensable to the main purpose of oxygenating the body. The pharynx acts as a passage for both air and food; two functions of the larynx are sound production and the prevention of liquids and solids from entering the trachea. The function of both the trachea and the bronchi is to provide a pathway for air to reach the lungs.

The respiratory system as a whole takes oxygen into the body and rids it of carbon dioxide. To carry out the main function of the respiratory system, air must be moved from the atmosphere to the terminal units of the lung, a process called **ventilation**, and gas must pass across tissue from air to blood and blood to air, a process called gas exchange or perfusion. The functional units for gas exchange are thin-walled alveoli. Each alveolus is supplied by a terminal pulmonary arteriole, which in turn gives rise to capillaries. **Perfusion** takes place at this point as each alveolus gives off its oxygen into the blood in the capillary surrounding it. Oxygenated blood can then be sent to various parts of the body to distribute its oxygen.

Since the diaphragm is attached to the thoracic wall, only the dome is able to move. As the dome contracts and pushes down, the abdominal organs are compressed, allowing the lungs to increase in length. At the same time, the ribs are expanded outward, which increases the width of the lung. This change in the shape of the lungs causes a decease in intrapulmonic pressure, causing air to rush into the lungs. At the end of inspiration, the pressure between the outside atmosphere and the lung is equal.

At expiration, the diaphragm relaxes and the chest cavity returns to its normal size. Air pressure within the lungs is now greater than outside, so air must be expelled again to equalize the two pressures.

Each alveolus is covered by a surfactant that assists in reducing the surface tension around the alveoli. This surfactant is a complex material composed of multiple phospholipids and proteins and is what allows the expansion of alveoli on inspiration. Without the surfactant the surface tension is so great that the alveoli will not be able to expand enough to prevent collapse on expiration.

The thorax plays a major role in the function of respiration. It is the changes in size of the thorax that actually bring about inspiration and expiration. The respiratory center in the brain controls the rhythmic movements produced by respiration. The nerves from the brain that pass down the chest wall and diaphragm to control respiration are the vagus nerve, the phrenic nerve, and the thoracic nerves.

Pathology

Congenital Diseases

Cystic fibrosis (CF) is a recessive genetic (inherited) disease of the exocrine glands involving the lungs,

pancreas, and sweat glands. The child inherits CF by inheriting one defective gene from each parent. The parents probably do not have the disease but have a single defective gene that is passed down to the child. CF has an incidence of 1 in 2,000 births. Heavy secretions of abnormally thick mucus are excreted into the lungs and cause progressive clogging of the bronchi and bronchioles, leading to frequent and progressive pulmonary infections. A main manifestation of this disease is chronic cough. As pulmonary dysfunction progresses and chronic infections occur, the patient may also suffer from pulmonary hypertension, bronchiectasis, and cor pulmonale. Pulmonary disease with repeated bouts of pneumonia and pancreatic insufficiency are the major clinical manifestations.

Recent advances in treatment have extended life expectancy. Over 90% of children diagnosed with CF will live to their teens. The estimated median survival age of children born in the 1990s will be 40 years or more. Radiographically, hyperinflation is present, with an interstitial pattern showing thickening around the bronchi and scarring from the pneumonia and repeated bouts of infection (Fig. 3-2). The radiograph may also demonstrate atelectasis due to mucus plugging of the bronchi, bronchiectasis, and consolidation in the middle and upper lungs.

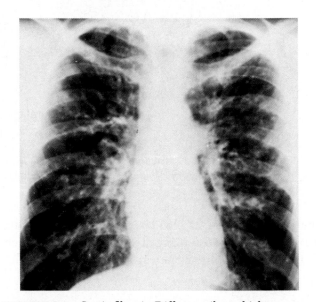

FIGURE 3-2   Cystic fibrosis. Diffuse peribronchial thickening appears as a perihilar infiltrate associated with hyperexpansion and flattening of the hemidiaphragms. (Eisenberg RL. *Clinical Imaging: An Atlas of Differential Diagnosis.* 5th ed. Philadelphia, PA: Lippincott Williams & Wilkins; 2010.)

Case Study

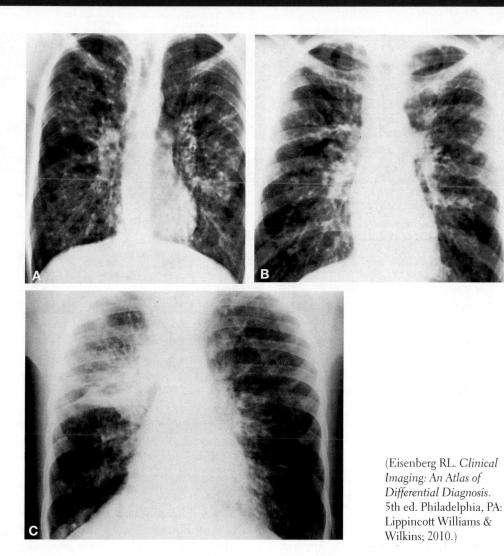

(Eisenberg RL. *Clinical Imaging: An Atlas of Differential Diagnosis.* 5th ed. Philadelphia, PA: Lippincott Williams & Wilkins; 2010.)

These images all show cystic fibrosis. Image (A) shows diffuse consolidation in both lungs near the perihilar region. The heart shadow is still normal for this patient's age. In image (B) the perihilar region has consolidated. The opacities seen in image (A) are becoming larger and more dense. Another PA image (C) was taken on another patient but shows the end stage of cystic fibrosis. Consolidation is detected in right lower lobe as well as in the upper and middle lobes. Atelectasis is persistent and the heart shadow is no longer distinct.

One of the more common indications for doing a chest radiograph on a newborn is **respiratory distress syndrome** (RDS). This is also known as *hyaline membrane disease*. A lipoprotein called surfactant coats the alveoli in the lung to reduce surface tension and prevents the collapse of the alveoli. In premature infants there is a deficiency in this surfactant, making inhalation difficult. Chest radiography shows increased density throughout the lung in a granular pattern known as a "ground glass" appearance. The granular pattern becomes diffuse,

Case Study

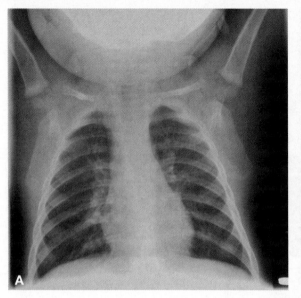 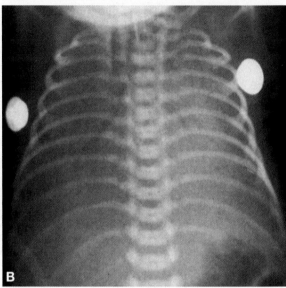

(A) A normal image of a baby in a Pigg-O-Stat. (B) "Ground glass" indicating RDS.

Chest image (A) is normal. Image (B) has the classic "ground glass" appearance indicative of respiratory distress syndrome in this premature infant.

presenting a homogeneous opacification of the lungs. The process may progress to form coalescent opacities with a well-defined "air bronchogram" sign. An air bronchogram sign is an area of fluid-filled tissue surrounding air in the bronchioles. RDS is the most common cause of death in premature infants due to failure to maintain aeration of the alveoli.

Inflammatory Processes

Lung abscesses are localized areas of diseased tissue surrounded by debris. Parenchymal necrosis that is due to inflammation is benign. When the abscess is caused by a tumor, malignancy is the usual cause. *Embolic abscesses* are caused by an infected blood clot being carried to the heart and then, by way of the pulmonary circulation, reaching the lung; a *pneumonic abscess* represents a complication of pneumonia; and inhalation abscess is caused by infected material being passed down the

trachea into the bronchi. An *inhalation abscess* is more common in the right lung, which has a more vertical bronchus. Foreign bodies may pass into the lung (especially in children) and cause this type of abscess.

Symptoms of an abscess are like pneumonia; however, the patient's coughed up sputum is infected with *Staphylococcus* or *Streptococcus*. Every time the patient coughs up the sputum (which is the destroyed tissue), a cavity is left. The chest image shows air-fluid levels within this cavity with a thick wall surrounding it known as an "air crescent sign" (Fig. 3-3). In the earlier stages, the image shows a consolidated area of dense pus (Fig. 3-4).

Adult respiratory distress syndrome (ARDS) is sudden respiratory system failure because of the inability of the alveolar capillary to exchange air and gases. It is similar to infant RDS, but the causes and treatments are different. ARDS can develop in anyone over the age of 1 year. ARDS is a life-threatening

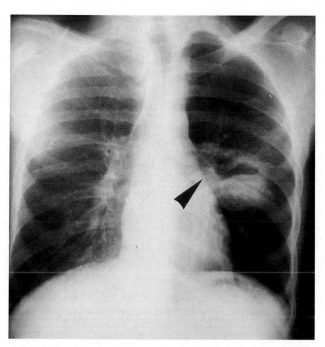

FIGURE 3-3   Lung abscess. *Arrowhead* points to a cavitary lesion with surrounding infiltrate. (Engleberg NC, Dermondy T, DiRita V. *Schaecter's Mechanisms of Microbial Disease*. 4th ed. Baltimore, MD: Lippincott Williams & Wilkins; 2007.)

condition. It is not a specific disease. It occurs in people with healthy lungs and can be caused by acute alveolar injuries such as toxic inhalation, septic shock, and near drowning. It starts with swelling of tissue in the lungs and building up of fluid in the

alveoli. This leads to low blood oxygen levels. ARDS usually develops in people who are already in the hospital being treated for any injuries listed above. However, only a small number of people who have these injuries actually develop ARDS. No one can predict who will get ARDS, but those who smoke, those with chronic obstructive pulmonary disease (COPD), or those over the age of 65 years and have the aforementioned injures are highly susceptible. The appearance on the radiograph (Fig. 3-5) is similar to that of pulmonary edema.

One common reason for obtaining a chest radiograph is a patient history of **asthma**. Asthma is a chronic disease that affects the lining of the bronchioles. They become inflamed and swollen. This hyperirritability of the airway causes reversible obstruction by bronchial muscle contraction, mucosal edema, and hypersecretion to the bronchial secretory cells. The underlying cause of asthma is not known, but factors that are thought to trigger an attack are respiratory tract infection, anxiety, exercise, and changes in the weather or allergies. For some people, no specific triggers can be identified. Also, what may cause an attack at one time may not affect a person with asthma the next time.

There are two types of asthma: extrinsic, which is an allergic form, and intrinsic. Extrinsic asthma occurs in childhood because of the immature system being hypersensitive to inhaled antigens. As the patient grows older

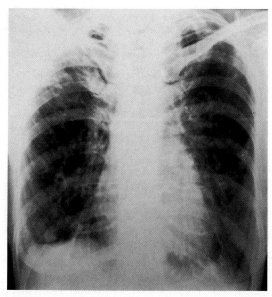

FIGURE 3-4   Lung abscess. No cavity is seen in the early stages.

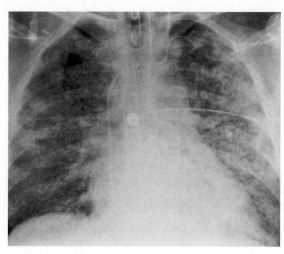

FIGURE 3-5   Adult respiratory distress syndrome (ARDS). Ill-defined areas of alveolar consolidation with some coalescence scattered throughout both lungs. (Eisenberg RL. *Clinical Imaging: An Atlas of Differential Diagnosis*. 5th ed. Philadelphia, PA: Lippincott Williams & Wilkins; 2010.)

and becomes immune to certain allergies, the asthma attacks may lessen in severity or frequency or both. Intrinsic asthma occurs in adults who have no immediate hypersensitivity but are prone to attacks caused by anxiety or exercise.

While symptoms will vary for each individual, wheezing, coughing, and a feeling of chest tightening characterize an acute asthma episode. With chronic asthma, forced breathing over a longer period of time may result in fatigue. There is secretion and edema of the bronchial mucosa and bronchiolar muscle spasm. This narrows the lumen of the bronchi, trapping air in the alveoli and causing labored breathing. When the patient breathes in, the lungs are overdistended because of this trapped air. The diaphragm appears low on the radiograph. The bronchial muscle may become hypertrophied and there is hyperplasia of the mucous glands in the bronchi, which is associated with increased mucous secretions.

Radiographic appearances in the majority of patients are normal. In severe or chronic asthma, the overall appearance of the lungs shows as opacity of the lung field because of this increased mucus. There is air trapping and hyperinflation leading to flattened diaphragm and increased retrosternal air space. As with COPD, there is limited diaphragmatic movement. Complications of severe asthma attacks include obstruction due to a mucous plug and pneumothorax or pneumomediastinum.

Obstructive

Compressive

Passive

Adhesive

Cicatrizing

The lung consists of millions of alveoli, interconnected to each other through small passageways or tubes. *Obstruction* of either large or small airways is the most commonly recognized cause of atelectasis. Since airway obstruction is produced by a wide variety of causes, this category may be subdivided into large and small airway obstructions. Examples of obstruction are a foreign body, aspiration, endobronchial tumors (Fig. 3-6), or inflammatory reactions such as tuberculosis. Bronchogenic carcinoma is one of the most important causes of large airway obstruction. Mucus plugging is another common cause of both large and small airway obstruction. An important iatrogenic cause of atelectasis is the improper placement of an endotracheal tube below the level of the tracheal bifurcation (Fig. 3-7). Lobar atelectasis in the absence of obvious explanations is an important sign of bronchogenic carcinoma and the patient may need to undergo computed tomography (CT) scan for further exploration.

Compressive and passive atelectasis differ from each other in causative factors. *Compressive atelectasis* is

TECH TIP

The technologist should try to ascertain if the patient is experiencing chronic episodes or if this is an acute occurrence. Remembering that in chronic asthma the patient will have hyperinflation and flattened diaphragms, the placement of the image receptor should be adjusted to assure the costophrenic angles and bases of the lungs are not "clipped" on the image.

Atelectasis is the collapse of a lung or a portion of it. It is not a disease in itself, but rather a condition caused by a pathologic condition. There are five major categories of atelectasis:

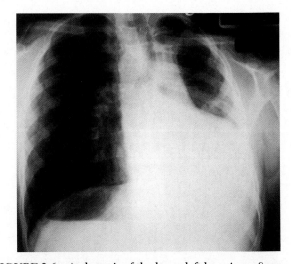

FIGURE 3-6   Atelectasis of the lower left lung in an 8-year-old boy. The collapse is caused by a right bronchial tumor. (Mulholland MW, Lillemoe KD, Doherty GM, et al. *Greenfield's Surgery Scientific Principles and Practice.* 4th ed. Philadelphia, PA: Lippincott Williams & Wilkins; 2006.)

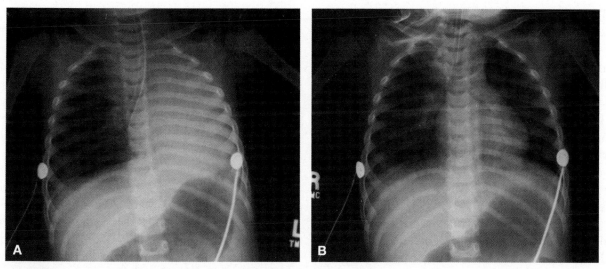

FIGURE 3-7   Improper placement of an endotracheal tube causes the left lung to collapse (A). Once the tube has been pulled back (B), the lung reinflates.

secondary to a compression of normal lung by a primary, space-occupying abnormality such as a tumor pressing on the lung. With compressive atelectasis the problem is intrapulmonary, whereas in the passive form the problem is intrapleural. Two of the most important causes of *passive atelectasis* are pleural effusion and pneumothorax. When the normal negative pressure within the chest wall is disturbed, either by a puncture wound or through a "blow out" in a weak spot in the lung, a portion of the lung collapses like a deflated balloon. In this passive form of atelectasis, the alveolar walls are opposed to each other and nothing separates them. Since the lung contains less air than normal, it is radiopaque (Fig. 3-8). The most common radiographic sign of atelectasis is a local increase in density caused by an airless lung that may vary from thin plate-like streaks to lobar collapse. When only a portion of the lung collapses, the remaining portion expands to fill in the collapsed area. This may cause a shift in the mediastinum. Indirect radiographic signs of atelectasis reflect an attempt by the remaining lung to compensate for the loss of the collapsed portion. These signs include elevation of the hemidiaphragm; displacement of the heart, mediastinum, and hilum toward the atelectatic segment; and compensatory overinflation of the remainder of the lung.

Adhesive atelectasis occurs when the surface of the alveolar walls stick together. This is an important component because it can occur in RDS or pulmonary embolism. In both of these processes there is presumed to be a deficiency of surfactant that normally allows the walls to slide next to each other.

Cicatrizing atelectasis is primarily the result of fibrosis or scar tissue formation in the interalveolar

and interstitial space (such as in interstitial pneumonitis). Because of the fibrosis, the lung loses elasticity and thus a reduced lung volume. Radiographically, cicatrizing and obstructive atelectasis may look similar. The differentiation between the two is due to their cause. If the cause of the atelectasis is determined, the type can be ascertained. For example, if the patient presents with tuberculosis and has atelectasis, it is most likely the cicatrizing type.

Bronchitis is a condition in which excessive mucus is secreted in the bronchi. This leads to severe

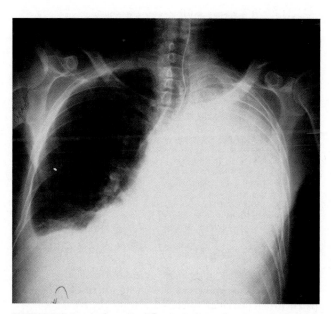

FIGURE 3-8   Atelectasis. The main bronchus was obstructed causing the lung to collapse.

coughing with the production of sputum. Bronchitis may be acute or chronic in form. The acute form usually involves the trachea as well as the larger bronchi. Causes include inhalation of tobacco smoke and industrial air pollution. When the irritant is removed, the inflammation subsides.

To qualify as chronic bronchitis, there must be a cough that produces thick sputum for at least 3 months during 2 consecutive years. In addition, there may be shortness of breath and wheezing, similar to the breathing problems experienced by people with asthma. The diagnosis of chronic bronchitis is based on clinical history. Chest radiographs add little information except to exclude other underlying abnormalities. To be signified as chronic bronchitis, all other causes of expectoration have to be ruled out.

The chief cause of chronic bronchitis is cigarette smoking. Repeated attacks of acute bronchitis may also lead to chronic bronchitis. People who live in smog-plagued areas, especially smokers, are even more susceptible to the disease. Occupational factors such as exposure to dust or noxious fumes also increase the risk of chronic bronchitis. The diagnosis is usually a clinical one, but the chest radiograph reveals hyperinflation and increased vascular markings (dirty chest) especially in the lower lungs (Fig. 3-9). These radiographic features are a very subjective finding, however. Clinical manifestations have caused the patients to be nick-named the "blue-bloaters." These patients have

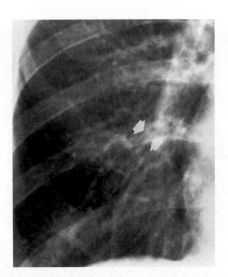

FIGURE 3-9   This "dirty chest" is indicative of chronic bronchitis and shows hyperinflation with increased parenchymal markings. (Brant WE, Helms CA. *Fundamentals of Diagnostic Pathology.* 4th ed. Philadelphia, PA: Lippincott Williams & Wilkins; 2012.)

tussive type of COPD (bronchitis), have episodic dyspnea due to exacerbation of bronchitis, and are young.

Bronchiectasis is the irreversible chronic dilation of smaller bronchi or bronchioles of the lung. Bronchiectasis can either be acquired or congenital. However, congenital bronchiectasis is rare. Cystic fibrosis plays an important part in congenital bronchiectasis. If the disease is acquired, the cause is probably repeated pulmonary infection (post-infectious, which is common) and bronchial obstruction. These cause a weakening of the wall of the bronchus, allowing the bronchi to become dilated. Bronchiectasis is also common in lung abscess cases. When the bronchus dilates, it forms an area where pus can collect. This leads to destruction of the bronchial walls. The patient with bronchiectasis typically has a chronic productive cough, often associated with recurrent episodes of acute pneumonia. The cough and expectoration are most often the major clues to bronchiectasis.

Although plain radiographic images may suggest bronchiectasis, bronchoscopy will accurately diagnose bronchiectasis and show dense pulmonary infiltrate and fibrosis usually occurring in the lower lobes.

Chronic obstructive pulmonary disease (COPD) is a disease in which the lungs have difficulty expelling carbon dioxide. Since all the space in the lungs is taken up by carbon dioxide, there is no room for the fresh oxygen. The term COPD is really a process that is characterized by the presence of either chronic bronchitis or emphysema. In chronic bronchitis, there is pathology of the airways but in emphysema the pathology is in the alveolar walls. These processes will eventually lead to airway obstruction. These diseases overlap and they share certain causes, therefore, they fall under the umbrella of COPD. Over 10 million people in the United States suffer from COPD with 25% listed as emphysema. Although changes to lung tissue differ with the two diseases, the causes and treatment are similar.

Emphysema is characterized by increased air spaces and associated tissue destruction leading to hypoxia. The condition causes dyspnea, particularly when the patient is lying down. The patient has a barrel chest and low diaphragm because of the permanent enlargement of the air spaces distal to the terminal bronchioles. The patients are nick-named "pink-puffers" because of the way they tend to puff out their cheeks when they blow out the air. Pink-puffers are elderly patients. The heart shadow is elongated because the diaphragm is being pushed down. This will cause the heart width size to be diminished (Fig. 3-10).

Emphysema is an irreversible, crippling disease that is known as "leather lung disease" by pathologists

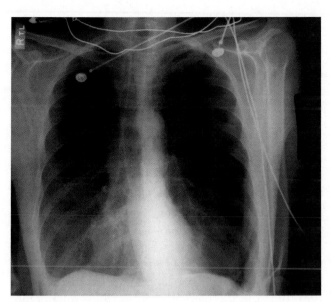

FIGURE 3-10   Posteroanterior chest image shows overinflation of the lungs and elongated heart shadow indicative of emphysema.

because the lungs become stiff and brittle. The alveoli lose their elasticity and remain filled with air during expiration. This may result in hyperinflation of the lung and reduced expiratory volume, and there is a chance that the alveoli will burst with the pressure of coughing. If a rupture occurs, the alveoli are destroyed and their numbers are reduced. An air-fluid level may appear signifying infection of a bulla. This will permanently hyperinflate the lung, trapping alveolar gas, essentially in expiration. Gas exchange is seriously compromised. Patients who are receiving oxygen have a very low administration level because their respirations are controlled by the carbon dioxide in their blood.

There are two basic types of emphysema: compensating and centrilobular. In *compensating* (or compensatory) emphysema, there is no air trapping. There are no clinical symptoms, and the condition is caused by the removal of one lung, or a portion of it, causing the overinflation of the other lung to compensate for the loss.

The second type contains three forms: *centrilobular* (also known as *centriacinar*) *emphysema* is found more in the upper lobes of the lung. It is second only to heart disease as a major cause of death and disability in the United States. It is associated with prolonged cigarette smoking, or occupational or environmental exposure to particles in the air. Panacinar and paraseptal are other forms of emphysema that trap air. *Panacinar* is found in the lower lobes and *paraseptal* is found

along the septal lines (periphery of lung and branch points of vessels). A major cause of all three types of air-trapping emphysema is smoking.

Once the diagnosis is made, follow-up radiographs are indicated only if there is clinical indication of supervening disease such as infection and congestive failure. In moderate to severe emphysema, the diagnosis can be made with chest radiography. For the detection of mild forms, a high-resolution CT (HRCT) is used. CT is excellent to differentiate between the different types but is not exclusive for diagnosis. Even though HRCT is currently the most sensitive method to detect emphysema, a chest radiograph should always be taken before the CT scan. A normal HRCT scan does not rule out the diagnosis of emphysema. Twenty percent of patients with emphysema have normal HRCT scans. X-ray and CT scans should complement each other. As emphysema becomes more severe with time, the CT differentiation of the three types becomes more difficult.

Radiographic features of emphysema are overinflation and flattening of the hemidiaphragm with less than 1.5 cm between the highest level of the dome and a line drawn from the costophrenic and vertebrophrenic junctions. There is decreased attenuation of the lung. The lateral image will show "tenting" of the diaphragm (Fig. 3-11) and invagination of thickened visceral pleura attached to septa. Less reliable signs are widely spaced ribs, anterior bowing of the sternum, and accentuated kyphosis (Fig. 3-12).

HRCT will show the central portion of the pulmonary lobule involved in centriacinar type and the whole acinus is involved and central arteries and bronchioles can be seen at the apices in panacinar. Paraseptal shows emphysematous changes adjacent to septal lines in the periphery and along the fissures.

TECH TIP

The radiographer must be careful to include the diaphragm and not to overexpose the lung field, which can be easily done because of the overdistention of the air spaces with trapped air. The image receptor should be placed lengthwise, not crosswise for chest imaging because the elongation of the heart and flattened diaphragms seriously increase the length of the lungs. The technical factors should be decreased when the patient is known to have emphysema.

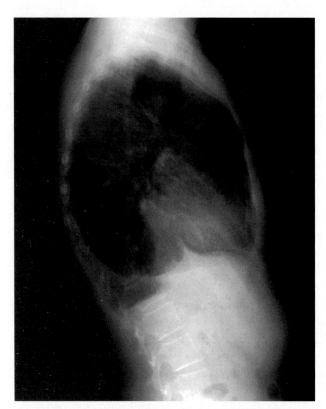

FIGURE 3-11   Lateral chest image shows flat hemidiaphragm with "tenting" indicative of long-term emphysema.

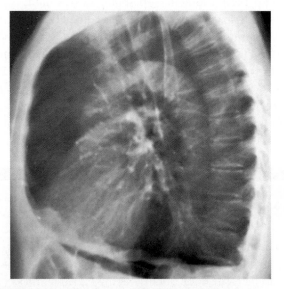

FIGURE 3-12   This lateral view of the chest demonstrates severe overinflation of the lungs, flattening, and concave configuration of the hemidiaphragm. There is increased size and lucency of the retrosternal air space and an increase in the anteroposterior diameter of the chest. (Eisenberg RL. *Clinical Imaging: An Atlas of Differential Diagnosis.* 5th ed. Philadelphia, PA: Lippincott Williams & Wilkins; 2010.)

Croup is primarily a viral infection, particularly of the parainfluenza viruses. It occurs most often in very young children, generally aged about 6 months to 3 years. The episode may begin in the evening after the child has gone to sleep. Labored breathing and a harsh, rough cough are characteristic. Fever does not always accompany croup. AP soft-tissue and lateral neck radiographs show spasm and constriction of the airway by demonstrating characteristic smooth, tapered narrowing of the subglottic airway. The key image is the AP soft tissue neck showing the subglottic narrowing known as the steeple sign or inverted "V" (Fig. 3-13). The lateral image is taken to rule out epiglottitis. (Epiglottitis occurs in 3- to 6-year-olds and is a life-threatening bacterial infection of the upper airway.)

Fluid in the pleural cavity is known as **pleural effusion**. Blood in the pleural cavity is called a hemothorax. The sources of fluid vary: congestive heart failure (CHF), infection, neoplasm, and trauma are all possible causes. The most common cause (about 40% of all cases) of bilateral or right-sided pleural effusion is CHF. When only one side is affected, it usually is the right side because people lie on their right side more commonly than the left. A pulmonary infarct, pancreatitis, or a subphrenic abscess may cause isolated left pleural effusion. The type of fluid (transudates vs. exudates) will help determine the cause of the effusion. Exudates are associated with infection, tumor, and embolism. Transudates are associated with CHF and renal failure or cirrhosis.

A large unilateral effusion causes pressure to be exerted on the lung. As pressure builds on the lung, the lung begins pushing on the mediastinum and eventually causes

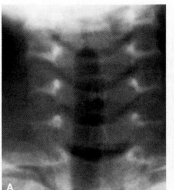
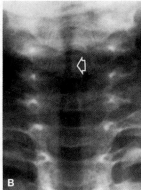

FIGURE 3-13   Croup. **(A)** Radiographic image of a normal trachea. **(B)** Smooth, tapered narrowing (*arrow*) of the subglottic portion of the trachea. (Eisenberg RL. *Clinical Imaging: An Atlas of Differential Diagnosis.* 5th ed. Philadelphia, PA: Lippincott Williams & Wilkins; 2010.)

a shift of the heart and mediastinum into the contralateral lung. If enough pressure is applied, the lung opposite the pleural effusion collapses, as it has nowhere to go. All this depends on the amount of fluid that accumulates within the pleural cavity. A large pleural effusion without a mediastinal shift is a significant indicator of malignancy.

Chest radiographs play an important role in the diagnosis of pleural effusion. Pleural fluid first accumulates in the posterior costophrenic angle that is viewed on the erect lateral view of the chest. This is the most dependent portion of the pleural space. A large quantity of fluid (more than 175 mL of fluid) is required for detection on the lateral image. On the PA view, the fluid can be seen at the lateral costophrenic angles. Less than 75 mL of fluid is required for detection. These opacities "blunt" or round off the normally sharp costophrenic angles by displaying an upper concavity known as the "meniscus" sign (Fig. 3-14A). A small amount of effusion is best shown with the patient lying with the affected side down in a lateral decubitus position (Fig. 3-14B). In this position, as little as 25 mL of fluid can be detected and the fluid is not superimposed by mediastinal shadows. Ultrasonography may disclose a small effusion that caused no abnormal findings during the chest radiographs. CT is very helpful if the lungs themselves are diseased.

If the cause of the pleural effusion can be determined and effectively treated, the effusion will clear and should not recur. If the effusion is large, a thoracentesis will make breathing easier. If heart failure can be controlled, then the pleural effusion should not recur.

Pneumonia (pneumonitis) is inflammation of the lungs. The lungs or certain sections of the lung are filled with fluid, causing opacity on the image. In this case, the technologist should slightly increase the technical factors to penetrate the lungs. There are various types of pneumonia. It can have over 30 different causes. Four of the main ones are bacteria, viruses, mycoplasmas, and other causes such as aspiration. Bacterial pneumonias are caused by *Streptococcus*, *Staphylococcus*, *Pseudomonas*, *Klebsiella*, or *Nocardials*. Viral pneumonias are caused by influenza, varicella, herpes zoster, rubeola, or respiratory syncytial virus (RSV). There is a 1% incidence of nosocomial pneumonias with a mortality rate of 35% of those acquired. Hospitalized patients who are in coma, are under anesthesia, have a seizure, have a tracheotomy, are under antibiotic treatment, or are immunosuppressed have a higher risk of acquiring pneumonia as a nosocomial infection.

Aspiration pneumonia results from the aspiration of a foreign object into the lungs, which irritates the bronchi

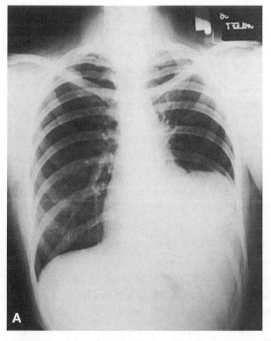
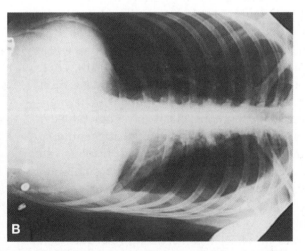

FIGURE 3-14   Pleural effusion. (A) PA projection showing blunting of the normally sharp costophrenic angles. (B) In this decubitus position, fluid goes to the dependent area and is not superimposed over other structures. (Crapo, JD MD. Gassroth J. MD, Karlensky JB, MD MBA and King TE jr., MD. *Baum's Textbook of Pulmonary Diseases*, 7th Edition, Philadelphia, Lippincott Williams & Wilkins 2004).

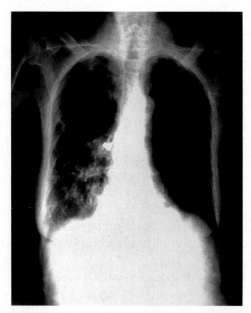

FIGURE 3-15   This elderly woman aspirated one of her teeth. It is lodged in a major bronchus, causing pneumonia.

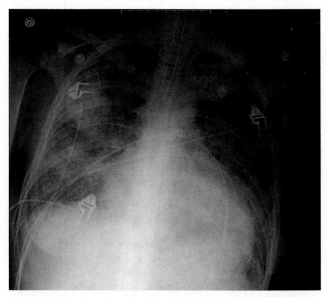

FIGURE 3-16   Bronchopneumonia involving several lobes on the right in a 57-year-old woman.

and results in edema. This type of pneumonia occurs in the upper portions of the lower lobes, as this is the most dependent area of the bronchi in the supine position. The segmental consolidation may lead to complete consolidation of the lobe. Radiographic images show multiple areas of opacity in this segment (Fig. 3-15). Small bronchioles containing air may also be visualized as the edema progresses causing the "air bronchogram" sign (see Fig. 3-17A).

Bronchopneumonia is actually bronchitis of both lungs, which can be caused by either the *Streptococcus* or the *Staphylococcus* bacteria. The bronchioles fill up with mucus and become infected, which leads to many small abscesses throughout the lungs and is seen as patchy pneumonic infiltrate (Fig. 3-16). There is volume loss as the bronchi fill with exudate. Bronchopneumonia and lobar pneumonia are synonymous. Bronchopneumonia that involves only a lobe or section of a lobe will be classified as lobar pneumonia.

Lobar (pneumococcal) pneumonia involves the alveolus in one or more segments or lobes of a lung and is caused by the bacteria *Streptococcus pneumococcus*. As in the other pneumonias, the bronchioles fill with fluid. As air in the alveoli becomes replaced by exudates, the affected part of the lung becomes consolidated. The bronchi are not involved and remain air-filled. There is no volume loss because the airways remain open. Because there is normal airway and fluid-filled bronchioles, the air bronchogram sign is seen. The patient presents with an upper respiratory

tract infection, cough, chills, and fever. The radiographic image shows the affected lobe as a radiopaque area (Fig. 3-17A, B, C). Lobar pneumonia is not as common as it once was because of early treatment.

Viral pneumonia is also called interstitial pneumonia because of its diffuse interstitial pattern on the radiograph. It is an inflammation of the alveoli and other supporting structures of the lung. Over 25% of all pneumonias are believed to be caused by viruses. It causes symptoms similar to lobar pneumonia. Patients have a fever and cough and may believe as having flu. Most of these pneumonias are short-lived and not serious. This virus-induced pneumonia shows infiltrate in the perihilar region.

Complications of pneumonia include empyema, fistula between the bronchus and pleural space, bronchiectasis, and pulmonary fibrosis. Eighty to ninety percent of pneumonias normally resolve within 4 weeks. In the older or diabetic patients (5% to 10%), it may take up to 8 weeks. Subsequent chest images should show progressive improvement compared to prior images. If the pneumonia does not show clearing within these time frames, there may be other issues such as antibiotic resistance, other pathogens (such as tuberculosis [TB]), recurrent infection, or obstructive pneumonitis due to tumors.

Pneumonia that occurs in children under the age of 3 years can be caused by a mycoplasma (less than 30% in this young age group); bacteria (only 5%); or by a virus (more than 65% in this age group). The viral pneumonia is known as **respiratory syncytial virus (RSV)**. The appearance on the chest image will most

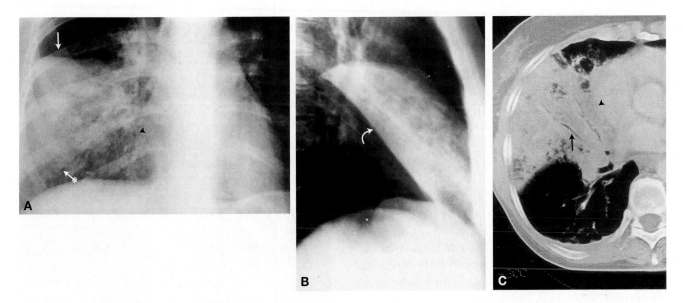

FIGURE 3-17 Right middle lobe pneumonia. (A) PA chest. (B) Lateral chest. Note the dense opacification throughout the right middle lobe, which is limited superiorly by the horizontal or minor fissure (*arrows*) and posteriorly by the oblique or major fissure (*curved arrow*). The right atrial heart border is obscured (*arrowhead*). Subtle radiolucent bronchi can also be seen within the consolidation (air bronchogram sign) (*crossed arrow*). (C) Computed tomography (CT) scan, axial chest. The air bronchogram sign can be seen in greater detail (*arrow*). Observe the contact of the alveolar infiltrate with the right atrial heart border (*arrowhead*). Terry R Yochum, Lindsay J. Rowe, Yochum and Rowe's *Essentials of Skeletal Radiology* Third Edition. Philadelphia. Lippincott, Williams & Wilkins, 2004.

commonly show bronchiolitis with parahilar and peribronchial opacities. There is a "dirty" appearance in the parahilar regions caused by inflammation. Also common is atelectasis. However, the chest radiograph may be normal and overaeration may be the only clue that the patient has RSV.

TECH TIP

When working with very young children, it is imperative that the radiographer take precautions not to spread this virus. It has a high rate of spread in the hospital (nosocomial infection) as the virus can live for long periods on a surface. Proper protective personal equipment must be used with diligent hand-washing.

The long-continued irritation of certain dusts encountered in industrial occupations may cause a chronic interstitial pneumonia known as **pneumoconiosis**. The dangerous element in the dust is silica. The inorganic dust particles overwhelm the normal clearance mechanism of the respiratory tract. Benign pneumoconiosis will show radiographic abnormalities yet there will be mild to no symptoms. Fibrogenic pneumoconiosis is symptomatic as are silicosis, asbestosis, and coal worker's pneumoconiosis (CWP).

Silicosis is the most widespread and the oldest of all occupational diseases. It is caused by inhalation of crystalline forms of silica and occurs in miners, sandblasters, and foundry workers. Phagocytes from the bronchioles carry very small crystalline particles of silica into the alveoli. There the dust acts as an irritant, which stimulates the formation of large amounts of connective tissue. At first, there are discrete nodules of fibrous tissue but over time, these coalesce to form large fibrous areas. These areas are well circumscribed and of uniform density. The bilateral masses are symmetrical and are almost always found in the upper lung area. Calcium salts are deposited in the periphery of the enlarged lymph nodes. These fibrous areas give rise to the radiographic hallmark sign of "eggshell," which denotes exclusively silicosis. The severity of the disease is related to the total amount of inhaled dust.

Asbestosis is disease caused by the inhalation of asbestos dust. The disease may be acquired either during the handling and crushing of asbestos rock or if the person was involved in the manufacture and installation of asbestos when it was being used as insulation. Asbestosis is associated with pulmonary fibrosis, bronchogenic carcinoma, and malignancy of the pleura. There are a number of thoracic manifestations. In the pleura, there is diffuse thickening, benign pleural effusion, and pleural calcifications directly above the diaphragm. The lungs show the same fibrous condition characteristic of silicosis as well as rounded atelectasis and fibrous masses. The determining factor between radiographs of asbestosis and silicosis is the involvement of the pleura (Fig. 3-18).

Berylliosis, another form of pneumoconiosis, had a ground glass pattern. Berylliosis was caused by inhalation of beryllium salt fumes or the absorption of the salt through the skin. Berylliosis is now a rare disease.

Coal worker's pneumoconiosis (CWP) is dependent on the type of coal that is inhaled. Anthracite is the cause of 50% of CWP. The radiograph is indistinguishable from silicosis with upper and middle lobe involvement. The diagnosis is made after the radiograph and a patient history of this type of work have been completed.

When free air gets into the pleural space through any route, it is known as a **pneumothorax**. Causes of a pneumothorax include penetrating chest wounds (e.g., stabbing, gunshots, and fractured ribs), surgery, biopsy, and pathologic conditions of the bronchi that cause a spontaneous rupture of an emphysematous bleb. The lung is displaced away from the chest wall.

An upright expiration chest radiograph shows a lung that is not expanded with air thereby making the pneumothorax more prominent (Fig. 3-19A, B). There are no lung markings seen in the area of the pneumothorax. The air in the pleural space is radiolucent. The white line of the visceral pleura is distinctly visible. There is volume loss of the underlying lung. In the erect position, air rises to the apex; therefore, a small pneumothorax, unless loculated, is first seen at the apex on the upright image with maximum expiration. The boundary of the lung, or "lung edge," should always be identified. On fluoroscopy, the heart seems to "flutter" because of the lack of stabilizing effect from the collapsed lung.

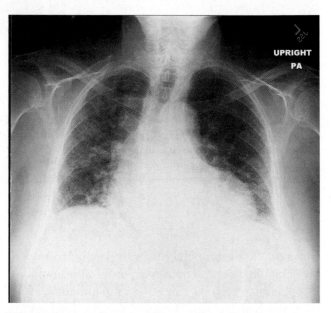

FIGURE 3-18   Asbestosis. There are dense fibrous areas throughout the pleura of the lungs.

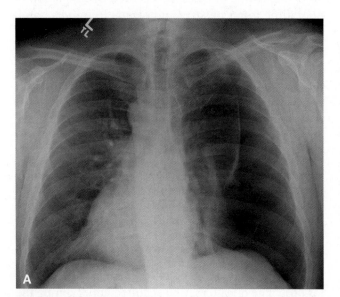 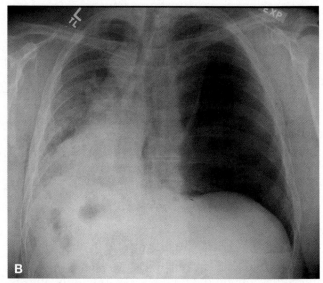

FIGURE 3-19   Pneumothorax. (A) Inspiration image shows a pneumothorax on the right side. (B) Expiration image shows the true size of the pneumothorax by allowing more room for the pleural cavity to expand.

T E C H   T I P

When performing portable chest radiography, the technologist must take care to pull the patient forward before inserting the image receptor behind the patient. There should be no excess skin that has been folded down when the IR is pushed down behind the patient. This excess skin produces an artifact known as a pseudopneumothorax, as the skin folds mimic a real pneumothorax.

T E C H   T I P

Chest images for pneumothorax should be taken with the patient in the upright position, as it may be very difficult to identify this condition if the patient is supine. If the patient is unable to be in the erect position, the radiographer should position the patient in a lateral decubitus position with the affected side up (not down as with pleural effusion). As little as 5 mL of air is detectable in the lateral decubitus position. In addition to routine full-inspiration images, a PA image should be obtained with the lungs in full expiration to identify small pneumothoraxes. The maneuver causes the lung to decrease in volume and become relatively denser. CT is the most sensitive if radiography is not distinct.

If air enters the pleural cavity during inspiration but does not leave upon expiration, a *tension pneumothorax* exists. This valve effect during inspiration/expiration leads to progressive air accumulation in the pleural cavity. The increased pressure causes a shift of the mediastinum and ultimately vascular compromise. The dome of the hemidiaphragm becomes depressed or inverted. This is a life-threatening situation and requires an emergency chest tube placement (Fig. 3-20).

Pulmonary edema is an accumulation of excess fluid in the extra-vascular space within the lung. About three-fourths of all cases are caused by pulmonary circulation obstruction. Pulmonary edema occurs quite suddenly when the left ventricle is inadequate to pump blood to the pulmonary vascular system due to coronary artery disease (CAD). This causes a backup of blood in the lungs (Fig. 3-21). Other cardiogenic causes of pulmonary edema include mitral

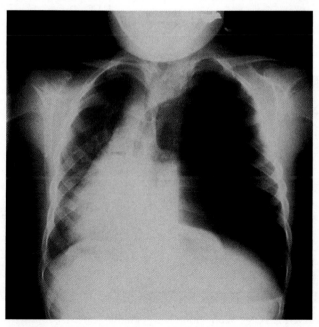

FIGURE 3-20   Chest radiograph of a 5-year-old girl demonstrates a left-sided tension pneumothorax. The patient was intubated, and a chest tube was placed which improved her status.

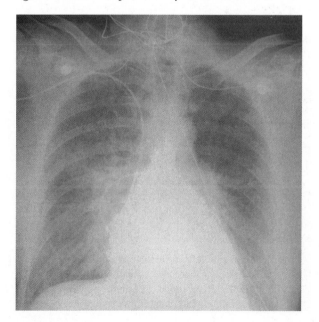

FIGURE 3-21   Diffuse alveolar pulmonary edema shows ill-defined opacification in both lungs that is most prominent in the perihilar regions. (Kahn GP, Lynch JP. *Pulmonary Disease Diagnosis and Therapy: A Practical Approach*. Philadelphia, PA: Lippincott Williams & Wilkins; 1997.)

regurgitation, ruptured chordae, and endocarditis. Renal causes include renal failure and volume overload. Other causes include septic shock, neurogenic shock, fat embolism inhalation of sodium, aspiration, or near drowning.

Patients will present with dyspnea, shortness of breath, rapid pulse, rapid breathing, and abnormal heart sounds. The neck veins are enlarged owing to the obstruction and causing a backup of blood. A chest X-ray is taken to confirm the clinical diagnosis. There is a diffuse increase in density of the hilar regions, which are homogeneous and fade toward the periphery of the lung. A classic radiographic sign is "Kerley B" lines (Fig. 3-22). These are thickened interlobular septa and are shown most clearly laterally above the costophrenic angles. They are fine, perfectly straight liners perpendicular to the chest wall and running 1 to 3 cm from the periphery. The chest radiograph will help rule out ARDS that has similar symptoms.

Pulmonary edema requires immediate treatment that includes oxygen and drug therapy to reduce the amount of fluid in the lungs, improve gas exchange and heart function, and, if possible, to correct the underlying cause. Patients who seek immediate medical attention will recover.

Pulmonary emboli (PE) are the most common pulmonary complication of hospitalized surgical patients.

Ninety-five percent of all cases of PE are caused by deep vein thrombus (DVT). They are fatal in more than 50% of cases. Acute pulmonary embolism is associated with significant morbidity and mortality, causing approximately 120,000 deaths per year in the United States.

Emboli, as discussed in Chapter 1, are blood clots that have traveled through the circulatory system, and in this case, lodged in one of the pulmonary vessels that have become too small in size to allow passage of the clot.

Risk factors for a PE include immobilization for longer than 72 hours (55%), recent hip surgery (40%), cardiac disease (30%), malignancy (20%), estrogen use (6%), and prior DVT (20%). Symptoms include a sudden onset of chest pain that may be worse with breathing or coughing, shortness of breath, tachycardia, anxiety, and syncope. However, no symptoms may be present. Most PE result in no abnormalities on the PA and lateral chest images. On rare occasions and with a massive pulmonary embolus, a focal hyperlucency may be present in the area supplied by the occluded vessel. The appearance of an infiltrate is usually delayed by 8–12 hours after the embolus has occurred. The involvement almost always occurs in the lower lung zones, especially the costophrenic angles. The radiographic appearance of an inverted wedge-shaped area of opacity (Hamptons hump) with the base at the pleural surface and the apex directed toward the hilum is suggestive of pulmonary infarct. The pleural-based nature of the infarct is even more graphically displayed by HRCT (Fig. 3-23). Nuclear medicine scans will

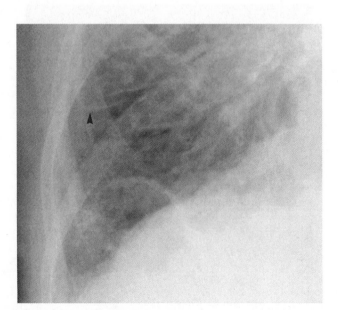

FIGURE 3-22   Kerley B lines in interstitial pulmonary edema. These are short opaque lines (*arrowhead*) seen best along the lateral aspects of the lungs. (Khan GP, Lynch JP. *Pulmonary Disease Diagnosis and Therapy: A Practical Approach.* Philadelphia, PA: Lippincott Williams & Wilkins; 1997.)

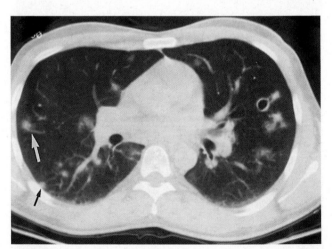

FIGURE 3-23   Septic pulmonary emboli. Scattered, mostly peripheral, poorly defined foci of air-space consolidation, many of which contain varying degrees of cavitation. (Eisenberg RL. *Clinical Imaging: An Atlas of Differential Diagnosis.* 5th ed. Philadelphia, PA: Lippincott Williams & Wilkins; 2010.)

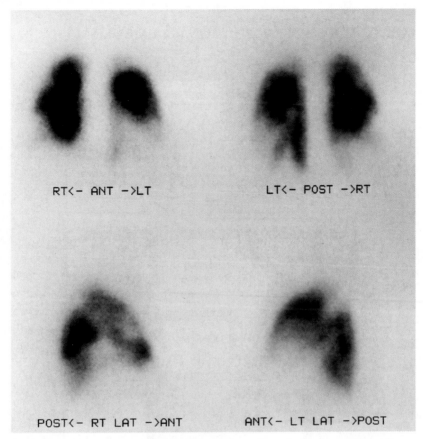

FIGURE 3-24   Nuclear medicine scan showing areas where air is not filling the lungs due to pulmonary emboli. (Daffner RH. *Clinical Radiology: The Essentials.* 3rd ed. Philadelphia, PA: Lippincott Williams & Wilkins; 2007.)

demonstrate which segment of the lung is not receiving blood (Fig. 3-24). This results in a ventilation–perfusion mismatch. Results of the ventilation study are normal, but the perfusion study shows abnormality.

The overall radiographic appearance of a pulmonary infarct may mimic pneumonia. Air bronchogram signs are often absent in a pulmonary infarct, whereas they are commonly present in pneumonia, which should be a differentiating characteristic. Other findings on the radiographic image are atelectasis, parenchymal infiltrates, and pleural effusion. However, these are not solely inclusive of a PE. The chest radiograph is necessary to exclude other common lung diseases and to permit the interpretation of the nuclear medicine ventilation–perfusion scan. It does not itself establish the diagnosis. Display 3-1 is a flow chart demonstrating the preferred imaging sequence for a pulmonary embolism.

Tuberculosis (TB) is caused by *Mycobacterium tuberculosis* or *M. bovis.* It is spread through inhalation of infected material from someone who already has

the disease. The tubercle does not grow very easily in a patient who is not immunocompromised unless there is constant or repeated contact with sputum-positive patients. General symptoms include fever, loss of weight, and weakness. Coughing and sputum production depend on the type of TB the patient has. Until cavities are formed, very little sputum is coughed up. The patient may also experience pain in the side from TB pleurisy.

Patients who are more likely to contract TB include homeless; alcoholic; immigrants from Mexico, Philippines, Indochina, or Haiti; the elderly; AIDS patients; and prisoners.

Although it generally affects the lungs, other areas of the body such as the spine may also be affected. The type of pulmonary TB determines the site of infection. *Primary tuberculosis,* also known as *childhood tuberculosis,* occurs in someone who has never had the disease before. It used to occur almost exclusively in childhood when TB was common, hence

DISPLAY 3-1 IMAGING SEQUENCE OF PULMONARY EMBOLISM

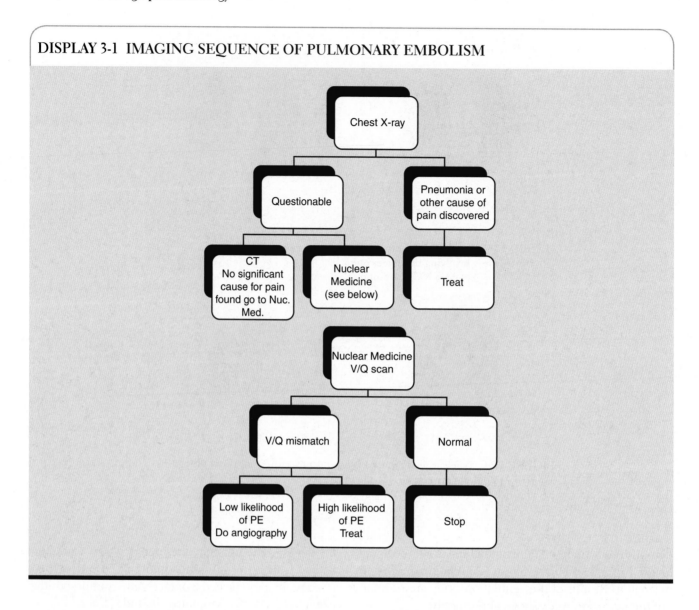

the second name. However, primary TB is now common in adults that fit the profile listed above. The lesions are small focal spots that can be found in the lower lobe (60%) and the upper lobe (40%) (Fig. 3-25). This contrasts sharply with secondary TB, which is found in the apices of the lungs. The disease is spread along the lymphatics; therefore, hilar enlargement is an important sign in primary TB. Again, this contrasts with what is found in secondary infection. Primary infection does not become chronic, nor is there any cavity formation. Recovery is marked by the disappearance of the lesions within the lung and along the lymph nodes, or the conversion of some or all of these lesions into fibrous tissue with calcification. This is known as miliary TB and occurs when the bacteria has spread through the entire lung by way of the blood stream. There will be an infinite number of small granulomas throughout the entire lung. Primary infection usually heals with little or no complications. Pleural effusion occurs in approximately 10% of the affected population.

Reactivation (secondary tuberculosis) usually develops in adults and is almost always found in the apical and posterior segments of upper lobes bilaterally. The right lung is attacked first more often than the left because of the right bronchus being more vertical and larger. The first radiographic signs of this type of TB are bilateral infiltrates, which are mottled, and calcifications, which are streaked. Figure 3-26 shows four different stages and types of TB.

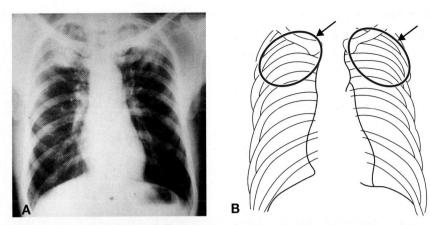

FIGURE 3-25   Pulmonary tuberculosis. (A) Chest radiograph from a young adult with tuberculosis involving the apices of both lungs. (B) The most affected areas are encircled. (Engleberg NC, Dermondy T, DiRita V. *Schaecter's Mechanisms of Microbial Disease*. 4th ed. Baltimore, MD: Lippincott Williams & Wilkins; 2007.)

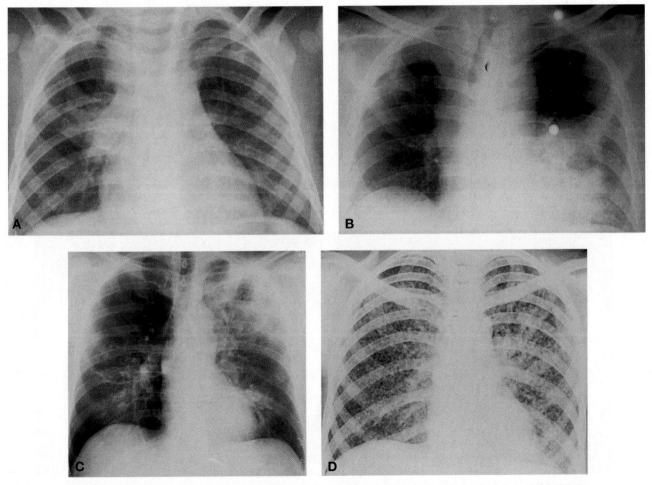

FIGURE 3-26   Chest radiographs of different presentations of tuberculosis. (A) Primary tuberculosis in a child. (B) Lower lung field tuberculosis infiltration and cavity with air-fluid level in lingula. (C) Reactivated tuberculosis, far-advanced disease with bronchogenic spread. (D) Miliary tuberculosis. (Gorbach SL, Bartlett JG, Blacklow NR. *Infectious Diseases*. Philadelphia, PA: Lippincott Williams & Wilkins; 2004.)

As reactivation heals, the hilar region retracts and the lung shrinks in size. Fibrous tissue surrounds and invades the lesion, leaving only a scar with calcification (Fig. 3-27). Cavities develop in approximately 40% of these cases that are clearly demonstrated on radiography (Fig. 3-28) and on CT. In either primary TB or reactivation TB apical lordotic chest views, or CT and magnetic resonance imaging (MRI) are helpful in demonstrating the cavitations and calcifications. Figure 3-29 shows the formation of a necrotic cavity involving the entire upper lobe of the lung. The apical lordotic projection allows the demonstration of the cavities without the superimposition of the clavicles or ribs.

Complications of secondary TB include loculated effusions, bronchopleural fistula, pneumothorax, bronchiectasis, or bronchial stenosis. Spread to the gastrointestinal tract may occur from swallowed secretions. TB will also be found in the genitourinary tract by spreading through the blood stream to the kidneys, ureter, bladder, and seminal

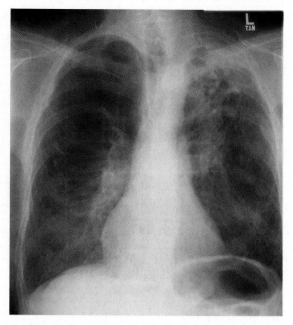

FIGURE 3-27   Scarring and calcification indicate healing in this tuberculosis case.

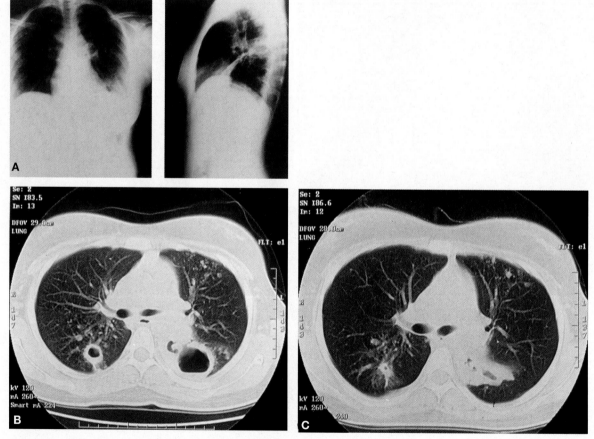

FIGURE 3-28   Chest radiograph (A) and CT scan (B), the latter of which more clearly demonstrates two cavitary lesions. A repeated CT scan (C) showed improvement after 1 month of treatment in a young woman with primary multidrug-resistant tuberculosis. (Gorbach SL, Bartlett JG, Blacklow NR. *Infectious Diseases*. Philadelphia, PA: Lippincott Williams & Wilkins; 2004.)

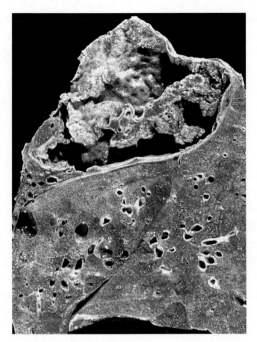

FIGURE 3-29   **Gross figure of reactivated** *tuberculosis* **with formation of necrotic cavity involving the entire upper lobe.** (Cagle PT. *Color Atlas and Text of Pulmonary Pathology.* Philadelphia, PA: Lippincott Williams & Wilkins; 2005.)

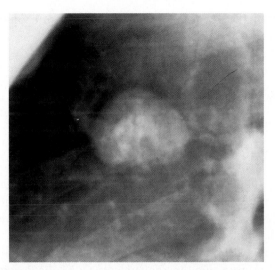

FIGURE 3-30   Hamartoma. Well-circumscribed solitary nodule containing characteristic irregular scattered calcifications (popcorn pattern) indicating a hamartoma. (Eisenberg RL. *Clinical Imaging: An Atlas of Differential Diagnosis.* 5th ed. Philadelphia, PA: Lippincott Williams & Wilkins; 2010.)

vesicles and epididymis in the male. Display 3-2 provides an easy method to compare primary TB to secondary TB.

Neoplasms

The only common benign lung lesion is a **hamartoma**. It is composed of cartilage, connective tissue, muscle, fat, and bone. It is rarely found in anyone under the age of 50 years and is diagnosed most effectively with HRCT. The radiographic indication that the tumor is a benign hamartoma is "popcorn" calcifications (Fig. 3-30). However, this is a rare occurrence found in less than 20% of the patients. CT will find a lesion filled with fat and this is the diagnostic indicator of the tumor. The radiographically important tumors in the lungs are malignant and those will be discussed in length in the following section.

Bronchogenic carcinoma is a broad term used to describe any carcinoma of the bronchus. The

DISPLAY 3-2 COMPARISON OF PRIMARY AND SECONDARY TUBERCULOSIS

	Primary TB	Secondary TB
Location	Lower lobe more than upper lobe	Upper lobes
Appearance	Focal lesions	Patchy pattern
Cavitation	No	Yes
Adenopathy	Frequent	No
Effusion	In 10% of those affected	Not common
Miliary pattern	Yes	Yes

use of the term is usually related to one of four types:

Adenocarcinoma (40%)

Squamous cell carcinoma (30%)

Small oat cell carcinoma (15%)

Large cell carcinomas (1%)

The highest risk factor for all types of bronchogenic carcinoma is smoking (for both men and women). Other factors include radiation and uranium miners, and asbestos exposure.

Adenocarcinoma is the most frequent primary lung cancer. *Bronchioalveolar carcinoma* is a subcategory of adenocarcinoma that does not arise from pulmonary tissue but rather comes from the major bronchus of one or both lungs. It is a slow growing tumor that grows into and surrounds one of the main bronchi, which results in narrowing and obstruction of the lumen. Obstruction of a bronchus results in atelectasis of the area of the lung that has lost its air supply. A second resulting condition is bronchiectasis and abscess formation. Secretions in the bronchus that cannot escape because of the blockage cause the abscess. The secretions stagnate and undergo putrefaction, causing the walls of the bronchioles to weaken and to dilate.

Squamous cell carcinoma is most directly linked to smoking but it carries the most favorable prognosis. Radiographically, the lung will show a cavitating mass or a peripheral nodule with central obstruction causing the lobe to collapse.

Small cell carcinoma is the most aggressive type of lung tumor and carries a poor prognosis. By the time the diagnosis is made, 80% of the patients have had the tumor metastasize most likely to the brain. *Large cell carcinomas* are extremely large lesions. This type of bronchogenic carcinoma is rare.

Symptoms of bronchogenic carcinoma include a persistent cough, bloody sputum, dyspnea, and weight loss. The chest image shows a rounded opacity without calcification in the lobes of the lung. The opacity represents the radiopaque lung nodule known as a "coin lesion" (Fig. 3-31). Malignant tumors rarely calcify; therefore, calcification in any type of lung tumor usually signifies that the tumor is benign. If the chest X-ray shows pleural effusion and adenopathy, the tumor cannot be surgically removed. Depending on the type of carcinoma, the tumor in the patient has varying prognoses. If left untreated, patients with primary lung cancer survive less than 1 year. The odds are low that a patient will survive 5 years even with treatment.

Metastatic carcinomas are more common than primary lung cancer. The routes of spreading cells are (from most frequent to least frequent) pulmonary arteries (hematogenous); lymphatic, direct extension (seeding); and endobronchial (inhalation).

Neoplasms that will spread through the vascular system most readily are renal cell carcinoma, sarcomas, testicular, and thyroid cancers. Other tumors will occur through lymphatic spread from the breast, stomach, pancreas, larynx, or cervix. If the primary source is the breast, the lung cancer is usually unilateral. If the primary source is the stomach, both lungs will usually be involved. The source of the cancer can be determined

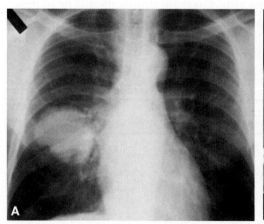
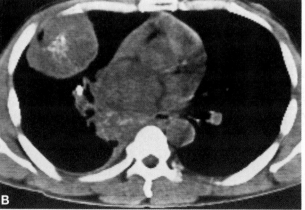

FIGURE 3-31   Primary bronchogenic carcinoma. This single nodule, known as a "coin lesion," is classic for adenocarcinoma of the lung. (A) shows the mass in the right upper lobe extending into the middle lobe. (B) The CT scan shows central calcifications within the lesion. (Eisenberg RL. *Clinical Imaging: An Atlas of Differential Diagnosis.* 5th ed. Philadelphia, PA: Lippincott Williams & Wilkins; 2010.)

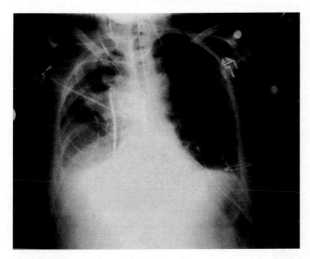

FIGURE 3-32 Pneumonic metastasis.

by the appearance of the cancer in the lungs. *Lymphangitic* is a diffuse form of metastatic cancer that appears as streaks and tiny nodules throughout the lungs. *Pneumonic processes* take on the appearance of localized areas of bronchopneumonia. The alveoli are filled with cancer cells just as they fill with fluid in pneumonia (Fig. 3-32).

Nodular metastatic disease is almost always multiple and appears as round masses of different sizes throughout the lung. These have the characteristic radiographic appearance known as "cotton ball" effect (Fig. 3-33).

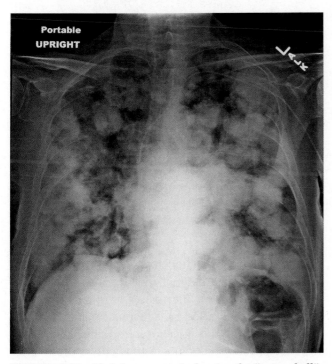

FIGURE 3-33 Nodular metastasis showing the "cotton ball" effect.

Imaging Strategies

Prior to discussing optional imaging modalities that allow the study of the lungs and their bronchi, a short review of the routine chest radiographic image is presented, as the chest is the most complex area examined. Not only are the lungs seen, but also the lower neck, the soft tissue of the thoracic wall, the mediastinum, the diaphragm, and the upper abdomen. Too much or too little soft tissue could indicate the presence of disease. Bony structures seen include ribs, thoracic spine, lower cervical spine, sternum, clavicles, scapulae, and shoulders.

All these may be present on the image, but if the patient is not positioned properly, good images still will not be obtained. Factors affecting the diaphragm height are rotation of the patient, obesity, scoliosis, loss of lung volume, and abdominal pressure due to a supine position. When the patient is completely upright, the diaphragm moves to a lower position during inspiration. Supine images are unacceptable, as the abdomen contents will raise the level of the diaphragm anywhere from 2 to 4 inches and obscure the lower lung fields. In addition to affecting diaphragm height, rotation will affect the hilar region, magnification of one lung, and heart size. Rotation on a chest image can be demonstrated by asymmetry of the sternoclavicular joint spaces. However, in patients with scoliosis, there are usually unequal distances from the medial ends of the clavicles to the sternum.

Deep inspiration is necessary to evaluate the heart size, as poor inspiration does not allow the heart to assume a more vertical position and chronic heart failure is simulated. On an adult, the 11th thoracic vertebra should be seen, and on a child, either six anterior ribs or eight posterior ribs should be visualized to verify deep inspiration. Also, 72-in source image distance is necessary to show true heart size. Other factors that affect cardiac size are posture and blood volume. A chest image taken during the systolic phase causes the heart to appear smaller than it would if the image had been taken during the diastolic phase.

All of these factors indicate that the "simple" chest X-ray, which is usually the first procedure students are taught to perform, actually has many components that must be remembered in order to make it a good image (Fig. 3-34A, B).

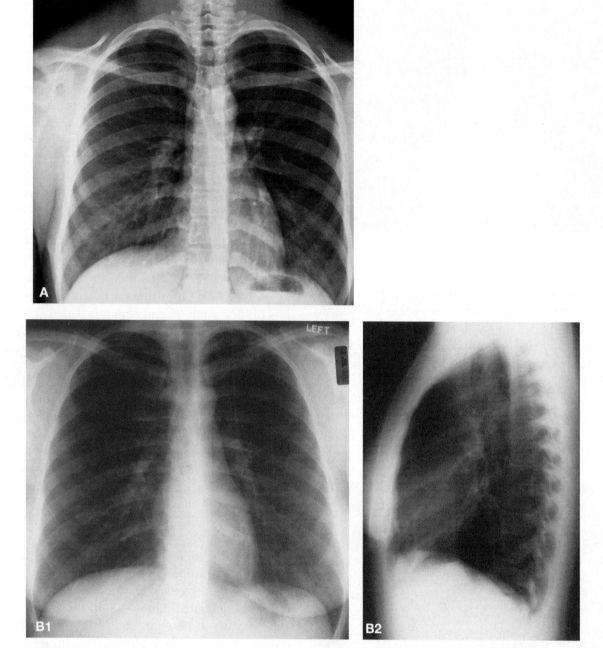

FIGURE 3-34   Normal chest radiographs (A) Posteroanterior projection (B1) Anterioposterior projection (B2) Lateral projection. (Richard H. Daffner, *Clinical Radiology, The Essentials,* 3rd Edition, Philadelphia; Lippincott, Williams & Wilkins, 2007)

Computed Tomography and Magnetic Resonance Imaging

Computed tomography (CT) of the chest is most often used in the evaluation of a mass involving the lungs or mediastinum. A central mediastinal mass is often shown better by CT than by plain-film tomography. A CT procedure may alleviate the need for mediastinoscopy in the evaluation of bronchogenic carcinoma. Small subpleural and paramediastinal metastasis can be shown clearly by CT even if the masses are not identifiable on a PA or lateral chest radiographic image. CT procedures following the injection of a radiographic contrast medium help differentiate an aneurysm from other mediastinal masses. The contrast agent causes a dramatic blush of the aneurysm, which is not found in a mass.

Fat has a characteristic appearance on CT attenuation coefficient. The ability to identify fat has dramatically aided in the evaluation of cardiophrenic angle "masses" that are often accumulations of fat. Diffuse widening of the mediastinum may be caused by the accumulation of fat and fat-containing mediastinal teratomas. These are clearly demonstrated by CT. CT is also useful in evaluating abnormalities of the thoracic cage.

Magnetic resonance imaging (MRI) scan of the chest gives detailed images of the structures from almost any angle. Abnormal growths are not only detected but also their size, extent, and degree of metastasis are determined for staging purposes. An MRI scan can distinguish between tumors, other lesions, and normal tissue. It can also provide visual guidance when doing an interventional procedure like taking a tissue biopsy. An MRI is very valuable when looking at the heart and the blood vessels within the

chest cavity. These will be discussed in the chapter on circulatory system.

Nuclear Medicine

Nuclear medicine lung imaging most commonly involves the use of a radionuclide to demonstrate ventilation and pulmonary perfusion. Ventilation scans require the patient to breath in an inert gas, usually xenon. The scan is performed while the patient holds his or her breath. In perfusion scans, a radionuclide material is injected into the venous system. It is carried through the pulmonary circulation around the alveoli where it is picked up by the gamma camera. The information gained from the images helps to differentiate diffuse and regional pulmonary disease. It also forms the basis for a noninvasive diagnostic procedure to diagnose PE.

RECAP

Anatomy and Physiology

- The right lung has three lobes, while the left has two lobes. Each lobe has a main bronchi that branches out in segmental bronchi, then bronchioles and then finally in the smallest form, the alveoli
- The alveoli are the functioning unit for gas exchange
- Each lung is encased in a "sac" that is composed of the visceral and parietal pleura. A small amount of fluid allows the two layers to slide over each other without pain
- The dome-shaped diaphragm moves with respiration. The right portion is higher than the left due to the liver pushing up from underneath
- The main purpose of the respiratory system is to take in oxygen and to rid the body of carbon dioxide

Congenital Pathologies

- Cystic fibrosis (CF)
  - Inherited disease of the exocrine glands
  - Causes progressive mucosal clogging of the bronchioles and bronchi

- Respiratory distress syndrome (RDS)
  - Also known as hyaline membrane disease
  - Chest image shows increased density throughout the lung in a granular pattern with a well-defined "air bronchogram" sign
  - Most common cause of death in premature infants

Inflammatory Processes

- Abscesses
  - Localized areas of diseased tissue surrounded by debris
  - Three types
    - Embolic abscesses are caused by an infected blood clot
    - Pneumonic abscesses represent a complication of pneumonia
    - Inhalation abscesses are caused by infected material being inhaled
      - Inhalation abscesses are more common in right lung
  - Most are the result of pneumonia or obstruction caused by foreign bodies breathed into the bronchial tubes

- Symptoms of an abscess are like those of pneumonia; however, the patient's coughed up sputum is infected
- The chest image shows air-fluid levels within a cavity
- Adult respiratory distress syndrome (ARDS)
  - Sudden inability of the alveolar capillary to exchange air and gases
  - This can be caused by toxic inhalation, septic shock, and near drowning
  - Appearance on the radiograph is similar to that of pulmonary edema
- Asthma
  - Common reason for obtaining a chest radiograph
  - Chronic process causing inflammation of bronchiole linings
  - Two types
    - Extrinsic
      - Childhood
      - Allergic reactions
    - Intrinsic
      - Adults
      - Anxiety or stress related
  - Symptoms are wheezing, coughing, and a tight chest
  - Edema of the bronchial mucosa and bronchiolar muscle spasm cause narrowing of the lumen of the bronchi, trapping air in the alveoli
  - Diaphragm appears low on the radiograph
  - Overall appearance shows as opacity of the lung field because of increased mucus
  - Many times the chest radiograph is normal
- Atelectasis
  - Collapse of a lung or a portion of it
  - Radiographic images show a local increase in density
  - Five major categories
    - Obstructive
      - Complete obstruction of a bronchus
    - Compressive
      - Intrapulmonary
      - Compression of the lung by tumor
    - Passive
      - Intrapleural
      - Pleural effusion or pneumothorax
    - Adhesive
      - RDS
    - Cicatrizing
      - Result of scar tissue or fibrosis
  - When only a portion of the lung collapses, the remaining portion expands to fill in the collapsed area

- Important iatrogenic cause of atelectasis is the improper placement of an endotracheal tube below the level of the tracheal bifurcation
- Bronchitis
  - Excessive mucus is secreted in the bronchi leading to severe coughing with the production of sputum
  - Two forms
    - Acute form usually involves the trachea as well as the larger bronchi
      - Bacteria, dust, or toxic fumes may cause it
    - Chronic form
    - Cough that produces thick sputum for at least 3 months
    - Must recur for at least 2 consecutive years
    - Diagnosis is usually a clinical one
    - Blue-bloater
    - The chief cause is cigarette smoking
      - Repeated attacks of acute bronchitis
      - People who live in smog-plagued areas
      - Occupational factors, such as exposure to dust or noxious fumes
- Bronchiectasis is the irreversible chronic dilation of smaller bronchi or bronchioles
  - Either congenital or acquired
    - If congenital, associated with CF
    - If acquired, caused by repeated pulmonary infection and bronchial obstruction that cause a weakening of the wall of the bronchus, allowing the bronchi to become dilated
  - Common in lung abscess cases
  - The patient typically has a chronic productive cough
  - Bronchoscopy will accurately diagnose bronchiectasis and show dense pulmonary infiltrate and fibrosis usually occurring in the lower lobes
- Chronic obstructive pulmonary disease (COPD) is really an umbrella process that is characterized by the presence of either chronic bronchitis or emphysema
  - Emphysema is characterized by increased air spaces and associated tissue destruction leading to hypoxia
    - It is irreversible
    - Patients are nicknamed "pink-puffers"
    - Known as "leather lung disease" because of the stiffness of lung walls
    - Alveoli lose elasticity and remain filled with air during expiration
    - Gas exchange is seriously compromised

- Causes dyspnea, particularly when the patient is lying down
- The patient has a barrel chest, low diaphragm, elongated heart shadow
- Radiographer must be careful to include the diaphragm and not to overexpose the lung field
  - Technical factors should be decreased when the patient is known to have emphysema
- Two basic types
  - Compensating (or compensatory)
    - No air trapping
    - No clinical symptoms
    - Condition is caused by the removal of one lung, or a portion of it, causing the overinflation of the other lung to compensate for the loss
  - Centrilobular emphysema is found more in the center of the lung
    - Two types
    - Panacinar emphysema found in lower lobes
    - Paraseptal emphysema found in periphery of lung
- Second only to heart disease as a major cause of death and disability in the United States
- Associated with prolonged cigarette smoking or occupational or environmental exposure to particles in the air
- After diagnosis, follow-up radiographs are indicated only if there is clinical indication of disease such as infection or congestive failure
- CT is rarely necessary but is excellent to differentiate between the different types
- Croup
  - Primarily a viral infection
  - It occurs in children of age about 1 to 3 years
  - Labored breathing and a harsh, rough cough are the characteristics
  - Soft-tissue AP and lateral neck radiographs show spasm and constriction of the airway
- Pleural effusion is fluid in the pleural cavity
  - Possible causes are congestive heart failure (CHF), infection, neoplasm, and trauma
  - Type of fluid (transudates vs. exudates) helps determine the cause
    - A large unilateral effusion causes pressure. As pressure builds, the lung pushes on the mediastinum and eventually causes a shift of the heart and mediastinum into the opposite lung

- If enough pressure is applied, the lung opposite the pleural effusion collapses
- A large pleural effusion without a mediastinal shift is a significant indicator of malignancy
  - Chest radiographs play an important role in diagnosis
    - Pleural fluid accumulates in the posterior costophrenic angle as viewed on the erect lateral chest X-ray
    - On the PA view, the fluid can be seen at the lateral costophrenic angles
    - These opacities "blunt" or round off costophrenic angles and are known as the "meniscus" signs
    - A small amount of effusion is best shown with the patient in a lateral decubitus position with the affected side down
- Pneumonia is inflammation of the lungs
  - The lungs are filled with fluid
  - Technologist should slightly increase the technical factors to penetrate the lungs
  - Various types of pneumonia
    - Aspiration pneumonia
      - Results from the aspiration of a foreign object
      - Occurs in the upper portions of the lower lobes
      - Radiographic images show multiple areas of opacity
    - Bronchopneumonia is actually bronchitis of both lungs
      - Caused by either the *Streptococcus* or the *Staphylococcus* bacteria
      - Bronchioles fill up with mucus and become infected which leads to many small abscesses
      - Seen as patchy pneumonic infiltrate
    - Lobar (pneumococcal) pneumonia
      - Involves one or more segments or lobes
      - Caused by the bacteria *Streptococcus pneumococcus*
      - Consolidation is usually confined to one or two lobes
      - The patient presents with an Upper Respiratory Infection (URI), cough, chills, and fever
      - Radiographic image shows the affected lobe as a radiopaque area
    - Viral pneumonia (also called interstitial pneumonia)
      - Inflammation of the alveoli and other supporting structures of the lung

- o Causes symptoms of fever and cough simulating the flu, hence its nickname of "walking" pneumonia
- o Shows infiltrate in the perihilar region
- o Respiratory syncytial virus (RSV) is viral pneumonia occurring in children under the age of 3 years
- Pneumoconiosis
  - o Caused by irritation of certain dusts encountered in industrial occupations
  - o There are three important types of pneumoconiosis:
    - Silicosis is the most widespread and the oldest of all occupational diseases
      - o Caused by inhalation of crystalline forms of silica
      - o Occurs in miners, sandblasters, and foundry workers
      - o Fibrous areas give rise to the radiographic hallmark sign of "eggshell," which denotes exclusively silicosis
    - Asbestosis is caused by the inhalation of asbestos dust
      - o Associated with pulmonary fibrosis, bronchogenic carcinoma, and malignancy of the pleura
      - o Lungs show the same fibrous condition characteristic of silicosis
    - Coal worker's pneumoconiosis (CWP)
      - o Major cause is anthracite
      - o Radiographic image similar to silicosis
      - o Diagnosis made by patient history to differentiate between silicosis and CWP
    - Berylliosis
      - o Caused chiefly by inhalation of beryllium salt fumes
      - o Now considered to be a rare disease
- Pneumothorax is free air in the pleural space
  - o Causes include penetrating chest wounds, surgery, and pathologic conditions of the bronchi that cause a spontaneous rupture of an emphysematous bleb
  - o Lung is displaced away from the chest wall
  - o Upright expiration chest radiograph shows an unexpanded lung with no lung markings seen in the area of the pneumothorax
  - o A small pneumothorax is first seen at the apex on the upright image with maximum expiration
  - o The "lung edge" should always be identified
  - o On fluoroscopy, the heart seems to "flutter"

- o In pseudopneumothorax, the skin folds mimic a real pneumothorax
- o Tension pneumothorax exists when air enters but does not leave the pleural cavity
  - The dome of the hemidiaphragm becomes depressed
  - Mediastinal shift and collapse of the opposite lung will follow
- o Chest images should be taken in the upright position
  - If the patient is unable to be in the erect position, the lateral decubitus position with the affected side up is used
  - A PA image should be obtained with the lungs in full expiration in addition to inspiration
- Pulmonary edema means excess fluid within the lung
  - o About three-fourths of all cases are caused by pulmonary circulation obstruction
  - o Usually occurs only when the left ventricle is inadequate to pump blood to the pulmonary vascular system
  - o Patients will present with shortness of breath, rapid pulse, rapid breathing, and abnormal heart sounds
    - The neck veins are enlarged
  - o Chest X-ray is taken to confirm the clinical diagnosis
    - A classic radiographic sign is "Kerley B" lines
    - Chest radiograph will help rule out ARDS that has similar symptoms
  - o Requires immediate treatment
    - Patients who seek immediate medical attention will recover
- Pulmonary emboli (PE)
  - o Most common pulmonary complication of hospitalized surgical patients
  - o Ninety-five percent are caused by deep vein thrombus (DVT)
  - o Fatal in more than 50% of cases
  - o Symptoms include a sudden onset of chest pain, shortness of breath, anxiety, and syncope
  - o Most result in no abnormalities on the PA and lateral chest images but may mimic pneumonia
  - o Nuclear medicine scans will best demonstrate a PE
- Tuberculosis (TB)
  - o Caused by *Mycobacterium tuberculosis*
  - o Spread through inhalation of infected material
  - o Symptoms include fever, loss of weight, and weakness

- Other areas of the body such as the spine may also be affected
- Two types
  - Primary TB (childhood) occurs in someone who has never had the disease before
    - Lesions can be found anywhere in the lung
    - Hilar enlargement is an important sign in primary TB
    - Does not become chronic and there is no cavity formation
    - Pleural effusion may occur
    - Recovery shows disappearance of lesions, or the conversion into fibrous tissue with calcification
  - Reactivation (secondary) TB usually develops in adults
    - Lesions almost always found in the upper lobes bilaterally
    - The first radiographic signs are bilateral infiltrates, which are mottled, and calcifications, which are streaked
    - As it heals, the lung shrinks in size
      - Fibrous tissue leaves a scar with calcification
      - Cavities commonly develop

Neoplasms

- Hamartoma
  - Benign
  - Rare under the age of 50 years
  - Diagnosed with high-resolution CT (HRCT)
- Bronchogenic carcinoma comes from the major bronchus of one or both lungs
  - Currently leading primary malignant tumor in males between the ages of 55 and 60 years
  - The incidence in women is rising
  - Smoking is the most important factor in causing the disease
  - Four types
    - Adenocarcinoma
      - Most frequent type
    - Squamous cell
      - Most favorable prognosis
    - Small oat cell
      - Most aggressive
      - Metastasize to the brain
    - Large cell
      - Rare

- Tumor grows into and surrounds one of the main bronchi resulting in narrowing and obstruction of the lumen
- Obstruction of a bronchus results in atelectasis of the area of the lung that has lost its air supply
- A second resulting condition is bronchiectasis and abscess formation
- Symptoms include a persistent cough, bloody sputum, dyspnea, and weight loss
- Chest image shows a rounded opacity without calcification in the upper lobes of the lung
  - The opacity represents the radiopaque lung nodule known as a "coin" lesion
  - Malignant tumors rarely calcify
  - If the chest X-ray shows pleural effusion and adenopathy, the tumor cannot be surgically removed
  - Left untreated, patients with primary lung cancer survive less than 1 year
  - Odds are low that a patient will survive 5 years even with treatment
- Metastatic carcinomas are more common than primary lung cancer
  - These are divided into three types:
    - Nodular is almost always multiple and appears as round masses of different sizes throughout the lung
      - Have the characteristic radiographic appearance known as "cotton ball" effect
      - In women, most often the primary source is uterine cancer
    - Lymphangitic is a diffuse form of metastatic cancer that appears as streaks and tiny nodules throughout the lungs
      - Occur from lymphatic spread from the gastric area
    - Pneumonic processes take on the appearance of localized areas of bronchopneumonia
      - Alveoli are filled with cancer cells just as they are filled with fluid in pneumonia
      - Breast cancer is commonly the primary source

Imaging Strategies

- Computed tomography (CT) is most often used in the evaluation of a mass
  - A central mediastinal mass is often shown better by CT
  - May alleviate the need for mediastinoscopy in the evaluation of bronchogenic carcinoma

- ○ Shows small subpleural and paramediastinal metastasis
- ○ CT following the injection of a radiographic contrast medium helps differentiate an aneurysm from other mediastinal masses
  - The contrast medium causes a dramatic blush of the aneurysm, which is not found in a mass
- ○ The ability to identify fat has dramatically aided in the evaluation of cardiophrenic angle "masses" that are often accumulations of fat
- ○ Diffuse widening of the mediastinum may be caused by the accumulation of fat and fat-containing mediastinal teratomas. These are clearly demonstrated by CT
- Magnetic resonance imaging (MRI) of the chest gives detailed images of the structures from almost any angle
- ○ Abnormal growth size, and extent and degree of metastasis are determined. MRI can distinguish between tumors, other lesions, and normal tissue
- ○ Provide visual guidance when doing an interventional procedure like taking a tissue biopsy
- ○ Very valuable when looking at the heart and the blood vessels within the chest cavity
- Nuclear medicine scan is most commonly used to demonstrate ventilation and pulmonary perfusion
- ○ Ventilation scans
  - Patient breaths in an inert gas
  - The scan is performed while the patient holds his breath
- ○ Perfusion scans
  - Radionuclide material is injected into the venous system
  - It is picked up by the gamma camera in the alveoli

CLINICAL AND RADIOGRAPHIC CHARACTERISTICS OF COMMON PATHOLOGIES

Pathologic Condition	Age (if known) Causal Factors	Manifestations	Radiographic Appearance
Cystic fibrosis	Inherited	Mucosal clogging of the bronchioles	
RDS (Hyaline membrane disease)	Inherited	Inability to breathe deeply and sufficiently to oxygenate body	Granular pattern and air bronchogram sign
Abscesses	Any age Embolic, pneumonic or inhalation	Symptoms are similar to pneumonia but with infected sputum	Air-fluid levels within a cavity
Asthma	Childhood—allergies Adults—stress or anxiety	Wheezing, coughing, and tight chest	Low diaphragm, slight opacity due to increased mucus May be normal
Atelectasis	Any age Multiple causes	Hypoxia and dyspnea	Increased opacity if cause is obstructive; look for lung edge in cases of pneumothorax
Bronchitis	Any age Tobacco smoke/industrial air pollution	Coughing with sputum, Shortness of Breath (SOB); wheezing	Hyperinflation and increased vascular markings (dirty chest)
Emphysema	Older patients Cigarette smoking	Hypoxia, barrel chest	Elongated heart shadow, low diaphragm, hyperinflation, tenting in long-term cases
Croup	Young children Viral infection	Labored breathing with harsh rough cough	Narrowing of the subglottic airway on soft-tissue neck image
Pleural effusion	Adults CHF, infection, trauma	Rales, difficulty in breathing	Blunted apices—meniscus sign; atelectasis
Pneumonia	Any age RSV in children under 3 y 30 causes; bacteria, virus, mycoplasmas, aspiration	Chills, fever	Areas of opacity depending on the location of the pneumonia or the cause

(continued)

CLINICAL AND RADIOGRAPHIC CHARACTERISTICS OF COMMON PATHOLOGIES *(continued)*

Pathologic Condition	Age (if known) Causal Factors	Manifestations	Radiographic Appearance
Pneumoconiosis	Adults (work related and caused by inhalation of dust particles)	Asymptomatic or only mild symptoms	Eggshell appearance pleural calcifications above diaphragm
Pneumothorax	Any age Chest wound, surgery, biopsy	Dyspnea, hypoxia	Atelectasis, lung edge, air in cavity is radiolucent, no lung markings
Pulmonary edema	Adults CHF; renal failure	Dyspnea, SOB, rapid pulse, rapid breathing	Kerley B lines, increased opacity in hilar region
Pulmonary emboli	Adults DVT	Sudden onset of chest pain, SOB, tachycardia, syncope or it may be asymptomatic	Hamptons hump, need HRCT and nuclear medicine for diagnosis
Tuberculosis	Any age *Mycobacterium tuberculosis*	Fever, weight loss, weakness, coughing, infected sputum, chest pain	Primary—lower lobes, no cavities Secondary—apical segment cavities
Carcinoma Primary Metastatic	Adults Smoking Primary elsewhere	Persistent cough, bloody sputum, dyspnea, weight loss	Single coin lesion Multiple nodules known as cotton ball

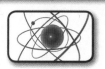

CRITICAL THINKING DISCUSSION QUESTIONS

1. Why are supine chest images unacceptable? Why is deep inspiration necessary on a chest radiograph?

2. Describe what should be seen on a well-positioned chest radiograph. Explain how to access rotation and inspiration. Why are all of these important?

3. Define emphysema. How is it related to COPD? What is emphysema characterized by? What manifestations will the patient present with? What must the radiographer be aware of when taking a chest radiograph? Why is this disease known as the "leather lung disease"?

4. Describe where fluid will be seen in a normally positioned chest series on a patient with pleural effusion. If the patient is unable to stand for upright images, describe how the images should be taken and explain why.

5. What does pulmonary edema mean? How are the lungs affected? What must the radiographer do to obtain a well-penetrated radiographic image?

6. Pulmonary emboli are best demonstrated by what modality? What causes pulmonary emboli in most cases? Why is it the most common process of hospitalized surgical patients? Why is it so urgent to diagnose?

7. A small pneumothorax requires both an inspiration and expiration PA radiograph. Explain why.

8. For the following conditions, explain if the process is additive or destructive. What the technologist should do to the technical factors and explain why.

   a. Pneumonia   c. Pneumothorax
   b. Emphysema   d. Pleural effusion

4

The Gastrointestinal System

● Goals

1. To distinguish the accessory organs from the main organs of the gastrointestinal system

   OBJECTIVE: List the accessory organs of the gastrointestinal system

2. To review the basic anatomy of the esophagus, stomach, small bowel, and large bowel

   OBJECTIVE: Identify anatomic components of the esophagus, stomach, small bowel, and large bowel in both radiographic images and illustrations

3. To review the basic physiology and function of the esophagus, stomach, small bowel, and large bowel

   OBJECTIVE: Explain the physiology and function of all organs of the gastrointestinal system

4. To understand the pathophysiologic and radiographic manifestations of all of the common pathologic conditions of the gastrointestinal system

   OBJECTIVE: Analyze how the different pathologies of the gastrointestinal system will affect the physiology and function of the gastrointestinal system

   OBJECTIVE: Identify the radiographic manifestations for common pathologies of the esophagus, stomach, and small and large bowels

● Key Terms

Achalasia
Adenocarcinoma
Aganglionic megacolon
Atresia
Barrett esophagus
Bezoar
Crohn disease
Diverticula
Dysphagia
Fistula
Gastritis
Gastroesophageal reflux disease (GERD)
Hernia
Hiatal hernia
Hirschsprung disease
Intussusception
Leiomyoma
Mechanical small bowel obstruction (MSBO)
Meckel diverticulum
Paralytic ileus
Peristaltic asynchrony
Pulsion diverticula
Pyloric stenosis

● Goals *continued*

5. To become familiar with how different imaging modalities serve to enhance and complement radiographic diagnosis of common pathologies of the gastrointestinal system

   OBJECTIVE: List and describe the various imaging modalities used in diagnosis of the gastrointestinal system

● Key Terms *continued*

Regional enteritis
Schatzki ring
Traction diverticula
Ulcer
Valsalva
Varices
Volvulus

The digestive tract of the body contains all the organs, ducts, and components necessary to start and complete the digestive process. Beginning where solid and liquid material enters the mouth, the components include the pharynx, esophagus, stomach, and small and large intestines (bowels). These areas are considered as the gastrointestinal system. Accessory organs to the system include the liver, gallbladder, bile ducts, and pancreas, and are known as the hepatobiliary system. Other accessory organs are the teeth and salivary glands. The accessory organs are studied in Chapter 5.

There are many interesting pathologies that occur in this area of the body; however, remembering that this text is intended for radiography personnel, many of the pathologic conditions that occur have not been addressed as that particular process may not be diagnosed with radiography or its subspecialties.

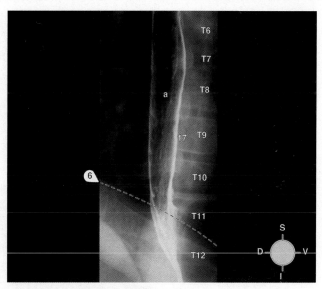

FIGURE 4-1   Esophageal sphincter and cardiac region of stomach. The esophagus is distended with air and coated with swallowed barium. Note how the mucosal lining of the esophagus is demonstrated. (Dean D, Herbener TE. *Cross-Sectional Human Anatomy.* Baltimore, MD: Lippincott Williams & Wilkins; 2000.)

Anatomy

Esophagus

The esophagus is a vertical tube approximately 10 inches long. It extends from the level of C6, inferior to the pharynx, to the stomach at the level of T11. The esophagus lies posterior to the trachea and heart and anterior to the spine. The descending thoracic aorta lies posterior to the esophagus. The esophagus lies in the thoracic cavity and pierces the diaphragm at an opening called the esophageal hiatus. It passes through this hiatus and opens into the medial side of the stomach. The opening of the esophagus into the stomach is termed the cardiac orifice (cardia) (Fig. 4-1).

The esophagus is not covered with peritoneum but rather has a covering of fibrous connective tissue. The esophagus is different from the trachea in that it is a completely collapsible tube, as it lacks the cartilage rings that the trachea contains.

Stomach

The stomach is a large collapsible sac that is located in the left upper quadrant of the abdomen. It is the most dilated portion of the digestive tract; it can hold almost 1.5 quarts (qt) of food and liquid. The fundus of the stomach is an enlarged, bulb-like portion located to the left and above the opening from the esophagus. The central portion is called the body. The greater curvature is along the lower border of the stomach and the lesser curvature is along the upper medial border. The incisura angularis, better known as the angular notch, is a sharp indentation along the lesser curvature.

The cardiac sphincter is located at the cardiac orifice to prevent regurgitation of the stomach contents into the esophagus. Located at the opening from the stomach into the duodenum, between the lesser curvature and the pyloric channel, is an area known as the pylorus (or pyloric orifice). It is guarded by the pyloric sphincter. Figure 4-2 shows radiographically the anatomy that must be demonstrated on an upper gastrointestinal (UGI) series.

When the stomach is empty, it collapses into many folds called rugae. These internal mucosal folds help to move the stomach contents into the duodenum. Rugae disappear when the stomach is full. The muscular coat of the stomach is actually three muscle layers. The innermost layer is known as the oblique layer. A circular layer of muscle is the middle section and a longitudinal layer of muscle is the outermost layer, which is visceral peritoneum.

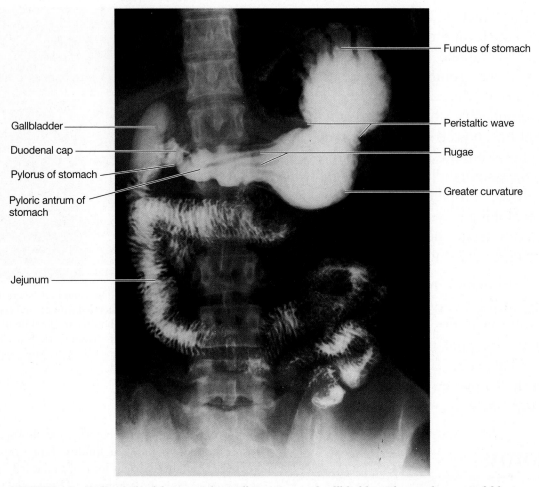

Gallbladder

Duodenal cap

Pylorus of stomach

Pyloric antrum of stomach

Jejunum

Fundus of stomach

Peristaltic wave

Rugae

Greater curvature

FIGURE 4-2   Radiograph of the stomach, small intestine, and gallbladder. Observe the gastric folds or rugae-longitudinal folds of the mucous membrane. Also observe the peristaltic wave that is moving the gastric contents toward the duodenum, which is closely related to the gallbladder. *Note*: The area marked as "Jejunum" is incorrect. That is the descending portion of the duodenum that makes up the "C" loop. (Moore KL, Dalley AF. *Clinically Oriented Anatomy*. 4th ed. Baltimore, MD: Lippincott Williams & Wilkins; 1999; courtesy of Dr. J. Heslin, Toronto, Ontario, Canada.)

Small Bowel

The small bowel (intestine) extends from the pyloric sphincter to the cecum. It is called the small bowel, not because it is short (it measures 18 to 23 feet), but because its lumen is smaller than that of the large bowel. There are three divisions of the small bowel: duodenum, jejunum, and ileum. The duodenum is the shortest, widest portion, being approximately 10 inches long. It is made up of four divisions to form a "C" shape. The superior portion is immediately adjacent to the pyloric opening. It includes the duodenal bulb. The descending duodenum connects with the superior portion and passes to the right of the median plane. The ampulla of Vater opens into this portion of the duodenum. The horizontal portion of the

duodenum courses over the median plane to the left and connects with the ascending duodenum, which travels upward to connect with the jejunum just posterior to the stomach.

The jejunum is the second portion of the small bowel and is approximately 8 feet long. The junction between the duodenum and jejunum is marked by the ligament of Treitz. The jejunum coils back and forth to fill the left upper quadrant of the abdomen. A loop is made in the right upper quadrant before the jejunum joins the third portion of the small bowel, the ileum. The ileum extends about another 13 feet before terminating at the ileocecal valve of the cecum. The ileum forms coils in the lower quadrants of the abdomen and in the pelvis.

Large Bowel

The large bowel averages 5 to 6 feet in length. It extends from the cecum to the anus. Many people mistakenly believe the colon to be synonymous with the large bowel. The colon along with the cecum and rectum is a part of the large bowel. The portion known as the cecum is an area that forms a sac-like structure inferior to the ileocecal opening in the right lower quadrant. The appendix is a long, narrow tube attached to the base of the cecum.

The colon is divided into the ascending colon located on the right side of the abdomen and extending to the liver; the transverse colon, which begins at the right colic (hepatic) flexure and extends horizontally across the abdomen, ending with the left colic (splenic) flexure; the descending colon, which is located on the left and continuing vertically; and the sigmoid colon, which is an S-shaped curved portion that attaches to the rectum (Fig. 4-3).

The last portion of the large bowel, which contains the anus, is known as the rectum. There are transverse folds located within the rectum known as Houston valves, as well as vertical folds called rectal columns. It is these columns that can enlarge to become hemorrhoids.

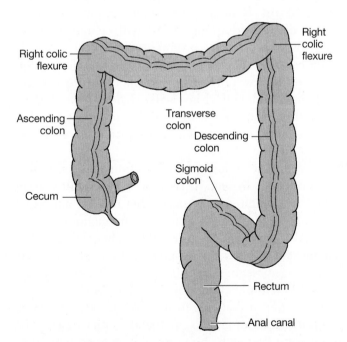

FIGURE 4-3   The anatomy of the large bowel. (Mulholland MW, Lillemoe KD, Doherty GM, et al. *Greenfield's Surgery Scientific Principles and Practice*. 4th ed. Philadelphia, PA: Lippincott Williams & Wilkins; 2006.)

The entire large bowel has three bands of muscle running its length. These muscle fibers are called teniae coli. (Teniae is also spelled taeniae. Tenia or taenia is the singular form.) They cause a puckering effect of the walls of the cecum and colon. The pouches that are formed by the puckering of the teniae coli are called haustra. Semilunar folds are located between each haustrum and are helpful in differentiating the large bowel from the small bowel.

Physiology and Function

Esophagus

The esophagus functions as a passageway from the mouth to the stomach. Since the esophagus is a fairly straight tube, liquids pass down mainly by gravity. Food passes by gravity also, but because it is a bolus of sold material, its passage is aided by peristalsis.

Stomach

As food and liquid pass from the esophagus through the cardiac orifice and into the stomach, digestion is initiated. The stomach secretes 2 to 3 qt of gastric juice that is a combination of pepsinogen, gastrin, and hydrochloric acid. The pepsinogen is converted to pepsin, an enzyme that digests food. Mucus and alkaline fluids are also produced to protect the stomach from auto-digestion. The stomach prepares the food so that it can be moved along the alimentary tract. By contracting the three muscular coats, the stomach breaks the food into small particles. As the action of the stomach wall breaks the food into smaller particles, it is mixed with the gastric juices. If the pyloric sphincter is closed, the stomach acts as a reservoir to store food until it is sufficiently digested to be moved, a bit at a time, into the duodenum. This semiliquid food is known as *chyme*. The stomach normally empties its contents into the duodenum within 2 to 6 hours. After 7 hours, it is assumed that retention has occurred that can be caused by a variety of pathologic conditions. The digestion process does not take place in the stomach. In fact, only a small amount of absorption of water and alcohol takes place there.

Small Bowel

The structure of the small bowel was designed to carry out the processes of digestion and absorption. The tiny tubes that are found inside the mucous membrane lining secrete an enzyme that acts on the food that is being passed through the bowel. When the food becomes liquefied by bile, digestive juices from the pancreas, enzymes from the stomach, and acid from the bowel, it is considered to be digested and is ready for absorption.

The finger-like projections, called villi, that are located in the bowel each have a blood vessel. When the liquid food passes these villi, nutrients are absorbed into the blood and lymph vessels of each villous. From there, the blood vessel transports the nutrients to the liver through the portal vein. From here, it is distributed to the organs of the body. It takes approximately 6 to 8 hours for food to go through the action of the small bowel.

Large Bowel

The mucous membrane of the large bowel does not contain any villi but is lined with tubular glands that are packed closely together. These glands do not secrete any digestive juices, as all digestion has been accomplished before material enters the large bowel. The large bowel aids in the regulation of the body's water balance by absorbing large amounts of water from undigested food back into the bloodstream. Bacteria found in the large bowel act on undigested food that produces acids, gases, and other waste products as well as vitamins K and D. With the water absorbed from undigested material and the bacterial action, the liquid matter that started out in the large bowel is now transformed into a semisolid form known as feces.

Pathology

Esophagus

Congenital Anomalies

Atresia is a congenital anomaly of the esophagus manifested as a lack of development of the esophagus at any point. The most common type, occurring in about 90% of cases, is the ending of the upper segment of the esophagus in a blind pouch near the level of the bifurcation of the trachea, with a lower segment from the stomach connected to the trachea by a short fistulous tract (Fig. 4-4).

A **fistula** (passageway) between the trachea and the esophagus is another anomaly that may occur. The most common is the congenital type III, where the esophagus appears to be in two parts. The lower end of the upper esophagus ends in a blind pouch and the upper end of the lower part is attached to the trachea. Air will be demonstrated in the bowel on the upright abdominal image (Fig. 4-4A).

Acquired Pathology

Achalasia refers to the combined failure of peristalsis to pass food down the esophagus and failure of relaxation of the cardia. The esophagus becomes dilated when food cannot pass into the stomach because of the spasm of the cardiac sphincter. Past the gastroesophageal junction (where the cardia is located), the esophagus is normal in size. Achalasia is seen in adults ranging in age from 20 to 40 years. Because of this, if achalasia is seen in an elderly patient, other causes of the stricture at the cardia (such as a neoplasm) should be explored. Symptoms include dysphagia and heartburn. Patients with achalasia feel that food gets stuck in the throat or chest and may experience regurgitation and weight loss. Radiographically, the esophagus shows as a dilated area (Fig. 4-5A) with a narrowing of the distal esophagus, producing the classic "rat tail" appearance. It has also been called a "beak" sign when the flow of barium is stopped during a spasm of the esophagus (Fig. 4-5B). Normal esophageal motility is absent in the middle and lower esophagus. Often, the trapped food particles are readily seen on the image.

When the esophagus suffers from peristalsis that is no longer in sync, it is known as **peristaltic asynchrony**, which simply means that there is abnormal motility. This presents as tertiary contractions causing a classic and readily identifiable radiographic image known as a "corkscrew esophagus" (Fig. 4-6A, B). The esophageal segment contractions are uncoordinated and therefore, nonpropulsive. This disorder is seen more often in patients in their 40s to 60s (vs. young adults) and sometimes in hiatal hernia cases. The patient suffers with chest pain and pressure, which are either caused by or increased with eating. The symptoms can occur spontaneously at any time and have been known to awake the patient at night.

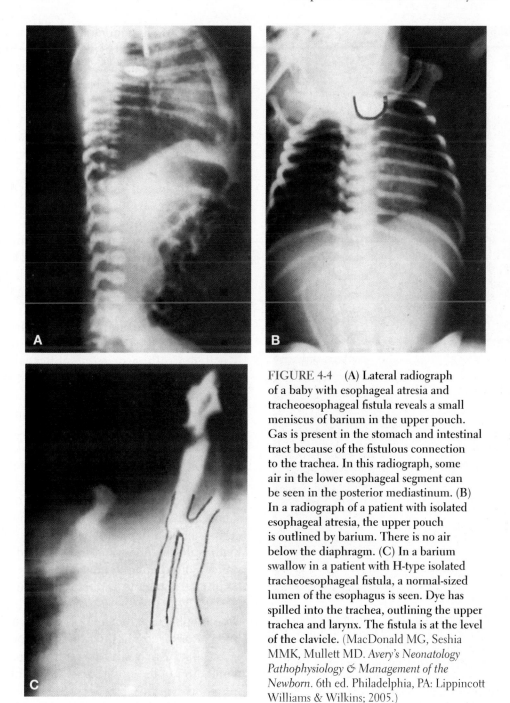

FIGURE 4-4   (A) Lateral radiograph of a baby with esophageal atresia and tracheoesophageal fistula reveals a small meniscus of barium in the upper pouch. Gas is present in the stomach and intestinal tract because of the fistulous connection to the trachea. In this radiograph, some air in the lower esophageal segment can be seen in the posterior mediastinum. (B) In a radiograph of a patient with isolated esophageal atresia, the upper pouch is outlined by barium. There is no air below the diaphragm. (C) In a barium swallow in a patient with H-type isolated tracheoesophageal fistula, a normal-sized lumen of the esophagus is seen. Dye has spilled into the trachea, outlining the upper trachea and larynx. The fistula is at the level of the clavicle. (MacDonald MG, Seshia MMK, Mullett MD. *Avery's Neonatology Pathophysiology & Management of the Newborn.* 6th ed. Philadelphia, PA: Lippincott Williams & Wilkins; 2005.)

Foreign bodies in the esophagus can cause dysphagia or can be asymptomatic. A radiopaque object (such as a coin or safety pin) (Fig. 4-7A) can be easily demonstrated without the use of a contrast agent. These types of objects in the esophagus usually result if a curious toddler accidently swallows the object. If the object poses no problem to the child's safety, it will be allowed to pass through the system ending up in the diaper. However, as in the case of Figure 4-7B, the object may need to be removed surgically.

Radiolucent objects, such as chicken bones, pose a problem. The object, especially if it is a small bone, can perforate the esophagus and an infection or abscess can occur. It is important that these objects be demonstrated radiographically. A barium swallow with a thick paste may be all that is required to visualize the object. On few

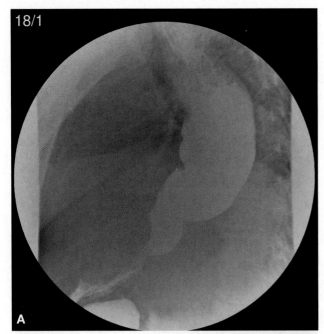

18/1

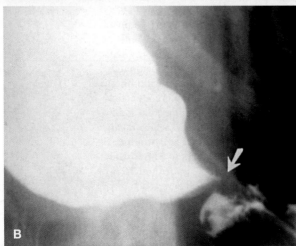

FIGURE 4-5   (A) Achalasia: the classic sign of a rat's tail can be imagined by looking at the stream of barium as it flows from the esophagus into the stomach. The enlarged esophagus is the "fat" rat's back side! (B) Achalasia: this does not show the flow of barium from the esophagus into the stomach but has been taken at the moment of a spasm. This image represents more of a "beak" image. (Eisenberg RL. *Clinical Imaging: An Atlas of Differential Diagnosis.* 5th ed. Philadelphia, PA: Lippincott Williams & Wilkins; 2010.)

instances, some material soaked in thin barium and then swallowed by the patient is necessary to try to locate the foreign body. Most of the times, shredded cotton is put into a cup with thin barium mixture and the patient is asked to swallow the entire contents of the cup. If there is a transparent object in the esophagus, the cotton will get hung up on the object and show its location.

When the stomach herniates through a defect in the diaphragm, it is known as a **hiatal hernia**. This condition can be found in approximately one-half of the population. There are two different types of hernias: a *sliding hernia* in which the stomach slides up into the esophagus, and a *rolling hernia* where the stomach pushes up alongside the esophagus. Figure 4-8 shows the difference between the two types of hiatal hernias.

The esophageal opening through the diaphragm can become weak, which allows a portion of the stomach and gastroesophageal junction to bulge up through the hiatus. A sliding type of hernia is by far the most common type. Small sliding hernias can be identified by the presence of an indentation at the distal end of the esophagus but above the diaphragm known as Schatzki ring (Fig. 4-9).

Another type of hernia occurs through the normal hiatus but is alongside the esophagus. This is called a rolling or paraesophageal hiatal hernia (Fig. 4-10). In this type, a portion of the fundus of the stomach slides above the diaphragm, through the same opening that the esophagus comes through, leaving the gastroesophageal junction in place. The distal esophagus will be displaced to the right and posteriorly to allow room for the fundus.

After a time, the hiatus becomes so large that the patient acquires a gastric volvulus or *intrathoracic stomach* (Fig. 4-11). In this condition, almost the entire stomach has herniated through the esophageal hiatus into the chest and has assumed an inverted or upside-down configuration. The greater curvature will be located superiorly and the lesser curvature inferior to that. This may be associated with a congenitally short esophagus if the condition exists at birth. Rarely, traction or torsion of the stomach at or near the level of the hiatus may lead to obstruction, infarction, or perforation of the intrathoracic stomach. Large hiatal hernia such as this may be seen on a plain chest X-ray. Figure 4-12A, B shows how the hernia has created an air-fluid level that can be indicative of an intrathoracic stomach. Patients with this condition often undergo emergency surgery because of their rapidly deteriorating clinical condition. There is an extremely rare type of hernia in which there is a completely separate congenital opening in the diaphragm next to the normal hiatus through which the fundus can herniate through.

A hiatal hernia can be demonstrated by placing the patient in a Trendelenburg position during a

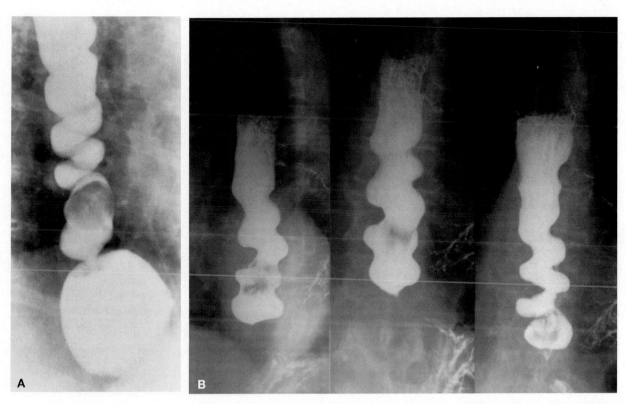

FIGURE 4-6　Peristaltic asynchrony of the esophagus produces the classic appearance of a corkscrew. (A) The contrast is able to flow nicely into the stomach but still shows the curling appearance of the corkscrew. (B) There is a spasm at the cardiac sphincter that is causing the upper esophagus to dilate. The radiolucencies represent food particles coated with contrast. (A: Eisenberg RL. *Clinical Imaging: An Atlas of Differential Diagnosis.* 5th ed. Philadelphia, PA: Lippincott Williams & Wilkins; 2010.)

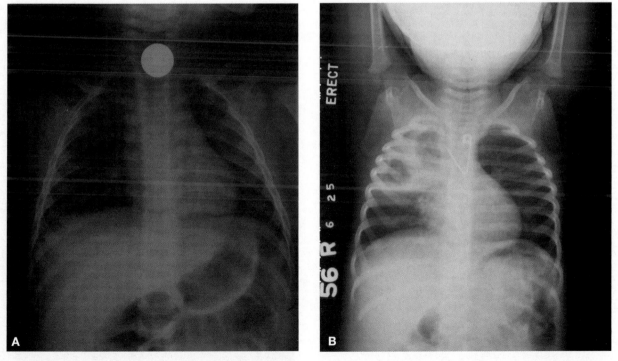

FIGURE 4-7　(A) A nickel is lodged in the esophagus of this toddler. (B) This young child swallowed a safety pin, which can be seen in the open position.

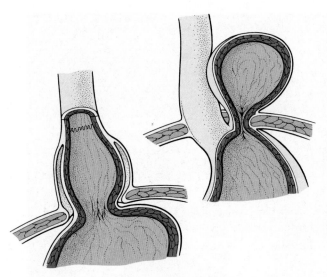

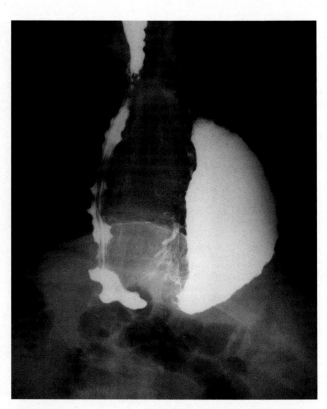

FIGURE 4-8   The figure on the left shows a sliding hernia. The figure on the right is a rolling hernia. (*Stedman's Medical Dictionary for the Health Professions and Nursing.* 6th ed. Philadelphia, PA: Lippincott Williams & Wilkins; 2008.)

series of upper gastrointestinal (UGI) radiographs. Asking the patient to perform a valsalva movement will help demonstrate the hernia. Symptoms of hiatal hernias are related to inflammatory changes of the esophageal mucosa caused by the action of gastric juices on it. These symptoms are heartburn and dysphagia.

FIGURE 4-10   This esophagram shows a paraesophageal hernia. The stomach can be clearly seen alongside the esophagus and above the diaphragm. Additionally, note the asynchrony of the peristalsis in the esophagus.

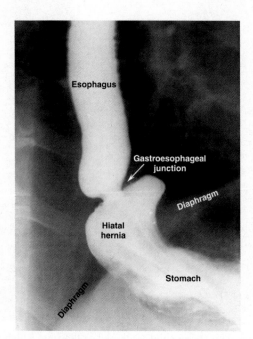

FIGURE 4-9   The constriction of the esophagus arising several centimeters above the diaphragm is known as Schatzki ring and is indicative of a sliding hiatal hernia.

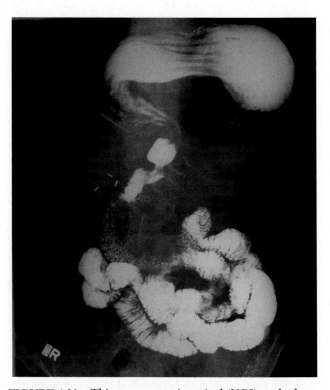

FIGURE 4-11   This upper gastrointestinal (UGI) study shows the stomach in an inverted configuration and located in the thoracic cavity.

Inflammatory Processes

Diverticula can occur anywhere in the body. They are herniations of mucosa and submucosa. There are two common types of diverticula of the esophagus: pulsion and traction. **Pulsion diverticula** are more common than traction ticks. Usually located at the esophageal–pharyngeal junction, they have a narrow neck with a round head protruding from the weakened esophageal wall. A *Zenker* diverticulum (Fig. 4-13) is located in the upper esophagus, and an *epiphrenic* diverticulum (Fig. 4-14) is located just above the hemidiaphragm. A *pharyngeal pouch* is another type of pulsion tick that occurs at the cricopharyngeal junction (Fig. 4-15). Food has a tendency to go into this pouch instead of down the esophagus. Eventually, enough food collects

to cause the diverticulum to be a noticeable mass on the outside of the neck.

Traction diverticula (Fig. 4-16) occur at the tracheal bifurcation, or at the middle third portion of the esophagus. These ticks are caused by scarring of the esophagus from a disease such as tuberculosis. They are triangular in shape, with the apex of the triangle being pulled by the scar tissue of the underlying disease process.

Diverticula may go unnoticed until they have reached a size large enough to cause a mechanical obstruction; or they may be discovered relatively early if a foreign object (such as medication) happens to go into the diverticulum. In addition, reoccurring pneumonitis may result from the contents of the diverticulum draining and being aspirated into the lungs while the patient is recumbent.

Case Study

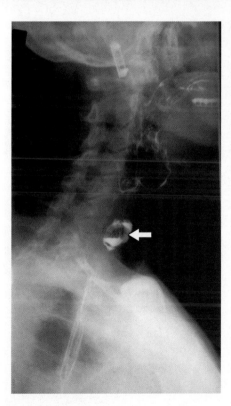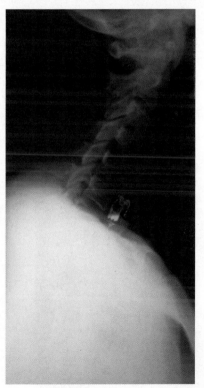

This 40-year-old female patient came into the emergency department (ED) in the late evening hours. She had been getting ready to retire for the night, had taken her medication and had gone to bed. She stated that she felt like she had something caught in her throat which persisted

for several hours and that is what brought her to the ED. This esophagram shows that the medication she had taken was trapped in a small Zenker diverticula. Both the oblique and lateral views demonstrate the round object outlined by barium that can be seen near the arrows.

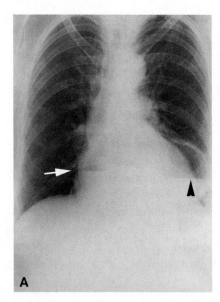
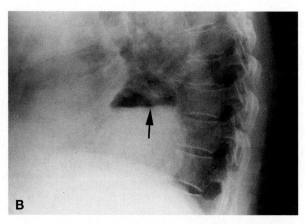

FIGURE 4-12   PA (A). An air -fluid level extends from near the right border of the heart (right atrium) (arrow) across the midline to the left lateral wall of the thoracic cage (arrowhead). These air-fluid levels represent gas in the fundus of the stomach after herniation through the diaphragm. Lateral (B) Note the air-fluid level (arrow) above the diaphragm in the retrocardiac space. (Yochum TR, Rowe LJ, *Yochum and Rowe's Essentials of Skeletal Radiology*, 3rd ed. Philadelphia: Lippincott Williams & Wilkins, 2004.)

Esophageal dysphagia is a symptom (vs. a separate disease entity) that gives the patient the sensation of food being stuck or getting "hung up" in the esophagus. Approximately 8% of the population over the age of 50 years has experienced dysphagia. The patient will have discomfort when he/she tries to swallow. The

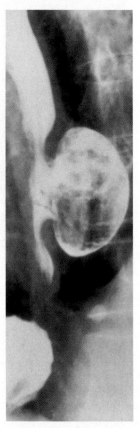

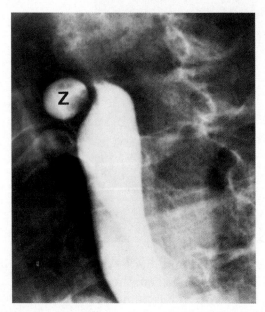

FIGURE 4-13   Zenker diverticulum of the proximal esophagus. (Daffner RH. *Clinical Radiology: The Essentials.* 3rd ed. Philadelphia, PA: Lippincott Williams & Wilkins; 2007.)

FIGURE 4-14   Epiphrenic diverticula. (Eisenberg RL. *Clinical Imaging: An Atlas of Differential Diagnosis.* 5th ed. Philadelphia, PA: Lippincott Williams & Wilkins; 2010.)

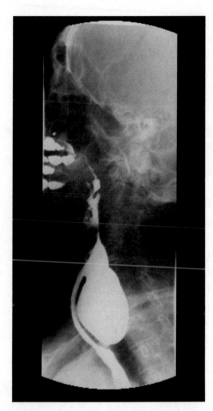

FIGURE 4-15   This large pulsion diverticulum has occurred at the cricopharyngeal junction. It is quite large and is considered a pharyngeal pouch.

the easiest to perform and can be completed during an UGI examination. Computed tomography (CT) is done if the patient is suspected of having esophageal cancer. Studies that are being done more frequently comprise video fluoroscopic swallowing study. In this study, the actual action of swallowing can be studied as the patient is asked to move in different positions and swallow different foods. The procedure is videotaped so that it can be studied later. The purpose is to determine if there are better positions for the patient to hold his/her head to facilitate swallowing.

Gastroesophageal reflux disease (GERD) is an inflammation of the mucosa and submucosa of the lower esophagus. Heartburn and pain are caused by reflux of gastric acid from the stomach into the esophagus. As the acid continues to rise into the esophagus it will eventually cause erosion of the protective mucosa. This gastric reflux is caused by increased abdominal pressure and incompetence of the sphincter at the cardiac orifice. Mild inflammation may be present but continued occurrences can result in ulcerations. The ulcerative areas of the esophagus are known as *Barrett esophagus* (Fig. 4-17). Adenocarcinoma may occur

patient may not even be able to swallow. Because the patient is usually in such distress there is loss of appetite and weight. The patient often wakes up at night with a cough and frequent clearing of the throat.

There are several procedures that the patient can undergo to make a diagnosis. A barium swallow (esophagram) is

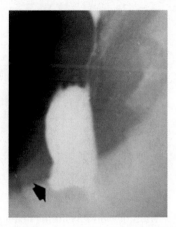

FIGURE 4-16   Traction diverticulum (*arrow*) of the esophagus caused by postoperative scarring after total laryngectomy. (Eisenberg RL. *Clinical Imaging: An Atlas of Differential Diagnosis.* 5th ed. Philadelphia, PA: Lippincott Williams & Wilkins; 2010.)

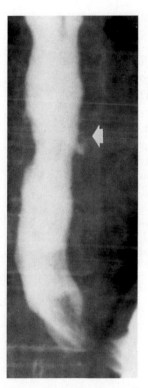

FIGURE 4-17   Ulcerations (*arrow*) have developed at a small distance superior to the esophagogastric junction. (Eisenberg RL. *Clinical Imaging: An Atlas of Differential Diagnosis.* 5th ed. Philadelphia, PA: Lippincott Williams & Wilkins; 2010.)

in these areas (Fig. 4-18). If persistent, the ulceration leads to scarring. Contraction of the scar tissue causes a stenosis and closure of the esophagus.

Reflux is readily identifiable with a contrast study and a water siphonage test. The patient is placed in the left posterior oblique position so that the fundus of the stomach fills with barium. With the use of fluoroscopy, the radiologist observes the gastroesophageal junction while the patient drinks water from a straw. Reflux is demonstrated if barium flows from the stomach back into the esophagus.

Varices are very important to diagnose, as fatal hemorrhage may result if they rupture. These dilated tortuous veins are located in the wall at the end of the esophagus and at the top of the stomach. They occur more frequently in alcoholic patients with portal venous hypertension and secondary to cirrhosis of the liver. The hardening of the liver restricts the blood flow and causes increased pressure in the portal venous system, which forces the veins to become enlarged and form a bypass. An enlarged spleen is associated with varices.

The best way to demonstrate small varices is by endoscopy. Varices that are large enough to displace barium and extensive are seen on a barium swallow done with the patient in the recumbent position will show multiple filling defects similar to "worm tracings" (Fig. 4-19A, B) or "rosary beads" (Fig. 4-20), which can be accentuated by the Valsalva maneuver.

TECH TIP

When looking for evidence of varices, the use of thin barium is recommended. Thick paste may cover the varice sign. Having the patient valsalva will put pressure on the portal system causing the tortuous veins to distend and make the filling defect larger. When trying to image varices, be sure to focus on the lower aspect of the esophagus.

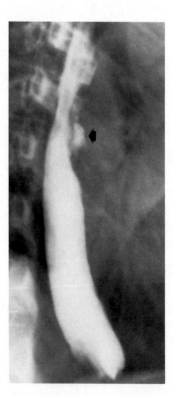

FIGURE 4-18   Squamous carcinoma of the esophagus. On this profile view, the lesion looks like an ulcer (*arrow*). (Eisenberg RL. *Clinical Imaging: An Atlas of Differential Diagnosis.* 5th ed. Philadelphia, PA: Lippincott Williams & Wilkins; 2010.)

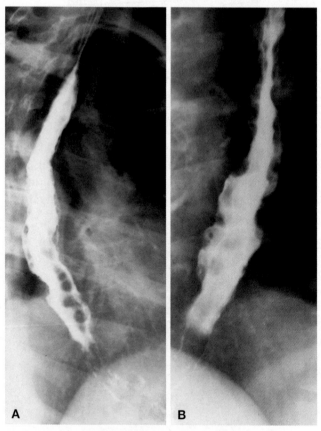

FIGURE 4-19   Multiple wormlike filling defects in two patients (A and B) with histories of chronic alcohol abuse. This is indicative of esophageal varices. (Daffner RH. *Clinical Radiology: The Essentials.* 3rd ed. Philadelphia, PA: Lippincott Williams & Wilkins; 2007.)

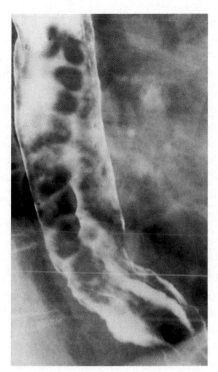

FIGURE 4-20   The multiple filling defects in this esophagus show the classic sign of "rosary beads" and are indicative of esophageal varices. (Eisenberg RL. *Clinical Imaging: An Atlas of Differential Diagnosis.* 5th ed. Philadelphia, PA: Lippincott Williams & Wilkins; 2010.)

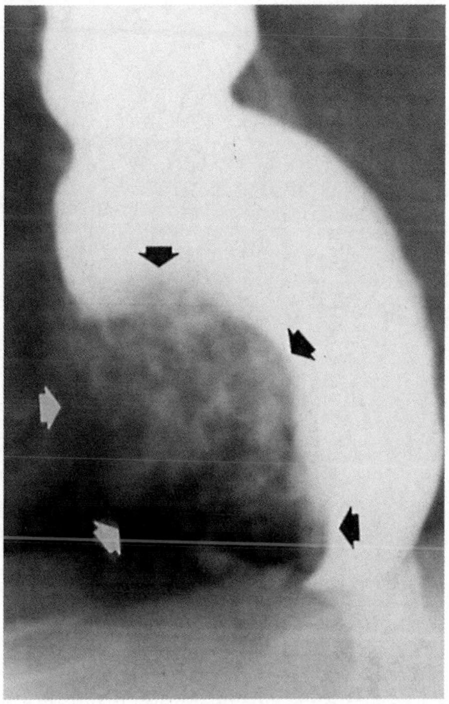

FIGURE 4-21   Calcification shown in this smoothly lobulated intramural tumor (*arrowheads*). (Eisenberg RL. *Clinical Imaging: An Atlas of Differential Diagnosis.* 5th ed. Philadelphia, PA: Lippincott Williams & Wilkins; 2010.)

Neoplasms

The esophagus can have both benign and malignant tumors. The most common benign esophageal neoplasm is a **leiomyoma** (Fig. 4-21). Radiographically, benign tumors within the esophagus characteristically produce an intraluminal polypoid defect with smooth narrowing of the lumen.

The most important tumors of the esophagus are *malignant neoplasms.* Esophageal carcinoma should be suspected until disproved when a 40-year-old or older patient is experiencing dysphagia. The incidence of squamous cell carcinoma (see Fig. 4-18) is higher in men than in women, and there is a strong correlation among excessive alcohol intake, smoking, and esophageal carcinoma. Two sites of carcinoma are at the middle of the esophagus, where it is crossed by the left bronchus, and in the lower third portion of the esophagus. These carcinomas usually stem from cancer of the stomach.

Malignant tumors demonstrate a definite division between normal tissue and tumor. This division is known as "shelving." The tumor grows into the lumen, causing narrowing and dysphagia.

Many of the esophageal pathologies just discussed can be seen in Figure 4-22.

Stomach
Congenital Anomalies

A narrowing of the lumen of the pylorus caused by hypertrophy of the muscle is called a **pyloric stenosis**. The cause of the hypertrophy is unknown. This is the most common cause of gastric outlet obstruction and it occurs almost four times more often in males. Symptoms of projectile vomiting after feeding begin 2 to 6 weeks after birth. This condition will cause the stomach to become dilated, as the contents cannot pass through to the duodenum (Fig. 4-23A). If the stomach contents have not emptied after 7 hours, retention is present. As the stomach continues to fill, the patient becomes greatly distressed and vomiting will result. The wall of the pylorus is thick which causes the stricture, as seen in the ultrasound image in Figure 4-23B. A simple surgical incision to cut the thickened pyloric muscle remedies the situation.

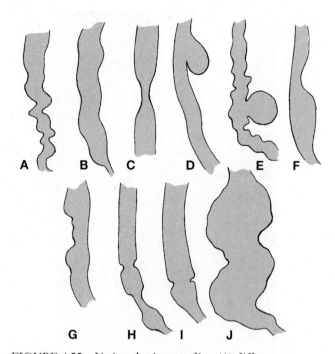

FIGURE 4-22   Various barium studies: (A) diffuse spasm,
(B) achalasia (moderate), (C) carcinoma: annular type,
(D) Zenker diverticulum, (E) diffuse spasm with epiphrenic
diverticulum, (F) leiomyoma, (G) carcinoma: fungating
type, (H) sliding hiatal hernia (type I) with Barrett esophagus
and esophageal stricture due to reflux, (I) Schatzki ring,
(J) achalasia (severe). (Blackbourne LH. *Advanced Surgical
Recall.* 2nd ed. Baltimore, MD: Lippincott Williams &
Wilkins; 2004.)

The radiographic appearance of pyloric stenosis is that of a distended stomach filled with contrast
medium with a small "string" of contrast trickling
through the pylorus to the duodenum. Figure 4-23C
shows an adult that presents with pyloric stenosis. This
is a somewhat confusing process. It could possibly represent a true congenital stenosis that was not discovered, or it may be the result of peptic inflammatory
disease. Most findings in adults have had some type of
peptic inflammatory disease; however, stenosis is rare,
thereby making the assumption that the stenosis was
congenital but undiscovered.

Acquired Pathology

The ability to determine pathology of the stomach is
dependent on recognizing its normal appearance on
an UGI study. Refer to Figure 4-24 to determine the
differences in appearances of the pathology processes
discussed below.

Foreign bodies usually pass through the stomach
without difficulty. There are several types of foreign
bodies that persist in the stomach however. **Bezoars**
are just such a type. These masses will cause chronic
gastritis if left untreated; however, they do not obstruct
the stomach outlet. Large masses may also cause the
feeling of being full before enough food has actually
been eaten.

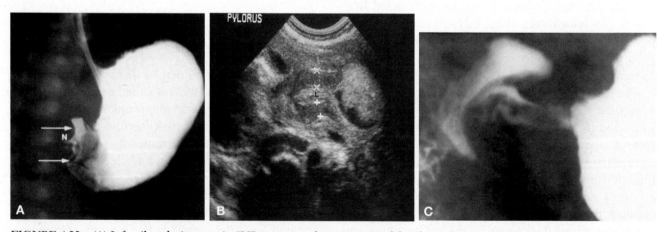

FIGURE 4-23   (A) Infantile pyloric stenosis. "N" represents the narrowing of the channel. Notice the enlarge stomach due to
nonpassage of barium into the duodenum. (B) Ultrasound examination of the pyloric region shows a narrowed lumen (L) and
thickening of the wall of the pylorus (sonolucent area between *white* × and +). (C) Adult pyloric stenosis. Here the string sign is
shown and only a small amount of barium is allowed to pass from the stomach into the duodenum. (A: Mulholland MW, Lillemoe
KD, Doherty GM, et al. *Greenfield's Surgery Scientific Principles and Practice.* 4th ed. Philadelphia, PA: Lippincott Williams & Wilkins;
2006. B: Daffner RH. *Clinical Radiology: The Essentials.* 3rd ed. Philadelphia, PA: Lippincott Williams & Wilkins; 2007. C: Eisenberg
RL. *An Atlas of Differential Diagnosis.* 4th ed. Philadelphia, PA: Lippincott Williams & Wilkins; 2003.)

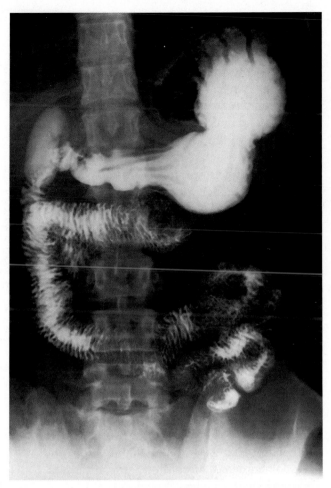

FIGURE 4-24   This is a normal UGI examination taken in the supine position. Since the fundus of the stomach is posterior, it is completely filled with barium. There rugae folds are identifiable but are normal in size.

There are two types of gastric bezoars: *phytobezoar* and *trichobezoar*. A phytobezoar is the most common type. It is an accumulation of organic material such as vegetable matter (Fig. 4-25). These are most often found after a gastrectomy, when the remaining stomach portion does not break the food down and prepare it for digestion. The food remains, collecting more material with each meal until it finally becomes a mass. The material is abrasive and often associated with ulcers.

Trichobezoars are collections of hair, food, and mucus that have congealed, not allowing the mass to pass through the pylorus (Fig. 4-26). When excised from the stomach, they are usually black in color and emit a foul odor. Such masses are usually found in patients suffering from mental or anxiety disorders, as

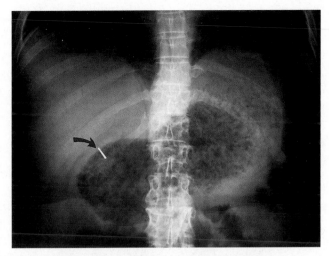

FIGURE 4-25   The patient has a phytobezoar, accounting for the mottled appearance of the stomach. There is a surgical clip (*arrow*) in the right upper quadrant following a cholecystectomy. (Daffner RH. *Clinical Radiology: The Essentials*. 3rd ed. Philadelphia. PA: Lippincott Williams & Wilkins; 2007.)

these patients have a tendency to chew their nails or eat their hair.

Bezoars were previously uncommon but are being identified more often as individuals attempt to smuggle illegal drugs into the country. The risk of a bezoar in these cases is slight compared to the risk of a ruptured condom and leakage of the drug into the person's system.

Inflammatory Processes

Gastritis is inflammation of the mucosa of the stomach. The most common cause is alcohol. Other causes

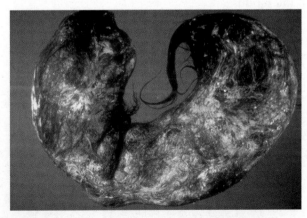

FIGURE 4-26   This excised trichobezoar had grown so large that it is actually a "cast" of the stomach. (Mitros FA. *Atlas of Gastrointestinal Pathology*. New York, NY: Gower Medical Publishing; 1988.)

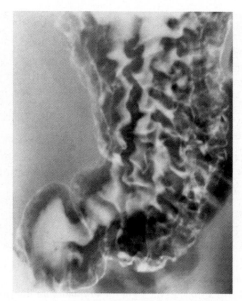

FIGURE 4-27   This patient has hypertrophic gastritis due to high hydrochloric acid output and peptic ulcer disease. Notice the increased rugae folds that displace the barium. (Eisenberg RL. *Clinical Imaging: An Atlas of Differential Diagnosis*. 5th ed. Philadelphia, PA: Lippincott Williams & Wilkins; 2010.)

are chemicals of corrosive nature and bacterial or viral infections. The mucous membrane of the stomach becomes red, swollen, and inflamed. Simple gastritis may be present without ulceration with the only finding being the enlarged gastric rugae folds seen on the UGI exam (Fig. 4-27). After repeated bouts of gastritis, the condition becomes chronic. The early signs of inflammation are gone, and the rugae become thin and atrophy, even to the point of becoming absent in the fundus.

Any **ulcer** of the stomach is called a peptic ulcer because of the digestive acid in the stomach, pepsin. A bacterium known as *Helicobacter pylori* is a major cause of peptic ulcers as it damages the protective mucus wall. Once the wall is damaged, the strong acid in the stomach can work on the sensitive lining causing the ulcer. The juice actually erodes and penetrates the muscle layer of the wall. Other cause of ulcers is the use of NSAIDs such as aspirin and ibuprofen. Ulcers are not caused by stress; however, stress can make the symptoms of the ulcer worse. In about 70% of all cases, the UGI study will show contrast material protruding outside the lumen of the organ. The other 30% of peptic ulcers are not demonstrated by radiography.

The ulcers may occur in two places. *Gastric ulcers* are most common along the lesser curvature of the stomach (Fig. 4-28). Gastric ulcers heal leaving very little scar tissue (regeneration), which allows normal peristalsis to resume. Ninety-five percent of gastric ulcers are benign. Five percent of all gastric ulcers are malignant and are found more often in the greater curvature of the stomach and in the fundus. Radiographically, benign ulcers display radiolucent mucosal folds running to the edge of the ulcer. Seen on edge, the appearance of the crater is round and smooth. Malignant ulcers show obliterated mucosal folds with irregular borders that continue into the ulcer crater and merge with its edges (Fig. 4-29).

Duodenal ulcers occur in the first portion of the duodenum (the bulb) (Fig. 4-30) in 95% of the cases. In only 5% of the cases are the ulcers located just postbulbar. As duodenal ulcers heal, scar tissue is produced, which narrows the lumen. As the ulcer becomes chronic, the lumen may actually close,

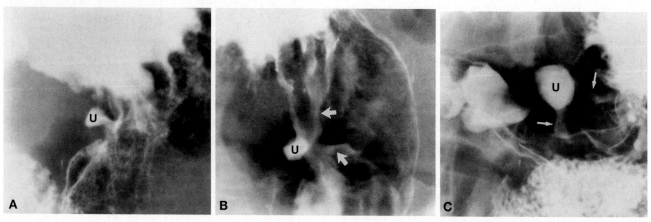

FIGURE 4-28   Three patients (A–C) with gastric ulcers of the lesser curvature. "U" marks the site of the ulcer. (Daffner RH. *Clinical Radiology: The Essentials*. 3rd ed. Philadelphia, PA: Lippincott Williams & Wilkins, 2007.)

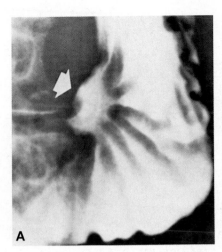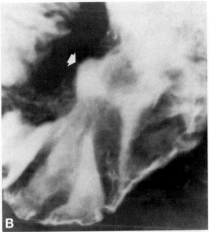

FIGURE 4-29   Fold patterns in gastric ulcers. (A) Small, slender folds (*arrow*) radiating to the edge of a benign ulcer. (B) Thick folds radiating to an irregular mound of tissue surrounding a malignant gastric ulcer (*arrow*). (Eisenberg RL. *Clinical Imaging: An Atlas of Differential Diagnosis.* 5th ed. Philadelphia, PA: Lippincott Williams & Wilkins; 2010.)

causing obstruction. This scarring will shrink the duodenal bulb, which will produce the classic radiographic appearance of a "clover-leaf" deformity. Duodenal ulcers are two to three times more common than gastric ulcers and occur more frequently in men between the ages of 30 and 50 years. Duodenal ulcers are almost always benign, and most respond to medical treatment.

Complications of ulcers can develop. Perforation occurs if the erosion goes through the muscle layer and into the peritoneal cavity. As the contents from the stomach pour into the abdominal cavity, peritonitis occurs, which can prove fatal unless surgery is undertaken to close the opening. An upright abdominal film shows free air in the abdomen.

A frequent complication is hemorrhage. Bleeding occurs when a vessel at the base of the ulcer has been eroded. The blood may be passed by vomiting or in the feces. A less common complication of ulcers is a benign stricture in the body of the stomach. As excessive scar tissue builds up, the stomach takes on the appearance of an "hourglass."

Neoplasms

Benign tumors of the stomach are usually a smooth muscle leiomyoma. While overall these tumors are not common when compared to malignant tumors, in terms of benign tumors of the gastric system, they are second only to gastric polyps. The average size is quite large at about 4.5 cm. As seen in Figures 4-31 and 4-32, the tumors grow at right angles to the wall of the stomach. Tumors will calcify in a small number of cases, making them visible without the use of a contrast medium.

FIGURE 4-30   Duodenal ulcers (*arrow*). Single-contrast study shows a small filling defect within the ulcer crater that represents a blood clot. (Daffner RH. *Clinical Radiology: The Essentials.* 3rd ed. Philadelphia, PA: Lippincott Williams & Wilkins; 2007.)

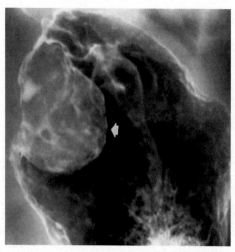

FIGURE 4-31   Leiomyoma of the fundus of the stomach (*arrow*). (Eisenberg RL. *Clinical Imaging: An Atlas of Differential Diagnosis.* 5th ed. Philadelphia, PA: Lippincott Williams & Wilkins; 2010.)

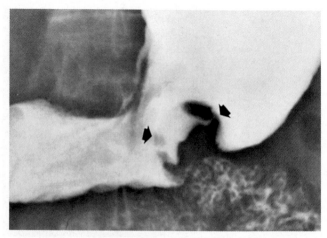

FIGURE 4-33   Polypoid carcinoma of the stomach. The polypoid tumor is causing a filling defect in the stomach (*arrows*). There is, coincidentally, a huge ulcer present within the wall of the mass. (Eisenberg RL. *Clinical Imaging: An Atlas of Differential Diagnosis.* 5th ed. Philadelphia, PA: Lippincott Williams & Wilkins; 2010.)

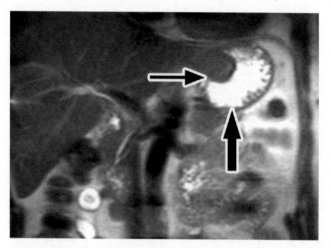

FIGURE 4-32   This MRI image shows a leiomyoma of the upper portion of the stomach at the gastroesophageal junction. The *thin arrow* points to the myoma, the *thick arrow* demonstrates water that was given to the patient to outline the benign tumor. (Leyendecker JR, Brown JJ. *Practical Guide to Abdominal and Pelvic MRI.* Philadelphia, PA: Lippincott Williams & Wilkins; 2004.)

The majority of stomach tumors are **adenocarcinomas**. Factors that are thought to be a predisposition to stomach cancer include the loss of gastric mucosa (this can occur in patients with pernicious anemia) and also individuals that have had previous peptic ulcer disease that led to a partial gastrectomy.

There are three types of primary cancer that are recognized. *Papillary* (*fungating*) tumors are polypoid masses that project into the lumen of the stomach (Fig. 4-33). They can occur anywhere but are more common near the cardioesophageal junction. Because these lesions are extremely difficult to demonstrate on conventional single-contrast barium studies, a double-contrast technique is essential for diagnosing them at the earliest possible stage. Papillary tumors are the least malignant type of the three. *Ulcerating* tumors show ragged mucosa and may be confused with benign ulcers. They have a predilection for areas of the stomach near the greater curvature and the pylorus (see Fig. 4-29). *Infiltrating* (linitis plastica) is the third type of adenocarcinoma. These tumors spread within the walls of the stomach, causing thickening of the walls and production of fibrous tissue. The tumor commonly begins near the pylorus and continues upward toward the fundus. Eventually, the thickening leads to an obstruction as the opening is closed off. The walls of the stomach become shrunken and rigid (leather bottle stomach) in the region of the tumor (Fig. 4-34). Figure 4-35 demonstrates not only the stomach malignancy which is the primary but also metastasis to the liver.

In the United States, the incidence of stomach carcinoma has been declining; however, it is estimated that roughly 22,000 Americans were diagnosed with stomach cancer during 2005 with an estimated 11,500 deaths. The cause of stomach cancer is unknown but dietary factors appear to be a determinant. Tumors present early symptoms of weight loss, loss of appetite, and vague abdominal discomfort. Later developments include weakness, anemia, and loss of blood through

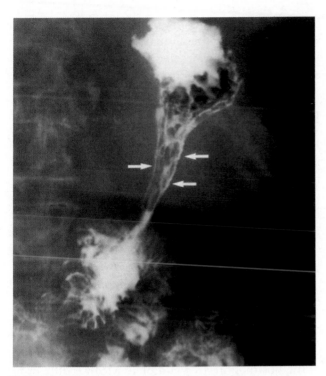

FIGURE 4-34 Barium contrast radiograph demonstrating extensive involvement of the gastric body by infiltrating adenocarcinoma (linitis plastica). The gastric silhouette is narrowed (*arrows*), and the stomach is nondistensible. (Mulholland MW, Lillemoe KD, Doherty GM, et al. *Greenfield's Surgery Scientific Principles and Practice*. 4th ed. Philadelphia, PA: Lippincott Williams & Wilkins; 2006.)

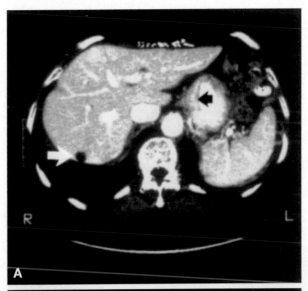

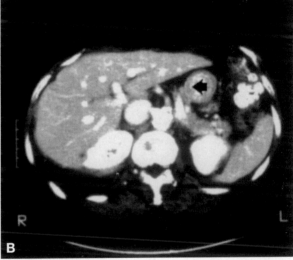

FIGURE 4-35 Computed tomography (CT) scans of the upper abdomen showing extensive thickening of the gastric wall (*black arrows*) caused by infiltrating adenocarcinoma and associated hepatic metastasis (*white arrow*). (A). While the liver metastasis can no longer be seen in (B), the thickened gastric wall of the primary cancer is still present. (Mulholland MW, Lillemoe KD, Doherty GM, et al. *Greenfield's Surgery Scientific Principles and Practice*. 4th ed. Philadelphia, PA: Lippincott Williams & Wilkins; 2006.)

the stool or by vomiting. Metastasis to lymph nodes along the greater curvature is frequent. The overall 5-year relative survival rate of people with stomach cancer is about 23% in the United States. This low rate is believed to be related to the fact that most cancers in the United States are diagnosed at an advanced stage and treatment is usually done for pain prevention rather than for curative purposes.

Small Bowel

Congenital Anomalies

Meckel diverticulum is a congenital diverticulum found in the ileum about 2 feet away from the ileocecal valve. It is a rounded sac that represents the persistence of the yolk sac. It occurs in 2% of the population before the age of 2 years. In contrast to an acquired tick, a Meckel diverticulum always contains all the muscular layers of the bowel wall (Fig. 4-36). This allows for rapid emptying on a barium study

that makes diagnosis of this type of diverticulum difficult. Fluoroscopy using careful compression is often required to see a Meckel diverticulum because overlapping bowel loops often obscure the diverticulum. Nuclear medicine studies are best for demonstrating this anomaly (Fig. 4-37). The technetium pertechnetate will penetrate in the normal and ectopic gastric mucosa to allow identification of the Meckel diverticulum. Most are asymptomatic but a clinical

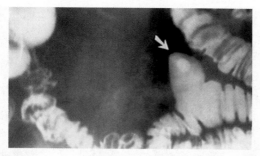

FIGURE 4-36 The *arrow* points to a small area of increased density indicating a Meckel diverticulum. (Eisenberg RL. *Clinical Imaging: An Atlas of Differential Diagnosis.* 5th ed. Philadelphia, PA: Lippincott Williams & Wilkins; 2010.)

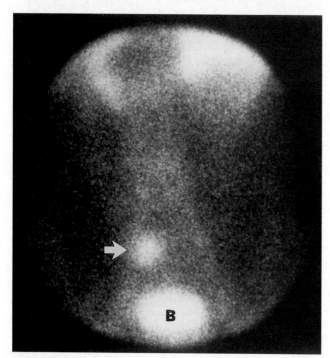

FIGURE 4-37 The increased uptake shown by the *white arrow* is caused by bleeding from a Meckel diverticulum. (Daffner RH. *Clinical Radiology: The Essentials.* 3rd ed. Philadelphia, PA: Lippincott Williams & Wilkins; 2007.)

indication of this type of diverticulum is usually unexplained painful, rectal bleeding. At times, there may be intestinal obstruction due to intussusception.

Acquired Pathology

A **hernia** occurs when a loop of bowel pushes its way through a weak spot or opening in the abdominal wall. The common sites for hernias are the groin and umbilicus. A strangulated hernia is one in which so much bowel has been forced through the opening

that the lumen of the bowel is closed off. The blood vessels that supply the herniated loop are also cut off. Unless the hernia is treated rapidly, gangrene develops and peritonitis sets in.

Inflammatory Processes

Diverticula can occur in any part of the small bowel but are more common in the duodenum. Ileal diverticula are often multiple and can become large (Fig. 4-38). Small bowel diverticula occur along the mesenteric side of the bowel where blood vessels penetrate through the muscular layer producing the defects. The concern of small bowel diverticula is that there may be bacterial growth because of the stasis of bowel activity.

Seventy-five percent of all **mechanical small bowel obstructions** (MSBO) are caused by fibrous adhesions. Other causes include volvulus, intussusception, and tumors. Distended loops of bowel can be demonstrated on an abdominal (KUB) image within hours of the obstruction. In a complete MSBO, little or no gas is found in the colon with much of the gas in the proximal small bowel as compared to the distal section. The upright radiograph shows air-fluid levels at different heights in the bowel (Fig. 4-39). This helps to differentiate it from adynamic ileus in which gas is seen within distended loops throughout the bowel. In acute cases of MSBO, a CT without contrast will demonstrate the obstruction as trapped fluid will act as the contrast medium.

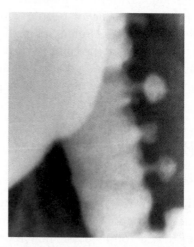

FIGURE 4-38 Ileal diverticula are located at or near the ileal valve. This, and the fact that there are multiple diverticula, helps to differentiate them from a Meckel diverticulum. (Eisenberg RL. *Clinical Imaging: An Atlas of Differential Diagnosis.* 5th ed. Philadelphia, PA: Lippincott Williams & Wilkins; 2010.)

pancreatitis may cause a sentinel loop in the duodenum, jejunum, or transverse colon.

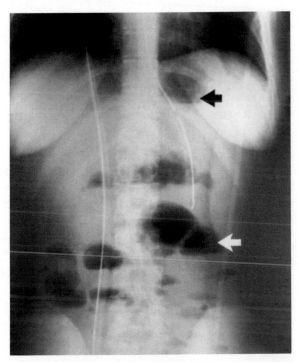

FIGURE 4-39 Upright abdominal film of a patient with mechanical small bowel obstruction (MSBO). Note the air-fluid levels in the stomach (*black arrow*), multiple dilated loops of small intestine (*white arrow*), and absence of air in the colon or rectum. (Mulholland MW, Lillemoe KD, Doherty GM, et al. *Greenfield's Surgery Scientific Principles and Practice*. 4th ed. Philadelphia, PA: Lippincott Williams & Wilkins; 2006.)

Paralytic ileus (adynamic ileus, nonobstructive ileus) is a common problem in which fluid and gas do not progress normally because of inactivity of the bowel. The bowel is not obstructed as in an MSBO. It is most often seen in postoperative patients or those receiving medications that decrease bowel activity. If it occurs in the neonate, lack of ganglions that promote peristalsis must be considered. Because of decreased motor activity, peristalsis cannot pass material from one portion of the bowel to the next. This causes a dilation of the whole bowel. Supine and erect projections of the abdomen demonstrate large amounts of gas and fluid in the small and large bowels. There is uniform dilation with no obstruction demonstrated. This classic radiographic appearance is called the "stepladder" sign (Fig. 4-40).

When inflammation of the bowel causes the distention, it is usually a localized ileus. The loop of distended bowel is known as "sentinel loop" (Fig. 4-41) and will occur in various locations depending on the inflammatory process causing it. For example, acute

Regional enteritis is more commonly known as **Crohn disease**. An idiopathic disease, it tends to begin at early ages (teens and 20s), and males are affected more often than females. It is a chronic inflammatory disease that occurs 80% of the time in the terminal ileum (Fig. 4-42). The condition may extend into the cecum and sometimes into the ascending colon. Early stages of the disease affect the bowel wall by causing it to become thickened. If the thickening continues, fibrosis can occur and that leads to an obstruction. As the wall thickens, the lumen will become narrowed. A segment of bowel with this narrow lumen is demonstrated by the

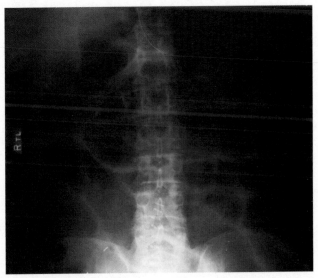

FIGURE 4-40 The classic stepladder sign can be seen on the patient with a paralytic ileus.

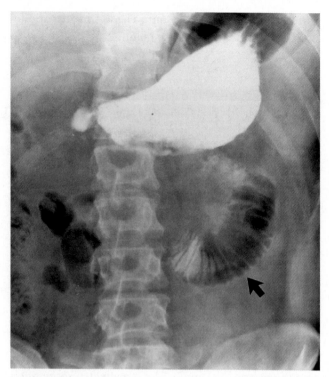

FIGURE 4-41   Small bowel sentinel loop in a patient with pancreatitis of the tail of the pancreas. A single dilated loop of jejunum (*arrow*) is present. Notice the increased distance between the jejunum and the contrast-filled stomach as the result of pancreatic phlegmon. (Daffner RH. *Clinical Radiology: The Essentials*. 3rd ed. Philadelphia, PA: Lippincott Williams & Wilkins; 2007.)

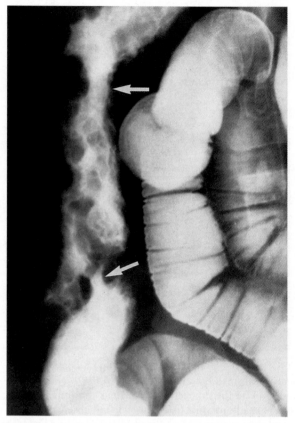

FIGURE 4-42   Small bowel strictures (*arrows*) in a patient with *regional enteritis* (Crohn disease). Notice the abnormal mucosa in the involved segment. (Daffner RH. *Clinical Radiology: The Essentials*. 3rd ed. Philadelphia, PA: Lippincott Williams & Wilkins; 2007.)

"string sign" on radiographic images. The combination of mucosal edema and ulcerations give the bowel a "cobblestone" appearance on the image (see Fig. 4-49A). Lesions affect only certain areas of the bowel, leaving unaffected areas in between. These normal areas of bowel are termed "skipped areas" (see Fig. 4-49B) and are characteristic of this disease. Medical treatment is mandatory, as the disease tends to become chronic.

Intussusception and **volvulus** can both occur in the small bowel. A description of each of these conditions can be found in the following section on colon pathology.

Large Bowel

Congenital Anomalies

Hirschsprung disease is also known as **aganglionic megacolon** because it is the congenital absence of

neurons in a segment of the colon that prevents peristalsis and passage of the colon's contents. This causes a greatly enlarged colon proximal to the affected area. The barium enema usually demonstrates a normal rectum, and an area of transition leading into the grossly dilated sigmoid area that seems to be the area that is affected most (Fig. 4-43). The entire bowel may also be involved but this is very rare.

Eighty percent of the patients with Hirschsprung disease are male and almost all of them become symptomatic within the first week of life. Symptoms include failure to thrive, constipation, abdominal distention, and episodes of vomiting. The newborn may fail to pass meconium in the first 24 to 48 hours after birth. A high incidence of complications, such as enterocolitis or perforation of the transverse colon or the appendix, is found. The important scout radiograph finding includes dilation of the entire small bowel, air-fluid levels on a decubitus view, and no evidence of air in the rectum.

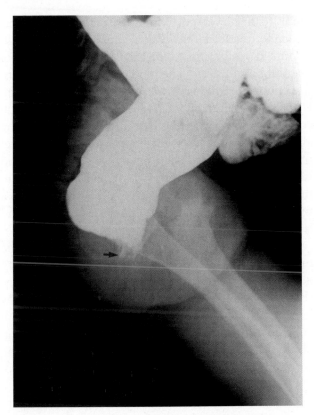

FIGURE 4-43   Lateral image shows a markedly large bowel proximal to the narrowed rectum (*arrow*) in Hirschsprung disease. (Daffner RH. *Clinical Radiology: The Essentials*. 3rd ed. Philadelphia, PA: Lippincott Williams & Wilkins; 2007.)

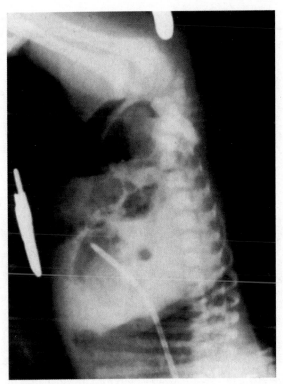

FIGURE 4-44   Upside-down radiographic technique of using a metal marker at the anus shows the distance between the rectal pouch and the anal skin. It is clearly above a line drawn between the pubis and lower border of the sacrum. There is a second gas-containing space anterior to the rectum. This indicates the presence of a rectourethral fistula with air trapped in the bladder. (MacDonald MG, Seshia MMK, Mullett MD. *Avery's Neonatology Pathophysiology & Management of the Newborn*. 6th ed. Philadelphia, PA: Lippincott Williams & Wilkins; 2005.)

The most significant finding on the barium enema is the "transition zone," the boundary between the normal dilated portion and the aganglionic portion of the bowel. The aganglionic colon is spastic, narrowed, and empty of stool. The normal (ganglionic) colon is dilated, hypertrophied, and filled with feces. This transition is found 80% of the time in the rectosigmoid area. If barium is forced in too rapidly, the transition zone or the spastic portion of the colon may not be recognized. Barium is often retained in the colon for as long as 48 hours after the procedure.

Two other congenital abnormalities are **imperforate anus** and **rectal atresia**. An imperforate anus is a condition that exists when there is no opening at the end of the anal canal (Fig. 4-44). Rectal atresia describes the failure of the distal rectum and anus to develop. Both of these abnormalities are causes of obstruction. While visual inspection will diagnose each of these conditions, radiography is performed to determine the extent to which they exist. Also, a complication of

imperforate anus or rectal atresia is a fistula into the genitourinary tract. These fistulas can be detected by contrast studies.

Acquired Pathology

A **cathartic colon** is one that develops after the prolonged (usually greater than 15 years) use of laxatives. The colon proximal to the splenic flexure is usually involved. As the patient becomes dependent on the laxative (because peristalsis is now no longer able to occur), mucosal atrophy and neuromuscular changes take place in the colon. There are likely to be "pseudostrictures," which are smooth tapered areas of narrowing. There is almost total loss of the haustral markings (Fig. 4-45); however, the walls of the colon remain distensible. The lack of rigidity, as well as the

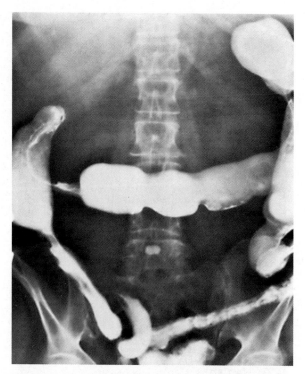

FIGURE 4-45   Bizarre contractions with irregular areas of narrowing primarily involve the right colon. Although the ileocecal valve is gaping, simulating ulcerative colitis, no ulcerations are identified. (Eisenberg RL. *Clinical Imaging: An Atlas of Differential Diagnosis.* 5th ed. Philadelphia, PA: Lippincott Williams & Wilkins; 2010.)

elongation of the colon, serves to differentiate this condition from ulcerative colitis. Because of the loss of haustral markings and the straightening of the colon, the appearance resembles a "stove pipe."

TECH TIP

Because the patient has lost the ability to expel material in the colon under normal circumstances, there will be poor evacuation of barium. This will require a change in technique and also excellent patient education on how to prevent the bowel from becoming blocked due to hardened barium. The patient should be instructed to increase fluid intake considerably and to contact the referring physician if a bowel movement has not occurred within 24 to 48 hours.

Intussusception is the telescoping of a proximal part of the bowel into a distal part because of peristalsis. It causes bowel obstruction and compromises the vascular

supply to the bowel wall. Ninety-five percent of all intussusception cases are *childhood intussusception*, which occurs idiopathically in males between the ages of 6 months and 2 years. The most common site for intussusception in children is near the cecum and ileum. Usually, the ileum spontaneously invaginates into the colon. In many cases, the barium enema reduces the affected parts of the bowel if it does not totally correct the situation. *Adult intussusception* is not common and is usually secondary to some type of mass located within the lumen of the bowel (Fig. 4-46). The presence of a mass is often obscured by the intussusception itself and is not shown until the intussusception is reduced.

Radiographically, the image is normal 50% of the times. With the use of contrast there is a convex filling defect giving the classic appearance of a "coiled spring" (Fig. 4-47), not unlike a Slinky toy, which is caused by barium being caught between the layers of bowel wall encased within the surrounding bowel. Ultrasonography has approximately 100% sensitivity in depicting adult intussusception. CT will show multiple concentric rings in the bowel on adult intussusception.

Classic signs are colicky abdominal pain leading to shock. Many times the condition temporarily corrects itself and the patient recovers and appears to be normal. However, since the self-correction is only temporary, the abdominal pain will continue.

Intussusception must be corrected early, as the portion of the bowel that is encased with the outside portion

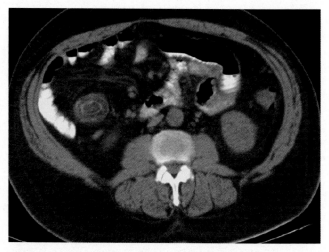

FIGURE 4-46   A 63-year-old man presented with a short history of abdominal pain that he described as similar to his pancreatitis pain. A CT scan demonstrated an ileal carcinoid tumor as lead point for an intussusception into the cecum. (Note the ringed appearance on the patient's mid-right side). (Mulholland MW, Lillemoe KD, Doherty GM, et al. *Greenfield's Surgery Scientific Principles and Practice.* 4th ed. Philadelphia, PA: Lippincott Williams & Wilkins; 2006.)

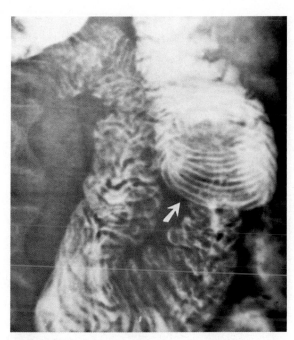

FIGURE 4-47   The *arrow* points to the coiled spring appearance in this intussusception case. (Eisenberg RL. *Clinical Imaging: An Atlas of Differential Diagnosis*. 5th ed. Philadelphia, PA: Lippincott Williams & Wilkins; 2010.)

may become strangulated, at which time gangrene may set in. Barium enemas administered under fluoroscopy are used to reduce the intussusception and are successful 80% of the times. The patient's bowel can be refilled up to three times during one examination before surgery should be considered. Once the invaginated portion is back into its normal position, a postevacuation image is taken along with a 24-hour image as there is recurrence rate (10%) within 48 hours of initial reduction.

A **volvulus** is a more commonly seen condition than intussusception. It generally occurs in the highly mobile sigmoid area and is the twisting of the bowel onto itself, producing an obstruction, which, like intussusception, can lead to gangrene if the blood supply from the vessels is shut off. It can also occur in the cecum and is associated with malrotation and a long mesentery. Volvulus of the cecum has an age peak of 20 to 40 years and occurs more often in males than females. Volvulus of the sigmoid usually occurs more often in the elderly.

The radiograph shows a large amount of air in the sigmoid colon because of the obstruction. The barium enema shows a classic hallmark sign called the "bird of prey" sign. The sign refers to a tapered narrowing at the site of the volvulus caused by twisting of the bowel and narrowing of the lumen which looks like the hook-like beak of a bird (Fig. 4-48).

TECH TIP

The request for the abdominal series must be reviewed to determine the reason for the examination. If the suspected diagnosis is a volvulus or intussusception, the technologist should not palpate the abdomen. The distended abdomen is very tender and extreme pressure could cause rupture on severely dilated bowels.

Inflammatory Processes

Colitis, as its name implies, is an inflammation of the colon. There are several types of colitis that should be recognized as they are indications for diagnostic imaging studies. The following disorders are part of a group of diseases generally known as irritable bowel disorder.

Granulomatous colitis (*Crohn colitis*) is the same process as regional enteritis in the small bowel and is similar to ulcerative colitis in its clinical manifestations. It begins near the terminal ileum, cecum, and ascending colon. Involvement of the rectum is rare. The cause is unknown but psychosomatic causes are believed to be linked to it.

All radiographic appearances described under regional enteritis (cobblestone, string sign, and skipped areas) are encountered in the large bowel (Fig. 4-49A, B). As the disease becomes chronic, the inflexibility of the bowel wall is compared to that of a "lead

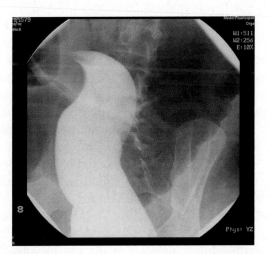

FIGURE 4-48   In this volvulus case, the beak sign can be clearly seen.

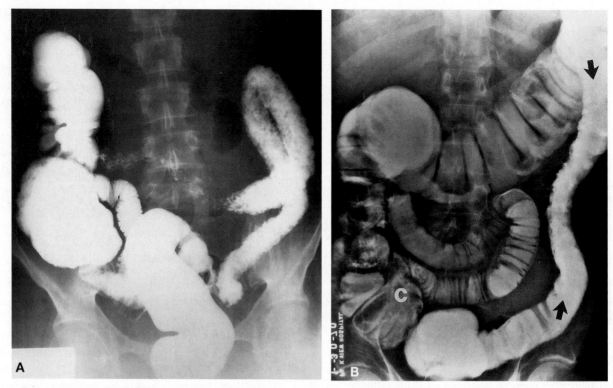

FIGURE 4-49   (A) "Cobblestone" appearance of the colon in a patient with ulcerative colitis. This typical pattern is best appreciated in the splenic flexure. (B) Crohn disease of the colon demonstrating skip lesions. The involved segment of bowel is the descending colon (*arrows*). C, cecum. (A and B: Daffner RH. *Clinical Radiology: The Essentials*. 3rd ed. Philadelphia, PA: Lippincott Williams & Wilkins; 2007.)

pipe." This is not the same as a "stove pipe" in a cathartic colon. In colitis, the colon wall becomes rigid like "lead." Carcinoma of the colon in association with this type of colitis is not often found.

Ulcerative colitis is a mucosal disease that begins in the rectosigmoid region in about 75% of cases and involves the ileum in about 25% of cases. It is first noticed in persons between the ages of 15 and 30 years. Ulcerative colitis is an autoimmune disease and the cause is believed to be linked to stress; however, this has not been proven. It usually starts with a series of attacks of cramping abdominal pain and is characterized by the passage of bloody mucus with stools and a large number of discharges of watery diarrhea almost daily. Toxic megacolon is a complication of ulcerative colitis.

Lesions of ulcerative colitis are located in the mucosa. Unaffected areas of mucosa become edematous and may appear as pseudopolyps. Such findings should not be confused with skipped areas, which are found in granulomatous colitis. The air contrast enema procedure reveals these pseudopolyps as multiple, ring-shaped filling defects. As the disease advances, the ulcerations in the bowel wall heal because of

fibrosis, which causes rigidity of the wall. This causes the appearance of the "lead pipe" as found in granulomatous colitis (Fig. 4-50). In most cases, the disease becomes chronic even though there are periods of remission. Chronic ulcerative colitis causes haustral folds to be irregular and asymmetrical (Fig. 4-50B).

Cancer of the colon is not an automatic consequence of colitis. The risk appears to be confined to those patients who have extensive ulcerative colitis for a period of 10 years or more. The risk of carcinoma is about 10% and increases with each decade of affliction. Again, this is unlike granulomatous colitis, in which the risk of cancer is low.

A final type of colitis that will be discussed is *ischemic colitis*. This usually occurs in patients over the age of 50 years who have a history of cardiovascular disease. It is characterized by abrupt onset of lower abdominal pain and rectal bleeding. The first sign seen radiographically is superficial ulcerations. As the disease progresses, the ulcerations become deeper and pseudopolyps, as seen in ulcerative colitis, are identified. The characteristic "thumbprint" sign is demonstrated (Fig. 4-51). Thumbprinting refers to well-defined indentations along the

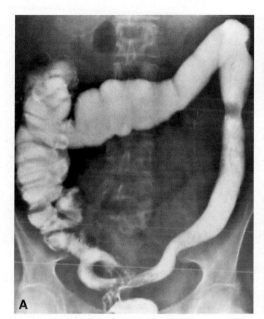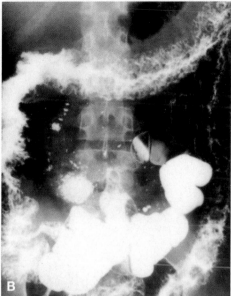

FIGURE 4-50   (A) In this case of chronic Crohn colitis (ulcerative colitis) there is foreshortening and loss of haustral of the descending colon depicting the lead pipe sign. (B) Severe ulcerative colitis: the mucosa appears granular, nodular, and edematous and is actively bleeding. (A: Eisenberg RL. *Clinical Imaging: An Atlas of Differential Diagnosis*. 5th ed. Philadelphia, PA: Lippincott Williams & Wilkins; 2010. B: Swischuk LE. *Emergency Imaging of the Acutely Ill or Injured Child*. 4th ed. Philadelphia, PA: Lippincott Williams & Wilkins, 2000.)

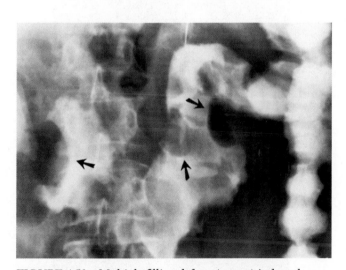

FIGURE 4-51   Multiple filling defects (*arrows*) indent the margins of the transverse and descending portions of the colon in this case of ischemic colitis. These indentations are known as the "thumbprint" sign. (Eisenberg RL. *Clinical Imaging: An Atlas of Differential Diagnosis*. 5th ed. Philadelphia, PA: Lippincott Williams & Wilkins; 2010.)

margins of the bowel wall that appear to have been made by a finger pressing in on it.

Diverticulosis of the large bowel is found in 60% to 70% of the population over 65 years of age, which makes it a common disorder of the bowel. There is evidence that the disease is occurring in younger patients. Patients who experience chronic irritable bowel syndrome (disease) appear to be at risk for diverticulosis.

Diverticula are outpouchings that occur through weakened areas of the bowel wall, especially along sites of vessel insertion in the sigmoid area. Without enough fiber and water in the digestive system, stool becomes hard, forcing the colon to squeeze more to move the harder stools through to the rectum. The extra pressure causes the lining of the colon wall to bulge out into pouches, usually about the size of a large pea. They rarely occur singularly. Rather, they are multiple protuberances found in clusters. These protruding points of mucosa contain fecal matter, which, if they become infected and perforate, may cause a pericolic abscess.

Diverticulitis occurs when the diverticula become infected or inflamed. The cause of these infections is unknown, but it is possible that they begin when fecal matter lodges in the opening of the diverticula. Infection can lead to complications such as swelling or rupturing of the diverticula. Symptoms often include pain, fever, and chills. In severe cases, peritonitis may result.

Radiographically, the diverticula are demonstrated as multiple barium-filled pouches off the outside of

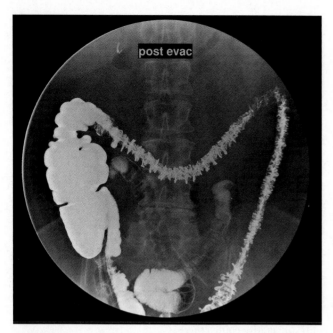

FIGURE 4-52   Multiple diverticula along the bowel wall demonstrate a "sawtooth" appearance.

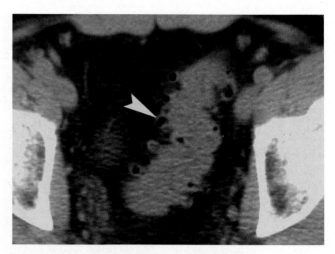

FIGURE 4-53   Diverticulosis. A noncontrast CT scan demonstrates air-filled outpouchings (*arrowhead*) representing diverticula in the sigmoid colon. Note the absence of soft tissue stranding or fluid in the adjacent fat indicating that no inflammation is present. (Brandt WE, Helms C. *Fundamentals of Diagnostic Radiology.* 4th ed. Philadelphia, PA: Lippincott Williams & Wilkins; 2012.)

the bowel wall (Fig. 4-52). The classic radiographic sign of "sawtooth" is best demonstrated on the postevacuation image because of the poor emptying capabilities of the diverticula. CT has replaced the barium enema study for the diagnosis of diverticula in many facilities due to the danger of rupturing a large "tick" and spilling barium and fecal matter into the peritoneal cavity (Fig. 4-53).

Neoplasms

The most frequent benign neoplasms of the gastrointestinal system are **polyps**. Polyps differ from diverticula in that they project into the lumen of the bowel. *Adenomatous polyps* are small, singular, sac-like projections that have a peduncle and rarely are cancerous (Fig. 4-54). However, if more than one polyp is found in a location, it should be suspicious for malignancy. Adenomatous polyps are more common than the villous polyps and the incidence increases with age. *Villous polyps* are usually over 2 cm in size, grow a broad base, and are not pedunculated (Fig. 4-55). About 20% contain cancer cells at the time of diagnosis. The likelihood that a polyp is malignant increases rapidly as the size increases.

Polyps are found in the descending colon and sigmoid and rectal areas. Any polyp that is larger than 2.5 cm or is thought to be a source of bleeding is

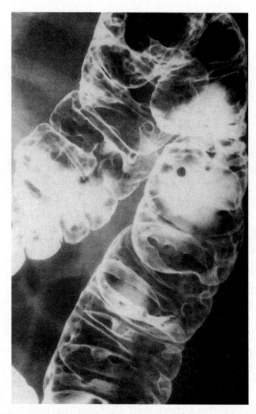

FIGURE 4-54   Small uniform polyps virtually carpet the colon. This patient had familial adenomatous polyposis. (Swischuk LE. *Imaging of the Newborn, Infant and Young Child.* 4th ed. Philadelphia, PA: Lippincott Williams & Wilkins; 1997.)

pattern and are highly suspected to be malignant. Radiographic appearance is not a reliable means of differentiating benign from malignant polyps.

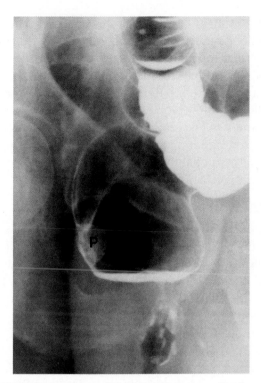

FIGURE 4-55   **Villous polyp (P) in the rectum.** (Daffner RH. *Clinical Radiology: The Essentials*. 3rd ed. Philadelphia, PA: Lippincott Williams & Wilkins; 2007.)

TECH TIP

Overall, the pathologies presented here require no change in technical factors in terms of the disease being an "additive" or "destructive" condition. Since all conditions require a contrast medium to enhance and image the area, the kVp and mAs will remain the same as in normal studies.

surgically removed. The most serious potential complication of the polyp is that it can undergo a degenerative change and become malignant.

Malignant neoplasms are almost exclusively in the form of **adenocarcinomas** (95%). They occur in the rectosigmoid area about 75% of the times. However, in severe cases, they spread to the entire colon. Colon cancer does not metastasize early, but if not diagnosed and treated in the first stages, it will metastasize to the liver and lungs. Colon cancer is the second most common cancer in both men and women. Those with polyps or ulcerative colitis have more of a risk for colon cancer than others.

There are different types of lesions that appear differently on the radiographs. *Annular lesions* slowly surround the bowel and cause gradual narrowing of the lumen and chronic intestinal obstruction. Radiographically, the colon has the unmistakable appearance of a "napkin ring" or an "apple core" (Fig. 4-56). The edges of the lesion tend to overhang and form acute angles with the bowel wall. *Polypoid lesions* project into the lumen as does a benign polyp (Fig. 4-55). Large polypoid colonic masses destroy the mucosal

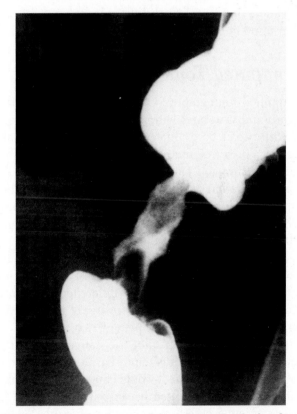

FIGURE 4-56   **Carcinoma of the colon. Note the localized concentric narrowing of the lumen in the sigmoid colon, creating an apple-core deformity.** *Comment:* **Barium enema remains a highly sensitive and specific study for identifying** *colon cancer* **and is frequently used when colonoscopy either fails or cannot be performed.** (Yochum TR, Rowe LJ. *Yochum and Rowe's Essentials of Skeletal Radiology*. 3rd ed. Philadelphia, PA: Lippincott Williams & Wilkins; 2004.)

Imaging Strategies

Ultrasonography

Endoscopic ultrasound is used in the diagnosis of gastrointestinal cancer through the use of an endoscope equipped with the ultrasound sensor and a retractable, hollow needle. The scope is placed into either the rectum or the esophagus and positioned to the suspicious area. The ultrasound transducer is able to show the proximity of any tumors and allow for biopsy of the tissue. The value of this procedure lies in the fact that many patients were undergoing exploratory surgery for pancreatic cancer which were discovered to be inoperable or esophageal cancer which was already terminal. Endoscopic ultrasound spares patients who have end-stage gastrointestinal cancer from the suffering brought by unnecessary surgery. Except abscess detection, there is relatively little role for conventional ultrasound in the evaluation of colonic abnormalities.

Computed Tomography

Computed tomography (CT) uses X-ray to view the organs and structures within the abdomen. Adjacent structures can be evaluated at the same time, making CT a preferred method of examination. CT scans show the stomach fairly clearly and can often confirm the location of stomach cancer and any possible lymph node involvement. It is also possible to perform CT-guided needle biopsy at this time. However, ultrasonography may be superior to CT in this respect.

The use of oral contrast material allows images to be taken without contrast and with contrast in the organs to highlight and create density differences. Contrast is essential to distinguish loops of bowel from a cyst, abscess, or neoplasm. The patient may be asked to drink water to help in imaging the stomach and small bowel. Conventional radiography barium suspension is not used in CT because it would cause artifact streaks. Barium cannot be diluted because it would settle in the system after ingestion and leads to irregular opacification of the bowel. Special contrast agents with a 1% to 3% barium suspension to be used in the gastrointestinal system have been developed exclusively for CT.

The role of CT has become important in colonic diagnosis and even replacing many barium enemas as a diagnostic procedure. It is more sensitive in evaluating diverticulitis than the barium enema. Abscesses are readily identified. CT colonography, also known as virtual colonoscopy, is a much less invasive procedure than visual (optical) colonoscopy. While both procedures need to have the bowel cleaned, the CT study does not require sedation for the insertion of a tube into the patient's colon. CT colonography uses the CT equipment to take multiple slices of the area and then uses a software to reconstruct the images to provide a three-dimensional image.

Magnetic Resonance Imaging

Magnetic resonance imaging (MRI) can provide very clear images of the body. Its advantage over CT is that MRI can provide sectional views of the body in different planes. The drawback to MRI is that it is more expensive than CT and takes longer to perform than other imaging methods do.

If the patient has kidney problems or is allergic to the CT contrast, an MRI procedure will be performed at some point during the evaluation. MRI, like CT, is used to better define something seen on the ultrasound procedure. While most physicians prefer CT scans to look at the stomach for cancer, MRI may sometimes provide some more information. It is used with limited scope in evaluating rectal tumors as a solo study but is used to stage the tumor.

Nuclear Medicine

Radionuclide imaging uses isotopes (a radioactive tracer) that are injected into the patient to image the organs of the gastrointestinal system. The radioactivity is detected by a gamma camera attached to a computer that generates an image. For each particular organ, an isotope that is "tagged" for that particular area is used. As the blood flows through the body, it carries the isotope to the designated organ. When the isotope arrives at its designated area, the gamma camera is positioned over that area which "counts" the radioactivity emitted from that spot. The following are procedures that can be performed by nuclear medicine: gastrointestinal bleeding detection and localization (commonly known as a gastrointestinal bleed); inflammatory bowel disease; ectopic gastric mucosa; gastric emptying half-time determination; gastroesophageal reflux and function; esophageal motility function; salivary glands; pancreatic scans and gallbladder and biliary ductal system; as well as liver scans.

Nuclear medicine is the only imaging modality that is able to determine the emptying rate of the stomach. After the patient eats a standard meal containing radioactive isotope, the patient will be monitored over a period of 1 to 2 hours to determine the time required for the radioactivity to decrease to one-half its original level. Although an UGI study using barium provides a gross indication of whether the stomach is emptying its contents, it does not provide quantification of the amount emptied. In addition, radiation exposure is quite high with the fluoroscopic UGI procedure.

RECAP

Anatomy, Physiology, and Function

- Esophagus
  - Straight tube that acts as passage way from mouth to stomach
- Stomach
  - Hollow organ that prepares food and liquid for digestion
  - Secretes gastric juice comprising pepsinogen, gastrin, and hydrochloric acid
  - Absorbs small amounts of water and alcohol
- Small bowel
  - 18 to 23 feet long
  - Carries out the process of digestion and absorption
  - Sends nutrients to the portal vein to go to liver
- Large bowel
  - Larger in diameter than the small bowel but only 6 to 8 feet long
  - Aids in the regulation of body's water balance by absorbing large amounts of water
  - Bacterial action in large bowel forms vitamins K and D

Pathology

- Esophagus
  - Achalasia
    - Dilated esophagus due to cardiospasm
    - Classic appearance of "rat tail"
  - Peristaltic asynchrony
    - Tertiary contractions
    - Classic appearance of "corkscrew"
  - Foreign bodies
    - May perforate the esophagus
    - Shown with barium swallow (thick or cotton ball in thin barium)

- Hiatal hernia
  - Two types are sliding and rolling (paraesophageal)
  - Sliding is accompanied by classic sign of Schatzki ring
  - Rolling is where stomach is alongside the esophagus (gastroesophageal junction is left intact)
  - Place patient in Trendelenburg and have patient valsalva in order to demonstrate hernia on the radiographic image
- Diverticula
  - Two types are pulsion and traction
  - Pulsion ticks have a narrow neck and rounded head and are more common than traction ticks
    - Types of pulsion ticks include Zenker, epiphrenic, and pharyngeal pouch
    - Pharyngeal pouch occurs at the cricopharyngeal junction and food will go into this pouch
  - Traction ticks have a triangular appearance
- Gastroesophageal reflux disease (GERD)
  - Heartburn and pain are caused by gastric acid that comes up from the stomach that eventually erodes the protective mucosa
  - Identifiable with a water siphonage test
- Varices
  - Dilated tortuous veins in the wall of the lower esophagus
  - Caused by portal hypertension and fibrosis of the liver
  - Two classic signs are "rosary beads" and "worm tracings"
  - Alcohol abuse is the most common cause

- Stomach
  - Pyloric stenosis is narrowing of the lumen of the pylorus
    - Common congenital anomaly occurring more often in males
    - Symptoms include projectile vomit
    - Classic radiographic sign is "string sign" from thin line of barium that is able to be passed through the narrowed pylorus
  - Bezoars are foreign bodies that persist in the stomach
    - Two types are
      - Phytobezoar which is vegetable matter and usually the result of surgical inactivity
      - Trichobezoar is usually found in mentally unstable patients or those with anxiety and is made up of hair, fingernails, and other nonorganic substances
  - Gastritis is most commonly caused by alcohol and is inflammation of the mucosa of the stomach
  - Ulcers are called peptic because they result from gastric juices of which pepsin is one
    - Benign gastric ulcers occur along lesser curvature
    - Heal leaving very little scar
    - Should be suspected for malignancy—especially if in the greater curvature
    - Duodenal ulcers occur in duodenal bulb or near the pylorus
    - Duodenal ulcers produce classic sign of "clover leaf" when healing
    - Complications of ulcers are hemorrhage or stricture leaving an "hourglass" appearance to the body of the stomach
  - Adenocarcinoma are of three types
    - Papillary (fungating) are polypoid masses that occur near the gastroesophageal junction, they are the least malignant of the three types
    - Ulcerating tumors may be confused with benign ulcers and appear most often in the greater curvature
    - Infiltrating tumor (linitis plastica) spreads within the walls of the stomach causing it to become shrunken and rigid (leather bottle stomach)
- Small bowel
  - Meckel diverticulum
    - Found in the ileum
    - Represents the persistence of the yolk sac
    - Difficult to diagnose because of rapid emptying
    - Seen best with nuclear medicine
  - Hernia
    - Occurs in the inguinal area and can cause gangrene if bowel becomes lodged in the opening, shutting off the blood supply to the wall
  - Mechanical small bowel obstruction
    - Seventy-five percent are caused by fibrous adhesions from surgery
    - Little or no gas found in the colon
    - Dilated loops of small bowel
    - Classic radiographic sign on upright image are air-fluid levels seen at varying heights and no air in the outer edges of the image
  - Paralytic ileus (adynamic ileus)
    - Caused by inactivity of the bowel to pass matter and gas, usually seen in postoperative patients
    - Classic sign is "stepladder" that is uniform dilation and no obstruction
  - Regional enteritis (Crohn disease)
    - Idiopathic disease that begins in the teens and 20s
    - Chronic inflammatory disease
    - Confined to the terminal ileum but may involve any part of the small bowel
    - Radiographic signs include "string" sign, "cobblestone," and "skipped areas"
- Large bowel
  - Hirschsprung disease
    - Congenital absence of neurons in the rectum
    - Causes megacolon
    - Eighty percent of the patients are male
  - Cathartic colon
    - Caused by taking too many laxatives for a long time period
    - Mucosal atrophy and loss of haustral marking
    - Wall remains distensible
    - Classic sign is "stove pipe"
  - Intussusception
    - Telescoping of proximal bowel into distal bowel
    - Classic radiographic sign is coiled spring
    - Adult intussusception is due to a mass located within the lumen
    - Childhood intussusception is idiopathic
    - Barium enema is used to diagnose and correct
  - Volvulus
    - Twisting over of the bowel unto itself
    - Can lead to gangrene

- Classic radiographic sign is "bird of prey" sign
- Usually occurs in highly mobile sigmoid area
- More common in elderly
  ○ Colitis inflammation of the colon but there are several types
    - Granulomatous colitis (Crohn colitis) is like regional enteritis but it starts near the terminal ileum
    - Ulcerative colitis begins near the rectosigmoid region
      ○ Risk of colitis becoming cancer is about 10% but increases with every decade of affliction
    - Ischemic colitis occurs in patients older than 50 years who have a history of cardiovascular disease
  ○ Diverticulosis: 60% to 70% of population over the age of 65 years have it
    - Multiple outpouchings in weakened areas of the bowel wall
    - If become inflamed, it is called diverticulitis
    - Cause by a diet low in fiber and high in fat
  ○ Polyps
    - Most common benign neoplasm of entire gastrointestinal system
    - Project into the lumen of the bowel
    - Adenomatous have a narrow neck and protruding round head
      ○ Most are found in the rectosigmoid area
      ○ Benign: usually solitary; malignant: multiple
    - Villous have a broad base and may contain cancer cells
  ○ Adenocarcinoma
    - Occur in the rectosigmoid area about 75% of the time
      - Annular lesion surround the bowel causing the "apple core" or "napkin ring" appearance

- Polypoid lesions look like a benign lesion so X-ray is not a reliable source to diagnose

Imaging Strategies

- Ultrasonography
  ○ Can determine tumors (solid vs. cystic), obstruction, and size and shape of the organ
  ○ Endoscopic ultrasound is used to diagnose stomach cancer and protects patient with end-stage carcinoma from having the pain of surgery
- Computed tomography (CT)
  ○ Best for large bowel
  ○ Can see any abnormal fluid collection
  ○ Can perform CT-guided needle biopsy
  ○ Is replacing barium enemas for diverticulosis
  ○ CT colonography is able to image polyps
- Magnetic resonance imaging
  ○ Advantage over CT is that it provides sectional views in different planes
  ○ Performed if patient is allergic to contrast media or has kidney problems
  ○ Does not provide much better answers than the CT scan
- Nuclear medicine
  ○ Uses isotopes that are monitored by a gamma camera
  ○ Is the only imaging modality that can study the function of the organs
  ○ Has multiple uses in the gastrointestinal system
    - Gastrointestinal bleed
    - Gastric emptying
    - Inflammatory bowel disease
    - Gastric prolapse
    - Gastroesophageal reflux

CLINICAL AND RADIOGRAPHIC CHARACTERISTICS OF COMMON PATHOLOGIES

Pathologic Condition	Age (if Known) Causal Factors	Manifestations	Radiographic Appearance
Achalasia	Esophageal stenosis	Dysphagia Heartburn Regurgitation and weight loss	Dilated proximal esophagus with narrow distal end—rat tail
Peristaltic asynchrony	More often in elderly Tertiary contractions Diffuse esophageal spasm More often in hiatal hernia cases	Severe intermittent pain while swallowing	Corkscrew

(continued)

CLINICAL AND RADIOGRAPHIC CHARACTERISTICS OF COMMON PATHOLOGIES *(continued)*

Pathologic Condition	Age (if Known) Causal Factors	Manifestations	Radiographic Appearance
Hiatal hernia Sliding (99%) Paraesophageal (1%)	Sliding is associated with diverticulosis, reflux esophagitis, or duodenal ulcer Incidence increases with age	Heartburn Dysphagia	Sliding: Schatzki ring
Esophageal diverticula	Pulsion: often associated with hernia; weakened esophageal wall Traction: response to pull from fibrous adhesions	Feeling of something stuck in the throat but usually asymptomatic	Pulsion: stalk with round head Traction: triangular in shape
GERD	Reflux of gastric acid from the stomach into the esophagus	Heartburn and pain	May lead to ulcerations and scarring
Esophageal varices	Portal hypertension	Vomiting with blood	Worm tracing Rosary beads
Esophageal malignancy	Males over females <40 y Excessive smoking and alcohol intake	Dysphagia	Shelving
Pyloric stenosis	Newborn males > females Hypertrophy of pyloric muscle	Projectile vomiting	String sign
Ulcer	Duodenal: females > males Gastric: males > females 30–50 y *H. pylori* bacteria and gastritis	Heartburn Pain May lead to bleeding	Duodenal: clover leaf
Stomach malignancy (primary)	Predisposing factors: pernicious anemia; partial gastrectomy Cause is unknown	Early: asymptomatic Pain after progression	Multiple appearance Leather bottle stomach
MSBO	Fibrous adhesions	Severe abdominal pain	Distended bowel loops proximal to obstruction No gas in large bowel
Paralytic ileus	Decreased bowel activity	Abdominal pain	Distended bowel loops throughout small and large bowel Stepladder sign
Regional enteritis	Teens and 20s Idiopathic	Diarrhea, cramping	String sign Skipped area Cobblestone
Hirschsprung disease	Congenital Males > females Absence of neurons in rectum	Failure to thrive Constipation, abdominal distention	Spastic narrow rectum with dilated proximal bowel Transition zone
Intussusception	Children: idiopathic Adult: mass	Bowel obstruction and pain	Coiled spring sign

(continued)

CLINICAL AND RADIOGRAPHIC CHARACTERISTICS OF COMMON PATHOLOGIES (continued)

Pathologic Condition	Age (if Known) Causal Factors	Manifestations	Radiographic Appearance
Volvulus	Cecum: males > females 20–40 y Sigmoid: <60 y Mobility of bowel	Bowel obstruction and pain	Bird-of-prey sign
Cathartic colon	<50 y Reliance on laxatives	Constipation due to neuromuscular incoordination	Diminished or absent haustrations Stove pipe
Granulomatous colitis (Crohn colitis)	20–30 y Idiopathic	Diarrhea and abdominal pain	String sign Skipped area Cobblestone
Ulcerative colitis	15–30 y Autoimmune	Crampy abdominal pain	Pseudopolyps Lead pipe
Ischemic colitis	<50 y History of cardiovascular disease	Lower abdominal pain Possible rectal bleeding	Thumbprint sign
Colonic diverticula	<60 y but increasingly seen in younger ones Lack of fiber and water in diet Weakened bowel wall	Many asymptomatic Cramping Abdominal pain on left side (left-sided appendicitis)	Multiple out pouchings Sawtooth sign
Polyps	Adenomatous: older ones	Watery diarrhea May cause rectal bleeding	Adenomatous difficult to see.on DCBE due to change in position
Colon cancer	Rectal: 50–70 y Polypoid: incidence increases with age Males > females	May cause rectal bleeding	Annular: apple core or napkin ring Polypoid: board base

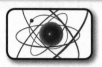 **CRITICAL THINKING DISCUSSION QUESTIONS**

1. List the functions of the small bowel. How do nutrients pass from the small bowel to the liver?

2. Describe the procedure performed to demonstrate radiolucent foreign objects of the esophagus on a radiograph. What complications can occur from foreign objects lodged in the throat?

3. What is the general definition of a hiatal hernia? What are the two types? What is the radiographic sign that is used to distinguish them? What is an intrathoracic stomach and what causes it?

4. Define bezoar. What are the two types and what are they composed of?

5. Compare and contrast gastric and duodenal ulcers. Include where they occur, what happens as they heal, their radiographic appearance (if any), which one is more common, who is more prone to acquiring them, and their predisposition to malignancy.

6. What causes mechanical small bowel obstruction and paralytic ileus? Describe how the radiographic image will appear differently so that processes are readily distinguished.

7. Describe the main difference between the cathartic colon "stove pipe" and the ulcerative colitis "lead pipe."

8. Describe intussusception. How is intussusception different from volvulus? What are the classic radiographic signs of each of these pathologies?

9. What is a Meckel diverticulum? How is it different than other diverticula of the bowel? What modality is best able to demonstrate this diverticulum?

10. How does Hirschsprung disease manifest itself in patients? Why will this manifestation occur? What will the radiographic image show?

11. How does diverticulosis occur? What imaging modality has virtually replaced barium enemas for this disease and why?

12. Describe how endoscopic ultrasonography is able to spare patients with end-stage gastrointestinal cancer from unnecessary surgery.

5

The Hepatobiliary System

● Goals

1. To review the basic anatomy of the liver, gallbladder, and pancreas

   OBJECTIVE: Identify anatomic components of the liver, gallbladder, and pancreas

   OBJECTIVE: Explain the relationship of each of these organs to each other in terms of cross-sectional anatomy

2. To review the basic physiology and function of the liver, gallbladder, and pancreas

   OBJECTIVE: Explain the physiology and function of all organs of the hepatobiliary system

   OBJECTIVE: Describe how each organ functionally affects the others

3. To understand the pathophysiologic and radiographic manifestations of all of the common pathologic conditions of the hepatobiliary system

   OBJECTIVE: Describe the pathology and manifestations of the liver

   OBJECTIVE: Describe the pathology and manifestations of the gallbladder

   OBJECTIVE: Describe the pathology and manifestations of the pancreas

4. To become familiar with how different imaging modalities serve to enhance and complement radiographic diagnosis of common pathologies of the hepatobiliary system

   OBJECTIVE: List and describe the various imaging modalities used in diagnosis of the hepatobiliary system

● Key Terms

Alcoholic liver disease
Ascites
Bile
Cholangitis
Cholecystitis
Cholelithisasis
Cirrhosis
Enzymatic necrosis
Fatty liver
Hemangioma
Hepatic encephalopathy
Hepatitis
Hepatoma
Jaundice
Pancreatitis
Pseudocysts

The gastrointestinal system cannot complete its processes without the accessory organs which are the liver, gallbladder, bile ducts, and pancreas. Together these are known as the hepatobiliary system. There are many interesting pathologies that occur in this area of the body; however, most of the diagnoses are made with the subspecialties of radiography and not by conventional X-rays. Therefore, all technologists should have an understanding of the pathologies and the modalities that will be used to diagnose the disease.

Anatomy

Liver

The largest organ in the body, the liver weighs about 3.5 pounds. It is roughly triangular in shape and is located immediately below the diaphragm in the right upper quadrant, with a portion extending to the left of midline.

The liver is divided into four lobes (Fig. 5-1). The two main lobes are the right and left lobes, which are separated by the falciform ligament. The inferior portion of the falciform ligament has a free border, which contains the ligamentum teres, a remnant of the fetal umbilical vein. Only the main right and left lobes can be identified anteriorly. On the posterior surface of the liver, the right lobe is divided into three segments called the right lobe proper, the caudate lobe, and the quadrate lobe, which bring the total number of lobes in the liver to four. A normal variant of the right lobe can sometimes be seen in women. This variant, known as Reidel lobe, often looks like an additional lobe located in the posterior, inferior aspect of the right lobe.

An important vessel to remember is the portal vein. Seen on the posterior surface of the liver, the portal vein is formed when the splenic vein and the superior mesenteric vein unite. Venous blood from the spleen and the gastrointestinal tract is sent to the liver for processing through this vital vessel.

Gallbladder

The gallbladder is a pear-shaped sac that lies in a shallow fossa on the posterior surface of the right lobe of

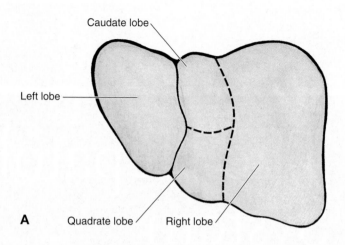

A

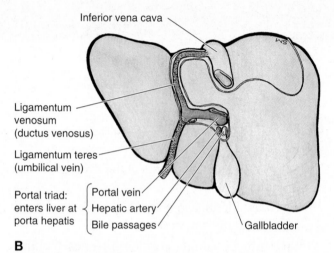

B

FIGURE 5-1 **Anterior and posterior views of the liver and its lobes.** (Moore KL, Dalley AF. *Clinically Oriented Anatomy.* 4th ed. Baltimore, MD: Lippincott Williams & Wilkins; 1999.)

the liver. It consists of three parts: fundus, body, and neck. In the posterior neck of the gallbladder, a small pouch is occasionally found that is known as a Hartmann pouch. This is a prime site for gallstones to collect, as it is the most dependent portion of the gallbladder. The neck merges with the cystic duct.

The wall of the gallbladder has three layers: an outer serous, middle muscular, and an inner mucous layer. The mucosal lining has rugae (folds) that help promote the passage of bile when the gallbladder contracts.

Bile Ducts

The minute bile ducts that are located in the lobules of the liver unite to form larger and larger bile ducts, which eventually form the right and left hepatic ducts that are located in the right and left lobes of the liver. The right and left hepatic ducts converge to form the common hepatic duct. Coming off the neck of the gallbladder is a small duct called the **cystic duct**. The lumen of the cystic duct contains membranous folds called the **spiral valves of Heister**. These valves help prevent the collapse or distention of the cystic duct. The common hepatic duct merges with the cystic duct and forms the common bile duct (CBD). Also known as the choledochus, the CBD descends posterior to the head of the pancreas. It joins the pancreatic duct near the duodenum and becomes the hepatopancreatic ampulla, better known as the **ampulla of Vater**. The hepatopancreatic sphincter, or sphincter of Oddi, is located at the opening of the ampulla into the C-loop of the duodenum.

Pancreas

The pancreas is divided into four areas: head, neck, body, and tail. The head sits in the C-loop of the duodenum. An inferior extension of the head that courses toward the midline is known as the uncinate process. The head constricts slightly to form the neck, and

then widens again to form the body. The body courses from the inferior vena cava toward the left across the midline. Part of the body is posterior to the stomach. The tail sits in the splenic hilum anterior to the left kidney. The entire organ is retroperitoneal.

The pancreas contains several types of cells. Beta cells, acinar cells, and the islets of Langerhans are all important as tumors may arise from these cells.

The main pancreatic duct, also known as the **duct of Wirsung**, runs the entire length of the pancreas. It unites with the CBD after it enters the head of the pancreas. It is at this point that the ampulla of Vater is formed. A minor accessory duct is sometimes found branching off the superior aspect of the duct of Wirsung. This duct is called the **duct of Santorini** and enters the duodenum superior to the ampulla of Vater.

Figure 5-2 is a cross section showing the relation of the pancreas to liver, gallbladder, and stomach in an oblique plane through the long axis of the pancreas.

Figure 5-3 shows the biliary ductal system beginning at the left and right hepatic ducts. The anatomic locations of the ducts within the pancreas are important to remember, as special diagnostic imaging procedures are done specifically for this area.

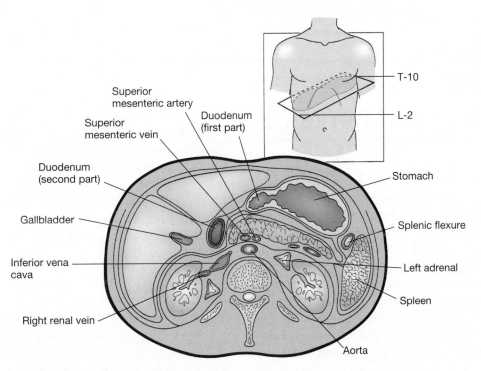

FIGURE 5-2   Cross-sectional relation of the pancreas to other abdominal structures in an oblique plane through the long axis of the pancreas extending from the level of L2 on the right to T10 on the left. (Mackie CR, Moossa AR, ed. *Tumors of the Pancreas.* Baltimore, MD: Williams & Wilkins; 1980.)

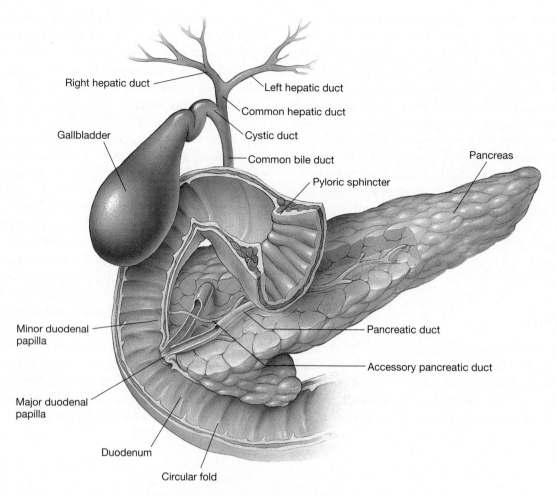

FIGURE 5-3   Pancreas, gallbladder, and duodenum in cross section.

Physiology and Function

Liver

In order to understand how pathology affects the body, the physiology of the liver must be understood, as the liver is one of the most important life-sustaining organs in the body. It is essential in keeping the body functioning properly. It produces bile and bilirubin. **Bile** contains bile salts, fatty acids, cholesterol, bilirubin, and other compounds. The components of bile are synthesized and modified in the liver cells. Bile is then taken to the gallbladder and small bowel through the biliary ducts to aid in the digestion process. Bilirubin is a yellow pigment that comes primarily from old red blood cells. It is taken from the blood, modified to a water-soluble form, and secreted into the bile.

The liver performs biochemical functions as well. Blood clotting factors are secreted from the liver. Albumin, the major protein in the blood, is also synthesized in and secreted from the liver. Many of the body's metabolic functions occur primarily in the liver including the metabolism of cholesterol and the conversion of proteins and fats into glucose. The liver is also where most drugs and toxins, including alcohol, are metabolized.

Gallbladder

The liver produces bile but has no place to store it. Bile is necessary to break down or emulsify fat into smaller fat globules to be digested. Bile passes through the bile ducts into the cystic duct and into the gallbladder where it is concentrated and stored. The liver produces 20 times more bile than the gallbladder can hold. The capillaries in the gallbladder wall extract the large amount of water that is a major component of bile (97%). The remaining 2% mineral salts and fatty acids and 1% bile pigments and salts are what remain to be stored in the gallbladder.

When food, particularly fat, is present in the duodenum, a hormone known as **cholecystokinin** (CCK) is released into the bloodstream. The hormone reaches the gallbladder and causes it to contract. At the same time, the sphincter of Oddi relaxes to allow the bile that is excreted from the gallbladder to flow into the ampulla of Vater and into the duodenum. The elapsed time between eating and gallbladder contraction is about 30 minutes.

Pancreas

The pancreas has both endocrine (ductless) and exocrine (secretion) functions. The endocrine functions include the production of the hormones insulin and glucagon. These are secreted directly into the bloodstream. Insulin exerts a major control over carbohydrate metabolism. Glucagon aids in this control. Two hormones are produced in the islets of Langerhans by two types of cells that comprise the islets: alpha-2 cells that secrete the glucagon, and beta cells that produce insulin.

The exocrine functions include the secretion of enzymes that digest carbohydrates, fat, and proteins. These three enzymes are amylase, lipase, and trypsin respectively, and are produced by the acinar cells of the pancreas. They travel along the main pancreatic duct and empty into the duodenum. Amylase, also called amylopsin, breaks down starch into maltose. Lipase is also known as steapsin. It works on fats to break them down into fatty acids and glycerol. Trypsin, or protease, will break down proteins into peptones and amino acids. Combined with the bile from the liver and gallbladder, these digestive juices further the process of digestion and absorption in the small intestine.

Pathology

Liver

Inflammatory Processes

Alcoholic liver disease is the result of direct toxicity of alcohol to the liver cells. When the alcohol enters the body, 95% of it will be metabolized in the liver. Here, it is turned into acetaldehyde, which is even more toxic to the liver than the original form of alcohol. This causes the entire liver to become inflamed. Long-term drinking causes the inflammation to become persistent and leads to fibrosis and cirrhosis.

Cirrhosis is one of the most common serious diseases. It represents the seventh leading cause of deaths in the United States, killing about 26,000 people each year. It is the third most common cause of deaths in adults 45 through 65 years of age. The term cirrhosis is used when changes occur in the structure of the liver as the result of any one of a number of chronic diseases. Normal tissue is destroyed and replaced by scar tissue, which diminishes the ability of the organ to function properly, hindering the circulation of the blood through the liver and reducing its power to remove toxins from the body.

It occurs twice as often in men than in women and in more than half of all malnourished chronic alcoholics. In Asia and Africa, most deaths from cirrhosis are due to chronic hepatitis B and D. As of 2005, cirrhosis is the leading cause of deaths among HIV-positive patients; with 30% of all HIV-positive patients infected with a hepatitis virus. This disease process may take anywhere from several months to several years to develop.

Cirrhosis is usually the result of alcoholism or hepatitis C (in the United States). Other causes include blocked bile ducts, drugs, toxins and infections, and some inherited diseases (such as a glycogen storage disease or an absorption deficit in which excess iron is deposited in the liver, panaceas, and other organs). Some studies have suggested that obesity should be recognized as a risk factor in nonalcoholic hepatitis and cirrhosis. Alcoholic cirrhosis usually develops after more than a decade of heavy drinking. Alcohol blocks the liver's metabolism of protein, fats, and carbohydrates. It is the end stage of most serious chronic liver diseases.

The liver takes on a characteristic appearance in the early stages of the disease known as a "fatty liver." This appearance is caused by the engorgement of the liver by fat, causing the liver to be enlarged. At this stage, the damage is reversible if the cause is removed. Many people with cirrhosis have no symptoms in the early stages. However, as the fat deposits continue, they interfere with normal function and cell death occurs. Damaged and dead liver cells are replaced by fibrous tissue which leads to fibrosis. Liver cells regenerate in an abnormal pattern primarily forming nodules that are surrounded by fibrous tissue. The patient experiences symptoms of exhaustion, fatigue, loss of appetite, nausea, weakness, weight loss, abdominal pain, and spider angioma on the skin. Hepatitis is triggered by necrosis. The liver and spleen are enlarged (Fig. 5-4A).

The last stage of cirrhosis is characterized by fibrous scars that disrupt the makeup of the liver cells. Scar tissue will pull on the liver parenchyma causing the appearance of a small liver. This interferes with blood flow to and from the liver because of obstruction of the portal vein. Portal hypertension causes ascites, jaundice, and esophageal varices. At this point, the liver is in failure and unable to detoxify ammonia, which can cause the patient to go into hepatic coma and die. In advanced cases, cirrhosis can cause abnormalities in the brain known as **hepatic encephalopathy**. This occurs when toxic metabolites, normally removed from the blood by the liver, reach the brain.

Complications of cirrhosis include edema and ascites (Fig. 5-4B), bruising and bleeding, jaundice, gallstones, portal hypertension, varices, diabetes, and liver cancer. Men may lose their chest hair and suffer from gynecomastia (enlarged breasts) with shrinkage of their testicles. Bleeding and bruising is a complication that technologists must be aware of so that during the course of an imaging procedure the patient is not injured. The liver may no longer be able to produce the proteins needed for blood clotting and a patient can bleed profusely. The ascites fluid in the abdomen often becomes infected causing peritonitis. Abnormalities in other systems such as immune system dysfunction and renal dysfunction and failure can be caused by cirrhosis as well.

Liver damage from cirrhosis cannot be reversed, but treatment can stop or delay further progression of the disease and may prevent complications. Treatment depends on the cause of the disease, as that must be treated first. Once complications have set in, then treatment will include remedies for those. Liver transplants are effective for treating end-stage cirrhosis and especially when encephalopathy, ascites, or bleeding varices are present.

The technologist should look for hepatomegaly, ascites, and air-fluid levels on the abdominal

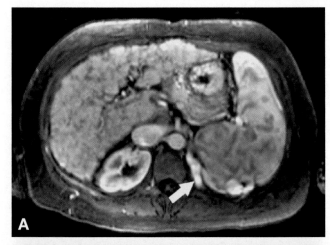
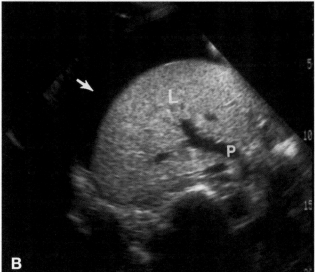

FIGURE 5-4   (A) Cirrhosis with regenerative nodules. Axial fat-suppressed, gadolinium-enhanced gradient echo image shows multiple small regenerative nodules throughout the liver associated with splenomegaly and varices (*arrow*). (B) Transverse scan shows a small, contracted liver (L) with increased echogenicity surrounded by ascitic fluid (*arrow*). P, portal vein. (A: Leyendecker JR, Brown JJ. *Practical Guide to Abdominal and Pelvic MRI*. Philadelphia, PA: Lippincott Williams & Wilkins; 2004; B: Eisenberg RL. *An Atlas of Differential Diagnosis*. 4th ed. Philadelphia, PA: Lippincott Williams & Wilkins; 2003.)

images. Ascites and edema are the most problematic for the radiographer as the increase in fluid in the abdomen requires an increase in kVp to penetrate and provide a quality image. Cirrhosis is considered an additive pathology process. The radiographer must be adept at understanding penetration and contrast of an image to avoid repeat radiographs.

TECH TIP

Supine radiographs of the abdomen will require an increase in kVp; but not as much as an upright image requires. In the supine position, the fluid and abdominal contents spread out to the sides; whereas in the upright position, the fluid falls to the most dependent portion allowed in the abdomen, concentrating the girth in the mid to lower sections of the abdomen. Usually, two images are taken crosswise (one high and one low). The lower image will usually require the maximum increase in kVp.

TECH TIP

It is easily discovered if the patient has ascites. If the abdomen is enlarged and does not "spread out" when in the supine position, the cause of girth is likely fluid. The technologist can gently push on the abdomen. Fluid in the abdomen will cause a tightness and inability to push the skin in very deeply. Also, the skin will blanche for a moment. If these are symptoms present, the probable cause is ascites and the technologist should increase the kVp to penetrate the fluid.

Case Study

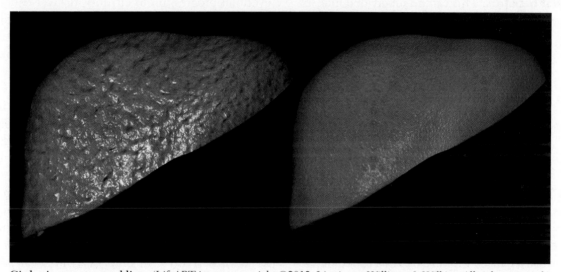

Cirrhosis versus normal liver. (LifeART image, copyright ©2013. Lippincott Williams & Wilkins. All rights reserved.)

As can be seen in these pictures, the normal liver on the right looks vastly different than the liver that is afflicted by cirrhosis. Notice the smaller overall size of the liver (compare the depth).

Also, the fibrotic scarring is easily seen as the lumpy surface. The parenchyma on the interior is being pulled and shrunken causing the bumpy appearance.

Fatty liver is not just caused by alcohol abuse. In fact, the most common cause is obesity. These fatty infiltrations form "masses" most commonly on the anterior and lateral aspect of the falciform ligament. The fat "tumors" are interspersed with normal liver tissue.

There is a rapid change in the liver with these lesions; appearance of lesions to complete resolution can occur within as few as 6 days. Sonography and computed tomography (CT) are best to make the diagnosis. In sonography, fat increases the echogenicity of the liver.

The intrahepatic vessel borders are not as bright and echo as on a normal liver or may not even be present. The same criteria is true for CT, where the vessel borders are indistinct and the liver is hypodense (normal liver on CT is hyperdense).

Hepatitis signifies inflammation of the liver cells. The cells die and are quickly replaced by new ones if the injury to the liver is slight. Cirrhosis results when the injury is more severe. Signs and symptoms of hepatitis include jaundice, fatigue, abdominal pain, loss of appetite, nausea, and vomiting. There are three types of hepatitis, any of which may result in cirrhosis:

1. **Deficiency hepatitis**: Chronic alcoholism is generally associated with malnutrition, or a deficient diet, which causes the liver to suffer damage.
2. **Toxic hepatitis**: One of the functions of the liver is to detoxify poisons that enter the system. However, certain drugs, taken illicitly or for medical purposes, can result in necrosis of the liver.
3. **Viral hepatitis**: This can be subdivided into six groups:
   a. Hepatitis A (formally known as infectious hepatitis)
   b. Hepatitis B (previously called serum hepatitis)
   c. Hepatitis C (previously known as non-A and non-B)
   d. Hepatitis D (sometimes referred to as delta hepatitis)
   e. Hepatitis E
   f. Hepatitis G

There is a seventh type of viral hepatitis known as hepatitis F, but it is only suspected and has not been confirmed.

Hepatitis A, caused by an RNA virus called hepatitis A virus (HAV), is the most benign form of viral hepatitis. The illness can lasts from 1 to 2 weeks to several months. It is rarely fatal and does not lead to chronic hepatitis, but convalescence is often prolonged. The virus is spread by fecal contamination through food handlers, shellfish harvested from contaminated waters, and contaminated produce such as lettuce and strawberries. Contaminated drinking sources or contaminated dishes from which food is eaten can spread the disease quickly. Adults will suffer with abrupt fever, malaise, anorexia, nausea, and abdominal discomfort followed by jaundice more than children will. No specific treatment other than rehydration is effective.

About 15% of the patients will experience symptoms for up to a year. Patients who have had hepatitis A cannot be reinfected with the same disease.

In contrast, *hepatitis B* is much more serious. Caused by a DNA virus known as HBV, that is found in all body fluids of an infected individual, it is transmitted from one human to another indirectly by use of contaminated syringes and needles for such things as tattooing, ear piercing, or intravenous injections. Hepatitis B is a major health problem in that 1 in every 1,000 individuals is a carrier. The hepatitis B vaccine is the best protection against the disease. Patients who do not get vaccinated run a risk of having chronic infections. Age is also a factor in chronic infections. The younger the patient is that has hepatitis, the higher the chance of infection being chronic. Chronic persistent hepatitis B is a mild illness that occurs when the first vaccination did not fully cure the disease. It causes no permanent liver damage and the patient can expect to eventually recover if revaccinated. Chronic active hepatitis causes the liver to undergo fibrosis and eventual progression to cirrhosis or liver cancer. This is the most severe form of hepatitis B, as it kills most liver cells and is eventually fatal in 15% to 20% of the patients. It is estimated that 1.25 million people in the United States are chronically infected with the HBV.

Hepatitis C is also caused by a virus, the HCV, and it spreads in the same fashion as hepatitis B. Most posttransfusion hepatitis is in the form of hepatitis C, particularly if the transfusion was prior to 1992. Unfortunately, hepatitis C has up to an 85% probability of becoming chronic active hepatitis. Of those chronically infected, approximately 70% will suffer from liver disease leading to cirrhosis in which 5% will die. Hepatitis C is the leading indicator for a liver transplant.

A rare cause of hepatitis is a delta agent or hepatitis D virus (HDV). In order to contract *hepatitis D*, the patient must already be infected with hepatitis B. Transmission of the HDV is through blood or body fluids. Another form of hepatitis not yet found in the United States (except in rare instances) is *hepatitis E*. It is most frequently seen in India, South Central Asia, and the Middle East. It was recently diagnosed in Mexico. The virus (HEV) is transmitted by eating food or drinking water that has been contaminated by feces of infected individuals or animals. Also there is no proven therapy or prevention for hepatitis E, it does not become chronic and the patient can fully recover.

Hepatitis G is a newly discovered form of liver inflammation caused by hepatitis G virus (HGV). HGV was first described early in 1996 and little is known about the frequency of the infection, the nature of the illness, or how to prevent it. People at risk are those with hemophilia or other bleeding disorders, people with kidney disease on hemodialysis, and those intravenous drug users. Sexual transmission is also a possibility. As of now, only costly DNA tests are able to make the diagnosis. These tests are not widely available. Since hepatitis G is blood-borne disease, prevention relies on avoiding possible contact with contaminated blood.

Hepatitis shows hepatomegaly and possible jaundice. The alert radiographer is able to identify an enlarged liver shadow on the abdominal radiograph. The radiograph may require an increase in mAs to increase the density of the image. Increasing the kVp will decrease the contrast and cause a gray image to be produced. If the liver is enlarged due to hepatitis, the image will be somewhat gray. Increasing kVp will only add to this. Technologists must be careful to be mindful of universal precautions so as not to become infected with the hepatitis B or C virus. Practicing good medical aseptic technique will alleviate this concern.

Jaundice denotes a yellowish cast to the skin and sclera of the eyes that is the result of excess bilirubin in the blood. It is not a disease itself, but is the result of another problem that causes the excess bilirubin. There are several ways in which bilirubin can excessively accumulate in the blood and thereby giving rise to jaundice:

1. **Medical jaundice** (non-obstructive): There are two forms of jaundice that fall under this category. *Hemolytic* jaundice occurs if an excessive amount of red blood cells are broken down, causing more bilirubin to be formed than can be excreted by the liver. The excess remains in the blood. *Hepatic* jaundice occurs when the liver is extensively diseased so that it is unable to excrete the normal amount of bilirubin, causing an accumulation in the blood.
2. **Surgical jaundice** (obstructive): The liver cannot excrete the normal amount of bile because of an obstruction, usually a gallstone. The bile is unable to drain into the duodenum. Under these conditions, bile backs up in the liver and is reabsorbed in the blood.

Patients who are jaundiced will usually undergo sonography to determine if the cause is from an obstruction.

An invasive procedure, endoscopic retrograde cholangiopancreatography (ERCP), may also be done if it is thought that the obstruction can be removed. The endoscopy also provides the physician the opportunity to place a stent in the patient.

Neoplasms

Hemangiomas are the most common benign hepatic neoplasms. They can occur at any age and are slightly more common in women than in men. The lesions are well seen on ultrasound as small, highly echogenic, well-circumscribed areas. They are usually single as seen in Figure 5-5.

Hepatomas are any tumor of the liver, but most often refer to malignant tumors of the liver originating in the parenchymal cells. Primary carcinoma of the liver presents as a massive, nodular, or diffuse appearance of the parenchyma (Fig. 5-6). The right lobe is more often affected in the massive and nodular types of hepatomas. The incidence of hepatomas is on the rise; currently they are seen in 20% of cases of cirrhosis. This highly vascular neoplasm is best demonstrated by CT and angiography. Clinically, there is an enlarging abdominal mass, pain in the right upper quadrant, and ascites. The changes in liver function result in an elevation of serum alkaline phosphate levels. Hepatomas have a high mortality rate.

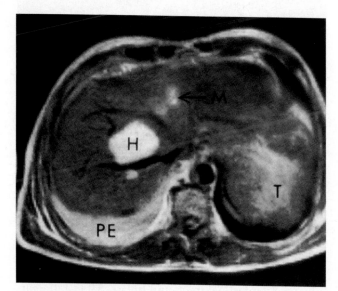

FIGURE 5-5   Hemangioma (H) of the liver as seen in this cross section of the abdomen. (Coexistant metastatic lesion (M), pleural effusion (PE), left renal tumor (T)). (Daffner RH. *Clinical Radiology: The Essentials.* 3rd ed. Philadelphia, PA: Lippincott Williams & Wilkins; 2007.)

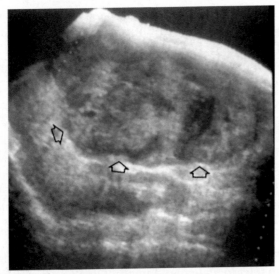

FIGURE 5-6   Complex mass (*arrows*) with a large echogenic component indicating a hepatoma. (Eisenberg RL. *Clinical Imaging: An Atlas of Differential Diagnosis.* 5th ed. Philadelphia, PA: Lippincott Williams & Wilkins; 2010.)

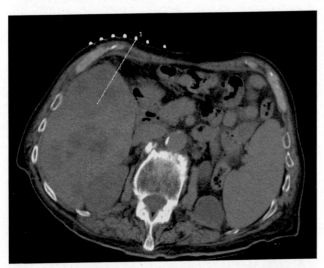

FIGURE 5-7   Computed tomography (CT)–guided biopsy of liver metastasis. Preliminary CT image used to calculate direction and depth of puncture. Notice the multiple metastatic lesions in the liver. (Daffner RH. *Clinical Radiology: The Essentials.* 3rd ed. Philadelphia, PA: Lippincott Williams & Wilkins; 2007.)

Metastatic carcinomas of the liver (Fig. 5-7) are far more common than the primary tumors. These tumors arise, as a rule from primary sources in the lung, gastrointestinal tract, and breast. Metastatic carcinoma usually involves both lobes of the liver, which becomes enlarged and easily palpable. Ultrasonography, CT, and angiography all can be used to make the diagnosis.

Gallbladder

Congenital Anomalies

Congenital anomalies should be considered under pathology, even though they may not cause damage or are rare. Duplication of the gallbladder is rare (Fig. 5-8), whereas a more common anomaly occurs with a variation in the shape of the gallbladder. A gallbladder with an internal septum dividing it into two chambers is called a bilobed gallbladder. Another shape deviation occurs when the body is narrowed in the middle, creating an hourglass gallbladder. The most common anomaly of the gallbladder occurs when the fundus folds over the body creating a "cap"-like appearance known as a Phrygian cap (Fig. 5-9).

Inflammatory Processes

Cholangitis is inflammation of the bile ducts. It is most often associated with gallstones of the CBD. This inflammatory process may spread into the intrahepatic biliary system, causing an abscess. **Cholecystitis** is inflammation of the gallbladder and is characterized by intermittent attacks of severe pain and belching. **Acute cholecystitis** should be suspected when the

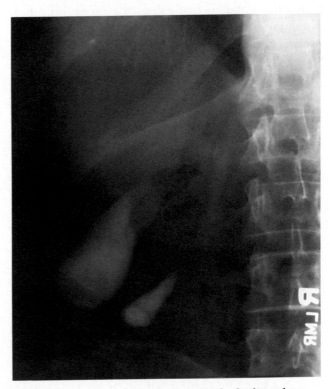

FIGURE 5-8   This congenital anomaly of a duplicated gallbladder can be seen on this image with contrast medium.

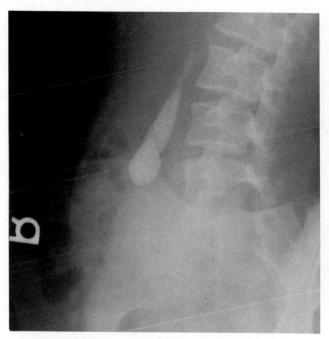

FIGURE 5-9   This image was taken after the patient ate in order to contract the gallbladder. The "Phrygian cap" can be seen at the fundus of the gallbladder.

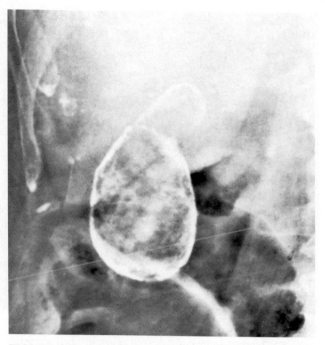

FIGURE 5-10   The white opacity around the gallbladder is the calcified walls of a porcelain gallbladder. (Eisenberg RL. *Clinical Imaging: An Atlas of Differential Diagnosis*. 5th ed. Philadelphia, PA: Lippincott Williams & Wilkins; 2010.)

gallbladder is not visualized with any type of imaging modality. A cystic duct obstruction is almost universally the cause. The patient experiences a very sharp, painful attack in the right upper quadrant, usually after eating a large fatty meal. This pain is accompanied by fever, nausea, and vomiting. *Chronic cholecystitis* is more common than acute cholecystitis, with the vast majority of patients having gallstones. Symptoms of chronic cholecystitis are vague but include intolerance to fatty food, belching, and pain after eating. As a result of chronic cholecystitis, the gallbladder wall may completely calcify becoming what is termed a *porcelain gallbladder* (Fig. 5-10).

Cholelithiasis (gallstones) is reported to afflict a large number of the adult population in the United States. Although anyone in the general population can develop gallstones, there are several groups who are at a higher risk. Those people who appear to be more prone to gallstones are women who are over 40 years of age and overweight. Also, pregnant women or women on oral contraceptives or estrogen therapy are more prone to develop stones. Any person who has lost a large amount of weight due to crash dieting is also susceptible. Native Americans and Hispanics are at a higher risk than others to develop cholelithiasis.

Gallstones are composed of constituents of bile (cholesterol) that have crystallized. Some are pure cholesterol, while others are pure bile pigment. These are radiolucent stones (Fig. 5-11). Other stones contain calcium carbonate and are radiopaque (Fig. 5-12). Of course a combination of any two or all three of these substances may comprise a stone (Fig. 5-13); however, radiolucent stones are the most common. About 80% of all stones are of mixed combinations of cholesterol, bile pigments, and small amounts of calcium. Only 10% of patients have enough calcium in their stones to make the stones radiopaque. Stones may not be readily visible during imaging so it is important to obtain multiple images in various positions. Regular X-ray has been replaced by better techniques such as ultrasound (Fig. 5-14) and CT scans. ERCP can not only find the stones but also remove them.

Although no cause is known for sure, it is believed that stones are associated with the inability of the gallbladder to absorb properly. In 90% of patients with gallstones, there is more cholesterol in the bile and a lower amount of chenodeoxycholic acid than normal. Ursodiol is a naturally occurring bile acid that lowers cholesterol levels in bile and slowly dissolves stones within 6 to 24 months, depending on the size of the

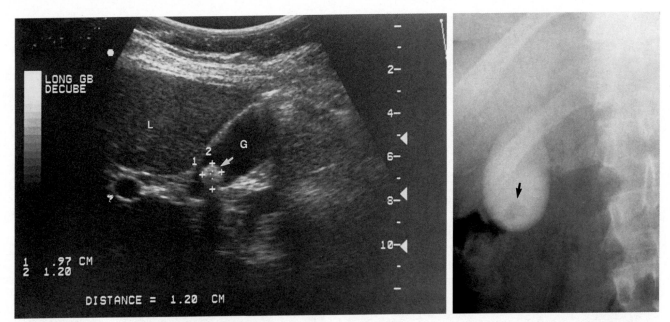

FIGURE 5-11   Radiolucent gallstone. The left image is a sonographic image demonstrating the classic appearance of a stone (*arrow*) with nontransmission of sound below it. The right image shows the gallbladder after oral cholecystography (OCG) demonstrating a filling defect (*arrow*) which is a single radiolucent gallstone. (Daffner RH. *Clinical Radiology: The Essentials.* 3rd ed. Philadelphia, PA: Lippincott Williams & Wilkins; 2007.)

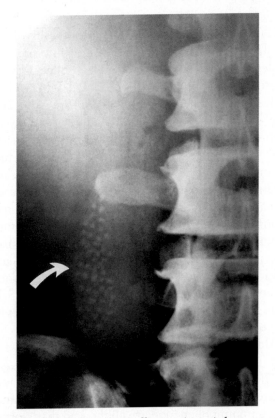

FIGURE 5-12   Radiopaque gallstones (*arrow*) demonstrated on a KUB. (Daffner RH. *Clinical Radiology: The Essentials.* 3rd ed. Philadelphia, PA: Lippincott Williams & Wilkins; 2007.)

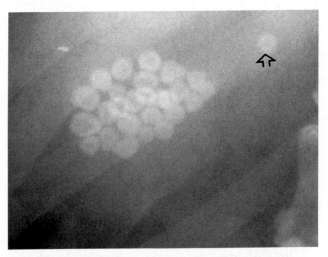

FIGURE 5-13   Gallstones that contain both calcium and bile. The thick opaque borders surround the radiolucent centers. The *arrowhead* is pointing to a stone in the cystic duct. (Daffner RH. *Clinical Radiology: The Essentials.* 3rd ed. Philadelphia, PA: Lippincott Williams & Wilkins; 2007.)

stone. Chenodiol is another medication that is used to dissolve stones and may be used in conjunction with ursodiol. Large stones may be crushed using intracorporeal electrohydraulic lithotripsy. In this procedure, a catheter wire is placed next to the stone to transmit a crushing force.

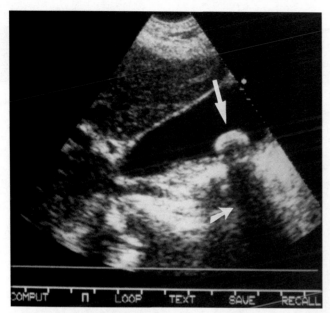

FIGURE 5-14   There is a hyperechoic stone (*large arrow*) in the dependent portion of the gallbladder, with a posterior shadow (*small arrow*). (Harwood-Nuss A, Wolfson AB, Lyndon CH, et al. *The Clinical Practice of Emergency Medicine.* 3rd ed. Philadelphia, PA: Lippincott Williams & Wilkins; 2001.)

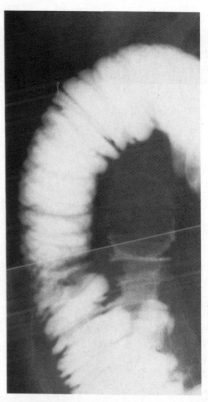

FIGURE 5-15   There is a fistula between the small bowel and the bile ducts. A large stone can be seen to have eroded through the bowel wall.

Most gallstones do not cause symptoms for a long time. If the stones remain in the gallbladder, they may never cause symptoms. If the gallstones cause a blockage in a bile duct, pain may occur intermittently. Complications of gallstones are rare; however, a large gallstone can erode through the wall of the bowel creating a fistula between the gallbladder and bowel (Fig. 5-15).

Neoplasms

Carcinoma of the gallbladder is the most common tumor of the biliary area even though it is a rare manifestation overall. It occurs more often in elderly women. An association with gallstones is believed to be a factor because of the chronic irritation from the stones and any ensuing infection. If the tumor is in the fundus of the gallbladder, it will frequently invade the liver and peritoneum (Fig. 5-16). Carcinomas found in the body and neck of the gallbladder often infiltrate the hepatic and biliary ducts, thus involving not only the liver but also the pancreas and the duodenum. Jaundice is associated as a late development of carcinoma that has spread to the ducts.

Pancreas
Congenital Processes

Cystic fibrosis is not solely related to the lungs. There is cystic fibrosis of the gastrointestinal tract and of the pancreas as well. Like the lungs, cystic fibrosis of the pancreas is an inherited autosomal disorder. The pancreatic ducts fill with thick mucus, which leads to dilation of the ducts and fibrosis of the pancreas. There is increased pancreatic lobulation, replacement of normal tissue by fat. The fibrosis will eventually lead to atrophy of the organ. Because the pancreas plays a vital role in digestion, malabsorption and weight loss are associated with cystic fibrosis of the pancreas. Pancreatic deficiencies eventually lead to death of the child.

Inflammatory Processes

Pancreatitis is inflammation of the pancreas and occurs when the enzymes released by the pancreas attack the organ itself instead of food. It can either be acute or chronic (as described in Chapter 1). *Acute pancreatitis* (Fig. 5-17) occurs suddenly causing the

Case Study

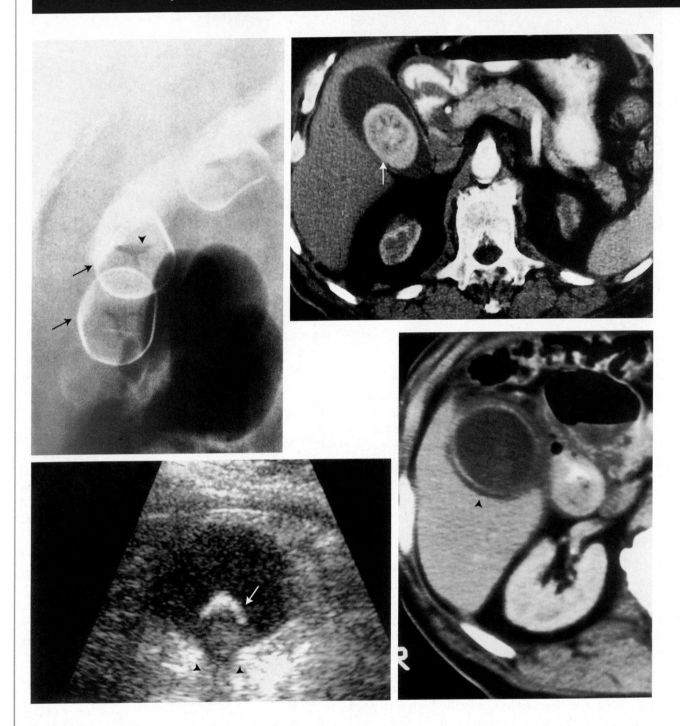

These four images show three different modalities that will demonstrate cholecystitis and cholelithiasis. (A) Collimated area of the right upper quadrant shows thin circular calcifications in the right upper quadrant of the abdomen, which are characteristic of multiple gallstones (*arrows*). There is a distinctive triadiate radiolucency representing gas in fissures within the sone (Mercedes Benz sign) (*arrowhead*) body (*arrowheads*) of the gallbladder. (C) Ultrasound is the most commonly used method for the detection of cholelithiasis, cholecystitis and biliary obstruction. Here, the arrow points to a density within the gallbladder with enhancement on either side below it. (*arrowheads*). (D) CT, axial abdomen: Note the low-density crescent of pericholecystic edema surround the gallbladder (GB) wall (*arrowhead*), a sign of cholecystits. (Yochum TR, Rowe LJ. *Yochum and Rowe's Essentials of Skeletal Radiology*, 3rd Ed. Philadelphia, PA: Lippincott Williams & Wilkins; 2004.)

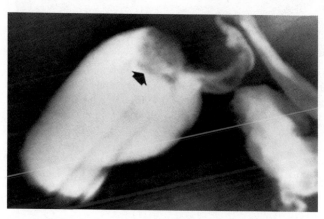

FIGURE 5-16 Carcinoma of the gallbladder. Irregular mural mass with tumor growth extending into the cystic duct (*arrow*). (Eisenberg RL. *Clinical Imaging: An Atlas of Differential Diagnosis*. 5th ed. Philadelphia, PA: Lippincott Williams & Wilkins; 2010.)

binge drinking, infections (such as viral hepatitis), and chemicals in the digestive tract. The symptoms include nausea and vomiting, fever, abrupt epigastric pain, and an increase in amylase and white blood cell count. A pseudocyst may be associated with acute pancreatitis (Fig. 5-18).

Chronic pancreatitis is a relapsing pancreatitis that causes progressive fibrosis and destruction of pancreatic cells. This is a permanent inflammation of the pancreas that, over time, will damage as much as 90% of the organ. The production of digestive enzymes and hormones is now impacted resulting in diarrhea and poor absorption of nutrients. This in turn can lead to diabetes. The pancreas increases in size. Late stages cause calcifications to form in the ductal system (Fig. 5-19). Most cases of chronic pancreatitis are due

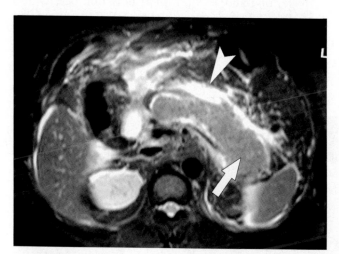

FIGURE 5-17 Acute pancreatitis. Fat-suppressed T2-weighted image demonstrates enlargement and edema of pancreatic body and tail (*arrow*) with peripancreatic fluid (*arrowhead*). (Leyendecker JR, Brown JJ. *Practical Guide to Abdominal and Pelvic MRI*. Philadelphia, PA: Lippincott Williams & Wilkins; 2004.)

pancreas to become enlarged and releasing enzymes into the duodenum. The exact cause is unknown but triggers include gallstones, blocked bile ducts, trauma,

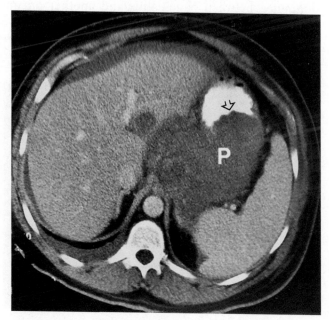

FIGURE 5-18 Pancreatic pseudocysts. CT image shows a large pseudocyst (P) compressing the posterior gastric wall (*arrow*). (Daffner RH. *Clinical Radiology: The Essentials*. 3rd ed. Philadelphia, PA: Lippincott Williams & Wilkins; 2007.)

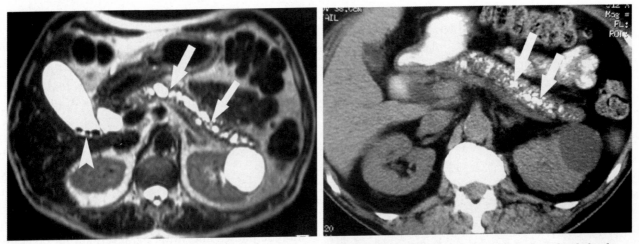

FIGURE 5-19   Chronic pancreatitis. (A) Heavily T2-weighted axial HASTE image through pancreatic body and tail clearly demonstrates parenchymal atrophy and dilated pancreatic duct (*arrows*) with multiple strictures. Note gallstones (*arrowhead*). (B) Noncontrast CT scan in same patient as (A) more clearly demonstrates pancreatic calcifications (*arrows*), but pancreatic duct is poorly seen. (Leyendecker JR, Brown JJ. *Practical Guide to Abdominal and Pelvic MRI*. Philadelphia, PA: Lippincott Williams & Wilkins; 2004.)

to a long history of alcoholism. Blockages from gallstones (rare), surgical scarring, tumors, or an abnormality in the pancreatic duct are responsible for the remaining cases.

Only 20% of people show radiographic sign of pancreatitis, which are a displaced stomach and effacement of bowel loops. CT scans will show swelling of the pancreas and any fluid in the abdomen. The difference between pancreatitis and another organ inflammation is that the powerful digestive enzymes secreted by the acinar cells may escape from the cells and start to digest the pancreas itself as well as the adipose tissue around it. This process is called *enzymatic necrosis*.

Pseudocysts are the most common cysts of the pancreas. These usually result from inflammation, but they have been known to develop following necrosis, hemorrhage, or trauma. Most often only one occurs at a time. Pseudocysts are identifiable on CT (see Fig. 5-18) and MRI (Fig. 5-20) scans. Pseudocysts are commonly found in the subhepatic region. They contain enzymes and are capable of dissecting tissue, which allow them

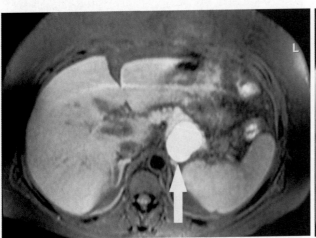
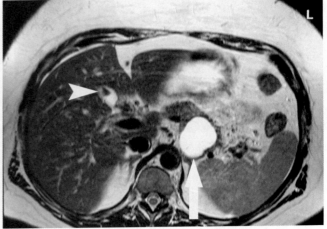

FIGURE 5-20   (A) Fat-suppressed, noncontrast-enhanced T1-weighted image shows high signal intensity collection (*arrow*) near tail of pancreas consistent with fluid containing blood products. (B) Respiratory triggered T2-weighted image shows collection (*arrow*) to be of very high signal intensity. Note gallstone (*arrowhead*). Hemorrhagic pseudocyst found at surgery. (Leyendecker JR, Brown JJ. *Practical Guide to Abdominal and Pelvic MRI*. Philadelphia, PA: Lippincott Williams & Wilkins; 2004.)

to travel anywhere in the body. Approximately 20% regress spontaneously and the remaining 80% are drained or left alone until they become so large that they begin to displace other organs.

> ## TECH TIP
>
> A careful review of the radiology request is always warranted. If the patient is determined to have acute pancreatitis, this is additive and the technical factors for a KUB may need to be increased due to an edematous pancreas. If there is a history of chronic pancreatitis, atrophy is likely which is destructive. The kVp should be reduced. This is also indicated so as not to overpenetrate the possible calcium that may be present with this process.

Neoplasms

Benign neoplasms of the pancreas are called islet cell tumors or adenomas. These occur in the beta cells and therefore contain high levels of insulin.

Carcinoma of the pancreas is not common; however, it ranks high among fatalities from malignancies in the United States. It was estimated to have killed approximately 29,000 Americans in 2001. It is rare before the age of 40 years and is more prevalent in men. **Adenocarcinoma** is the most common cancer; 99% of them arise from the ductal system (exocrine) and 1% from the acinar cells (endocrine). The head of the pancreas is involved in 75% of all cases of carcinoma.

Cancer of the head of the pancreas is an infiltrative process and frequently occludes the CBD, causing jaundice (Fig. 5-21). As bile backs up through the ductal system, the gallbladder can become massively distended. Causes of cancer are unknown but smoking seems to be the major cause that is preventable. Patients with chronic pancreatitis appear to be at a greater risk for cancer. Pancreatic carcinoma metastasizes to the liver in over 80% of the cases.

Pancreatic cancer often has a poor prognosis, even when diagnosed early. Pancreatic cancer typically spreads rapidly and is seldom detected in its early stages, which is a major reason why it is a leading cause of cancer deaths. Signs and symptoms may not appear until pancreatic cancer is quite advanced and surgical removal is not possible. Because of this, pancreatic cancer is considered a destructive process.

Imaging Strategies

Many of the images seen during the discussion of the gallbladder were performed with radiographic procedures that are no longer done now. Oral cholecystography

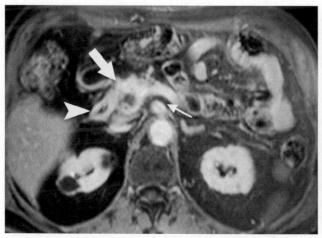
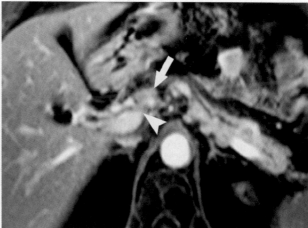

FIGURE 5-21 Ductal adenocarcinoma of pancreas deemed unresectable at surgery. (A) Fat-suppressed, gadolinium-enhanced T1-weighted gradient echo image of abdomen demonstrates enhancing pancreatic head mass (*thick arrow*). Note intact fat plane (*thin arrow*) around superior mesenteric artery. *Arrowhead* denotes duodenum. (B) Image of slightly higher resolution than (A) shows tumor (*arrow*) surrounding hepatic artery and involving anterior surface of portal vein (*arrowhead*). Findings were confirmed at surgery. (Leyendecker JR, Brown JJ. *Practical Guide to Abdominal and Pelvic MRI.* Philadelphia, PA: Lippincott Williams & Wilkins; 2004.)

(OCG) was one procedure in particular that was helpful in diagnosing gallstones. Because the images demonstrated the pathology so well, the decision was made to include them in this chapter in addition to the current methods of imaging described below.

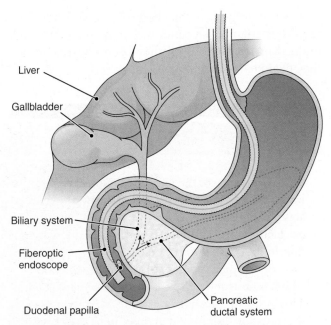

FIGURE 5-22   The course of the endoscope and fiberoptic tube in an ERCP. (Cohen BJ. *Medical Terminology*, 4th ed. Philadelphia Lippincott Williams & Wilkins 2003.)

Endoscopy

A common procedure used to visualize the CBD is endoscopic retrograde cholangiopancreatography (ERCP). This procedure is used to help locate and treat blockages in the duct, find the source of pain, and aid in the planning stages of surgery. In addition, pancreatic pathology can be located during this procedure. ERCP is more accurate than CT in diagnosing pancreatic cancer and is also highly accurate at diagnosing more rare pathology such as a choledochocele (which presents as repeated attacks of acute pancreatitis and jaundice).

The procedure normally takes anywhere from 30 to 90 minutes. The patient is placed in the supine oblique position and the throat is numbed. An endoscope is then placed into the mouth, through the upper digestive tract to the sphincter of Oddi (Fig. 5-22). Here a small cut (papillotomy) may be made in order to remove stones. As stones and other blockages are located and removed, contrast medium is injected and radiographs are taken. If stones are found in the duct, a small catheter is fed above the stone and a balloon is inflated. Retracting the catheter with the balloon inflated will gently pull the stone out of the duct and into the duodenum. Passing through the digestive tract, the stone is able to leave the body in the fecal matter.

Even though the procedure is done in the radiology department, the actual procedure is performed by a gastroenterologist aided by nurses from the floor and/or the department. The radiographer must be present to aid in the use of fluoroscopy. A radiologist may also be present but may only come in when the gastroenterologist has questions. Figure 5-23A and B demonstrates how the ERCP can identify the hepatobiliary anatomy.

While the most common blockages of the CBD are stones, there may be strictures of the duct that will slow down the passage of bile. In this instance, the endoscope will allow the physician to place a stent into any narrow places to allow the bile to flow freely.

ERCP carries a small amount of risks. These include pancreatitis, irritation of infection, bowel perforation, and allergic reaction to any of the medications or contrast media administered during the procedure. Since a papillotomy may be done, it is important to determine if the patient has avoided taking any blood-thinning medications (such as aspirin) during the last week as this may cause internal bleeding.

Ultrasonography

Ultrasonography uses sound waves to provide images of the liver, gallbladder, and biliary tract. The test is

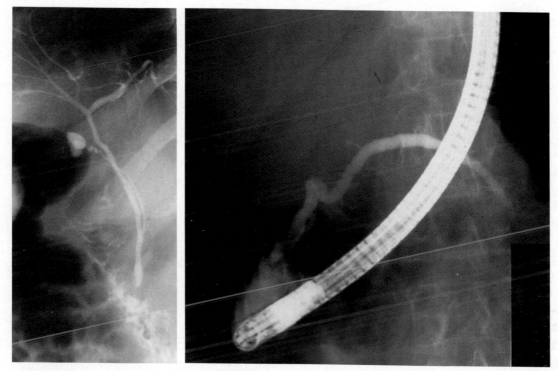

FIGURE 5-23   **(A) This image was taken after the endoscope was removed following an ERCP. The bile ducts and small bowel are visualized.** (Moore KL and Aqur A. *Essential Clinical Anatomy*, 2nd Ed. Philadelphia: Lippincott Williams & Wilkins 2002.) **(B) This image shows the endoscope still in place and demonstrated the main pancreatic duct.**

better for detecting structural abnormalities, such as tumors, than diffuse abnormalities, such as cirrhosis. It is the least expensive and safest technique for creating images of the gallbladder and biliary tract. By using ultrasound, gallstones can be easily detected. Obstructive jaundice can be distinguished from medical jaundice. Vascular Doppler ultrasound can show the flow of blood in the vessels of the liver. Ultrasound is also used to guide the needle placement when doing biopsy or a percutaneous transhepatic cholangiogram.

Computed Tomography

Computed tomography (CT) uses X-ray to view the organs and structures within the abdomen. CT looks at the patient's liver, gallbladder, spleen, pancreas, kidneys, and the vessels important to the liver, but also looks at the bowel and any abnormal fluid collections.

CT is a multiphase scan using oral and intravenous contrast material to take images in three phases: without contrast; with contrast in the arterial system; and finally, with contrast in the venous phase. The patient is asked to drink water, to help image the stomach

and small bowel. Some warmth may be noted by the patient during the injection of the contrast; however, this is normal.

CT provides excellent images of the liver. Doctors find it particularly useful for detecting tumors. It can also detect diffuse disorders, such as a fatty liver, abscesses, and an abnormally dense liver due to iron overload. Because CT is more expensive than ultrasound, and involves exposure to radiation, it is not as widely used, even though it provides more information regarding the liver. It is, however, the preferred method of assessing the severity of pancreatitis.

Magnetic Resonance Imaging

Magnetic resonance imaging (MRI) can provide very clear images of the body. The drawback of MRI is that it is more expensive than CT and takes longer to perform than other imaging methods do.

If the patient has kidney problems or is allergic to the CT contrast, an MRI procedure will be performed at some point during the evaluation. MRI, like CT, is used to better define something seen on the ultrasound procedure.

Nuclear Medicine

Radionuclide imaging uses isotopes (a radioactive tracer) that are injected into the patient to image the organs of the digestive tract. The radioactivity is detected by a gamma camera attached to a computer that generates an image. For each particular organ, an isotope that is "tagged" for that particular area is used. As the blood flows through the body, it carries the isotope to the designated organ. When the isotope arrives at its designated area, the gamma camera is positioned over that area and it "counts" the radioactivity emitted from that spot.

Liver, spleen, and pancreas scans are usually done following blood work that indicates an abnormality. Based on normal anatomy, the static scans are read for differences in size, shape, or position, or nonhomogenous uptake of the radioisotope. It is most often used to further evaluate masses or tumors. A gallbladder scan can detect gallstones, tumors, or defects within the gallbladder as well as blockages of the bile duct. Although all these can be detected by ultrasonography, nuclear medicine is able to determine the function of the gallbladder, which no other modality is able to do.

Nuclear medicine is the only imaging modality that is able to determine the emptying rate of the stomach. After the patient eats a standard meal containing radioactive isotope, the patient is monitored over a period of 1 to 2 hours to determine the time required for the radioactivity to decrease to one-half its original level. While an upper gastrointestinal (UGI) study using barium provides a gross indication of whether the stomach is emptying its contents, it does not provide quantification of the amount emptied. In addition, radiation exposure is quite high with the fluoroscopic UGI procedure.

Interventional Radiography

Interventional radiography is any procedure where an invasive technique is used to study the organs and radiographic images are taken. Such a procedure for the hepatobiliary system would be percutaneous transhepatic cholangiography (PTC). This procedure has also been called a "skinny needle" study because of the size and shape of the needle that is used to perform the procedure.

PTC is performed in the radiology department under sterile conditions. The patient is mildly sedated and a local anesthetic is administered so that the radiologist

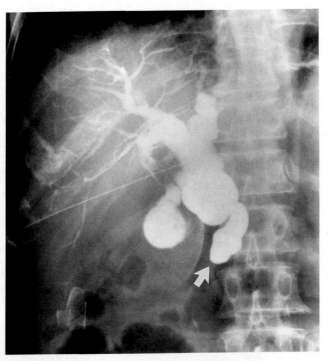

FIGURE 5-24   **PTC shows massive dilation of the common bile duct (CBD) and hepatic ducts in this patient with obstruction near the distal CBD (*arrow*). Note the skinny needle to the left on the image.** (Daffner RH. *Clinical Radiology: The Essentials*. 3rd ed. Philadelphia, PA: Lippincott Williams & Wilkins; 2007.)

can insert a long, thin-walled needle intercostally through the liver into a bile duct (Fig. 5-24). Contrast media is then injected directly into the duct and spot images are obtained. This procedure demonstrates the site of obstruction, particularly if it is in the CBD. It may also distinguish between obstructive and nonobstructive jaundice as well as pancreatitis. It is predominantly now performed as a therapeutic technique. There are less-invasive means of imaging the biliary tree including transabdominal ultrasound, CT, and MRI. If the biliary system is obstructed, PTC may be used to drain bile until a more permanent solution for the obstruction is performed (e.g., surgery). Additionally, stents can be placed across malignant biliary strictures to allow palliative drainage. Percutaneous placement of metal stents can be utilized when therapeutic ERCP has been unsuccessful, anatomy has been altered precluding endoscopic access to the duodenum, or where there has been separation of the segmental biliary drainage of the liver allowing more selective placement of metal stents.

This test has been mostly replaced by an ERCP test, which can also treat the blockage. This test may be done if an ERCP procedure cannot be performed or has failed. It is generally accepted that percutaneous biliary procedures have higher complication rates than therapeutic ERCP. There is a possibility that the liver may get damaged or that bile will spill into the peritoneum. However, the success rate of this procedure many times outweighs the risks involved. A magnetic resonance cholangiopancreatography is a newer, non-invasive imaging method based on MRI. It provides similar views of the bile ducts, but is not always possible to perform. It cannot be used to treat the blockage.

RECAP

Anatomy, Physiology, and Function

- Liver
  - Life-sustaining organ
  - Removes or neutralizes poisons from the blood
  - Produces immune agents to control infection
  - Removes harmful agents from the blood
  - Makes proteins that regulate blood clotting
  - Produces bile to help absorb fats and fat-soluble vitamins
- Gallbladder
  - Pear-shaped organ on posterior aspect of liver
  - Concentrates bile by removing water
  - Stores bile until cholecystokinin (CCK) stimulates gallbladder to contract
- Pancreas
  - Retroperitoneal organ that lies across the midline of the body
  - Head sits in the C-loop of the duodenum; tail sits near the spleen
  - Has both endocrine (ductless) and exocrine (secretion) functions
  - Endocrine system produces hormones: insulin and glucagon
  - Exocrine system secretes enzymes: amylase, lipase, and trypsin that digest food

Pathology

- Liver
  - Cirrhosis
    - Seventh leading cause of death in the United States
    - Leading cause of death in HIV-positive patients
    - Usually result of alcoholism or hepatitis C
    - Early stages: liver is "fatty," which interferes with liver function
    - Late stages: liver is scarred and small causing portal hypertension
    - Edema and ascites signal liver failure and present challenges for the radiographer
    - Complications include jaundice, portal hypertension, varices, diabetes, and liver cancer
  - Fatty liver
    - Most commonly caused by obesity
    - Also a result of cirrhosis
    - Seen best on ultrasound or CT
  - Hepatitis
    - Inflammation of liver cells
    - May result in cirrhosis
    - Three types
      - Deficiency
        - Due to poor diet and malnutrition (usually owing to alcoholism)
      - Toxic
        - Caused by drug or other toxic chemicals that destroy liver cells
      - Viral
        - Six subgroups include A, B, C, D, E, and G
          - A, D, and E are not as much a concern to the healthcare worker as B and C
          - All are caused by a virus
          - A and E are transmitted through fecal contamination of food or water that is ingested
          - B, C, and D are transmitted through blood and body fluids
          - Hepatitis B and C can become chronic and may be fatal
          - Hepatitis C is the leading indicator for liver transplant
          - Hepatitis G is most recently described, which is a blood-borne virus

- ○ Jaundice
  - Denotes a yellow cast to skin and sclera
  - Result of excess bilirubin in blood
  - Two types are medical (nonobstructive) and surgical (obstructive)
    - ○ Medical jaundice has two types: hemolytic or hepatic
- ○ Hemangioma
  - Most common benign tumor of the liver
- ○ Hepatomas
  - Any primary tumor of the liver but usually refers to malignant tumors
- Gallbladder
  - ○ Cholangitis is inflammation of the bile ducts
  - ○ Cholecystitis is inflammation of the gallbladder
  - ○ Cholelithiasis is the medical term for gallstones
    - Composed of bile, cholesterol, calcium carbonate, or all three
    - Most stones are radiolucent as only about 10% have enough calcium to be seen on X-ray
    - Best seen on ultrasound but CT and nuclear medicine will also show
- Pancreas
  - ○ Pancreatitis occurs when enzymes attack the organ not food
  - ○ Acute pancreatitis causes enzymes to be released into duodenum
    - Pseudocyst may be associated with acute pancreatitis
  - ○ Chronic pancreatitis is permanent inflammation that damages about 90% of the organ leading to calcifications
  - ○ Unique in that enzymatic necrosis occurs only in pancreatitis
  - ○ Best seen on CT
  - ○ Pseudocysts are most common cysts of pancreas
    - Contain enzymes and are capable of dissecting tissue

- ○ Adenocarcinoma
  - Ranks high for malignant deaths in the United States but is not a common cancer
  - Seventy-five percent occur in the head
  - Metastasizes to liver 80% of the times

Imaging Strategies

- Endoscopy
  - ○ Scope that is passed through the mouth and stomach into the duodenum to view the biliary ducts
  - ○ Contrast media is injected to highlight the pancreatic and biliary ductal system
- Ultrasonography
  - ○ Can determine tumors (solid vs. cystic), obstruction, and size and shape of the organ
  - ○ Endoscopic ultrasound is used to diagnose stomach cancer and keeps patient with end-stage carcinoma from having the pain of surgery
- Computed tomography (CT)
  - ○ Looks at liver, gallbladder, spleen, pancreas, kidneys, and bowel
  - ○ Can see any abnormal fluid collection
  - ○ Can perform CT-guided needle biopsy
- Magnetic resonance imaging (MRI)
  - ○ Performed if patient is allergic to contrast media or has kidney problems
  - ○ Does not provide much better answers than the CT scan
- Nuclear medicine
  - ○ Uses isotopes that are monitored by a gamma camera
  - ○ Is the only imaging modality that can study the function of the organs
- Interventional radiography
  - ○ Percutaneous transhepatic cholangiography (PTC) or skinny needle
  - ○ Injection of contrast directly into a bile duct
  - ○ Now done primarily for therapeutic reasons

CLINICAL AND RADIOGRAPHIC CHARACTERISTICS OF COMMON PATHOLOGIES

Pathologic Condition	Causal Factors to Include Age, if Relevant	Manifestations	Radiographic Appearance
Cholelithiasis	Women, 40 y and over	May be asymptomatic or may have pain upon eating fatty foods	Radiolucent, radiopaque, or a combination
Cirrhosis	25–65 y, usually ETOH, viral hepatitis	Ascites, jaundice, esophageal varices	Hepatomegaly; ascites, air-fluid levels

(continued)

CLINICAL AND RADIOGRAPHIC CHARACTERISTICS OF COMMON PATHOLOGIES *(continued)*

Pathologic Condition	Causal Factors to Include Age, if Relevant	Manifestations	Radiographic Appearance
Fatty liver	Obesity and ETOH		Fatty masses on anterior surface of liver
Hepatitis Deficiency Toxic Viral A B C D E G	ETOH Drug use Fecal contamination Blood and body fluid RNA virus Blood/body/hepatitis B Contaminated food Not yet fully determined	All types may lead to jaundice	Hepatomegaly
Jaundice Medical Surgical	Hepatic/hemolytic Obstruction	All types lead to yellow skin and sclera of eyes	
Pancreatitis Acute Chronic	ETOH or gallstones Long history of ETOH; recurring acute pancreatitis	Fever; epigastric pain Nausea/vomiting	May have a pseudocyst Calcifications; displaced stomach and effaced bowel

ETOH, ethyl alcohol.

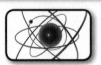 **CRITICAL THINKING DISCUSSION QUESTIONS**

1. Describe the anatomic relationship of the pancreas to the duodenum, IVC, stomach, splenic hilum, and left kidney. Where is the entire organ located?

2. Explain the composition of bile. Where is bile made? How is the gallbladder able to hold the amount that is produced? Describe this process.

3. Describe why cholecystokinin (CCK) is released and what impact it has on the digestive process.

4. List the functions of the pancreas. Define each.

5. What does ERCP stand for? Describe the procedure. What are the indications for it? What instructions should the technologist tell the patient regarding care after the procedure?

6. Describe the composition of gallstones. Which type is more common? Which population of people is more prone to gallstones?

7. List and describe the two types of pancreatitis. What causes them and what will radiographs of each demonstrate?

8. Define jaundice. What are some of the possible causes of jaundice? What modalities will help identify the cause?

9. Describe the liver's appearance in the early stages of cirrhosis. How will cirrhosis affect other organs in the body? What are some of the modalities that will show the disease?

6

The Urinary System

● Goals

1. To review the anatomy and basic physiology of the urinary system

   OBJECTIVE: Identify and describe the basic anatomy of the kidney, ureters, and bladder

   OBJECTIVE: Describe the process of urine production and its passage

2. To learn pathologic conditions related to the urinary system

   OBJECTIVE: Describe the radiographic appearance of selected urinary pathology

3. To understand the impact that pathology of the urinary system has on other systems of the body

   OBJECTIVE: Describe the etiology, sites, and complications for selected pathologic processes

4. To discover how various imaging modalities will demonstrate pathology

   OBJECTIVE: Identify and describe imaging procedures and interventional techniques appropriate for urinary pathology

● Key Terms

Bacteriuria
Bifid system
Dysuria
Extracorporeal shock wave lithotripsy
Glomerulonephritis (Bright disease)
Horseshoe kidney
Hydronephrosis
Hypernephroma (Grawitz)
Nephroblastoma (Wilms tumor)
Nephron
Nephroptosis
Nephrosis
Nocturia
Polycystic renal disease
Pyelonephritis
Pyuria
Renal agenesis
Renal calculi
Renal cell carcinoma
Renal ectopia
Renal failure
Struvite stones
Ureterocele
Uric
Vesicoureteral reflux

The urinary system is one of the four excretory pathways of the body, the other three being the large bowel, lungs, and skin. The urinary system consists of two kidneys, two ureters, a urinary bladder, and one urethra. While thinking in anatomical terms, the urinary system is not complicated, but the kidneys have the ability to shut down the entire body and may cause death if pathology disrupts the physiology of the renal system in any manner.

Anatomy

The kidneys are bean-shaped organs that lie behind the peritoneum (retro-peritoneal). Only the anterior surface is covered with peritoneum. They are not fixed in the abdomen and therefore are moveable with respiration.

The kidneys are about 4.5 inches in length and are found around the level of T12 to L3. The right kidney is slightly lower than the left because of inferior displacement by the liver. The inferior vena cava (IVC) lies medial to the right kidney and the aorta lies medial to the left kidney.

The renal capsule is the fibrous connective tissue that encloses the kidneys. Inside the kidney, the parenchyma is the pale-colored functional tissue of the kidney, extending from the capsule to the base of the pyramids. Here, the renal columns (columns of Bertin) are found between two minor calyces and their corresponding medullas. Each minor calyx has a darker-colored triangular-shaped area directly above it. This is known as the medulla. Inside each medulla, 8 to 12 renal pyramids that contain many collecting tubules are found. Each pyramid follows the shape of the medulla by being triangular, with the base toward the cortex and the apex fitting into the minor calyx.

The rounded medial ends of each renal pyramid are called the renal papillae. These ends fit into the cup-shaped end of a minor calyx. Minor calyces are a division of the major calyx. There can be as many as 12 minor calyces to 1 major calyx. One end receives the papilla while the other becomes the major calyx. There are approximately four major calyces per kidney. The major calyces are short and fat tubes that arise from the renal pelvis.

As the minor calyces unite to become major calyces, the major calyces merge together to form a sac-like collecting portion of the upper end of the ureter called the renal pelvis. The renal pelvis is found both inside and outside the actual kidney. As the renal pelvis becomes narrower and exits the kidney, it becomes the ureter. This point of transition is known as the ureteropelvic junction. Figure 6-1 shows the anatomy of the renal system that was described above.

Along the external medial border of each kidney is a depression called the hilum. The renal artery, vein, nerves, lymphatic vessels, and renal pelvis enter/leave the kidney at the hilum. This group of structures is collectively known as the renal pedicle.

There should be one ureter exiting each kidney (one on each side of the body). Anything other than this configuration is considered an anomaly. Each ureter is a hollow tube that extends from the kidney to the urinary bladder, which is about 10 to 12 inches. The urinary bladder lies posterior to the pubic symphysis. There are four coats to the bladder, the outer mucosal, submucosal, muscular, and the inner serosal. The three openings into the bladder consist of the

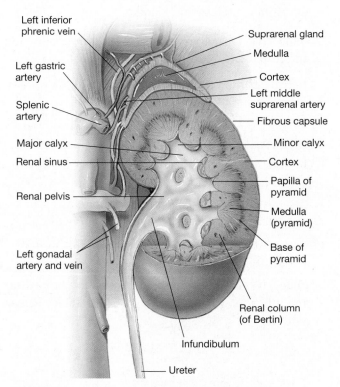

FIGURE 6-1   Cross section of the left kidney and adrenal gland. (Asset provided by Anatomical Chart Co.)

two ureteral and one urethral opening. The trigone is a band of musculature that connects these three openings.

The urethra is a hollow tube that is the single passage to the outside of the body from the bladder. The female urethra is short, only about 1 to 1.5 inches long, while the male urethra extends approximately 8 inches through the prostate gland and penis before reaching the outside. The opening to the outside is known as the urinary meatus.

Physiology and Function

The main function of the kidneys is to excrete urine so that the body maintains its hemostatic state, but also the kidneys regulate the fluid content of the blood and regulate the concentration of various electrolytes. To do this, the kidneys must filter all blood to remove waste products, reabsorb selected substances needed by the body, and secrete what is not needed by the body in the form of urine. Effective renal function depends upon adequate blood flow through the renal arteries. The speed at which the blood is filtered, reabsorbed, and secreted through the kidneys is affected by the blood pressure. About 1,200 mL of blood flows through the kidney of a normal adult each minute.

The functional unit of the kidney is the **nephron** which contains the Bowman capsule, the glomerulus, and the tubules. Over 1 million nephrons are located in the cortex of each kidney. It is within the glomerulus of the nephrons that the filtration of waste materials from the blood takes place so these can be excreted in the urine. The tubules select substances needed by the body and reabsorb them to be returned to the blood. Without this ability, the body would soon be drained of all fluids. Secretion takes place in the distal tubule and collecting ducts.

The kidneys also maintain the pH level of the blood so that it does not become too acidic or too alkaline. Regulation of the acid–base balance of the body fluids and the maintenance of normal concentrations of electrolytes are important to urine production and the body's ability to maintain a healthy state.

After passing through the tubules, urine enters the collecting ducts of the renal pyramids and then passes through the papillae into the minor and major calyces, the renal pelvis, and finally the ureter, whose only function is to convey urine from the kidney to the bladder. This is accomplished by peristalsis and gravity. The bladder acts as a holding tank for urine until enough has been collected that pressure upon the stretch and retention receptors signal the need to urinate. The bladder can hold as much as 500 mL of urine, but 250 mL should be enough to cause distention and discomfort.

Pathology

Congenital Anomalies

Duplication of any part of the urinary system, except the bladder, is the most common congenital anomaly. A **bifid system**, or double collecting system, can appear in many forms. A double renal pelvis or ureter (or even both) may appear in either one or both kidneys (Fig. 6-2A, B). The upper ureter is usually the "interloper" and it may insert into the bladder below the trigone, outside the bladder in the urethra, or, in the male, into the seminal vesicles. Occasionally, a complete double kidney will appear on one side. Usually the condition presents no symptoms and is found only when another condition is being investigated. When anomalies do cause problems, it is usually in the form of an obstruction to the upper pole collecting system or reflux.

A **horseshoe kidney** is a condition in which both kidneys are joined at their lower poles across the midline of the body (Fig. 6-3A–C). Because the lower poles are pulled together, the upper pole and hilum of each kidney is anatomically affected. The renal pelvis is now more anteriorly located causing a more horizontal angle, allowing urine to sit for longer periods of time. As the urine sits, it stagnates and collects the heavier potassium and calcium waste products. Renal calculi are more common in horseshoe kidneys because of this change in anatomical positioning.

Renal ectopia is the condition of a misplaced kidney and presents in several different manners. Usually, these kidneys are found in the pelvis and are associated with a congenitally short ureter. On an intravenous urogram (IVU), the kidney may be located by following the ureter up from the bladder (Fig. 6-4A, B). *Crossed ectopy* exists when one kidney (usually the lower one) lies either partially or completely across the

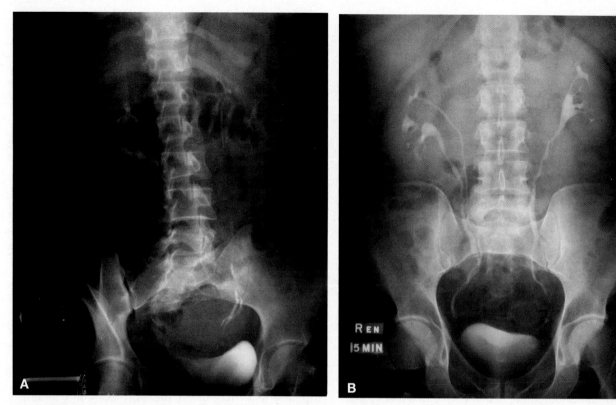

FIGURE 6-2   (A) A bifid system containing two complete and separate ureters on the same side. (B) A bifid or double collecting system each with its separate renal pelvis but leading to only one ureter.

midline and is fused with the upper kidney at its lower pole (Fig. 6-5). Both kidneys demonstrate various anomalies of position, shape, fusion, and rotation with this condition. Stone formation and reflux are more likely to be present than in a normal system.

For a better idea of where these anomalies are and how they appear, Figure 6-6 depicts several of the anomalies just discussed.

A floating kidney is termed **nephroptosis**. Remembering that the kidneys are retroperitoneal and that only the anterior surface is attached to the peritoneum, the kidneys will normally be displaced inferiorly about 1 inch (several centimeters) upon deep inspiration. When a person assumes the upright position, a descent of as much as 2 inches can be expected. Nephroptosis occurs when the anterior surface of the kidney is not attached to the peritoneum. As the person stands upright, the kidney will fall quite a distance, sometimes into the pelvic region. Nephroptosis is considered to be a variation of normal anatomy without significance; however, it must not be confused with an ectopic kidney. The determining factor is the length of the ureter (Fig. 6-7).

TECH TIP

When performing the post-void imaging following an IVU (which is usually done upright), do not center the beam as would be done for an abdominal series. The central ray must be positioned so that top of the pelvic crest is in the middle of the image as would be done for a KUB. If too much diaphragm is included, a "floating kidney" may not be identified on the upright post-void image.

Polycystic renal disease (also known as polycystic kidney disease or PKD) is an inherited renal cystic condition. If one parent carries the gene, the children have a 50% chance of developing the disorder. The exact cause of the formation of the cysts is unknown. It is thought that approximately 1 in 1,000 Americans suffer from this disease. Patients with polycystic renal disease should have their liver, pancreas, and spleen

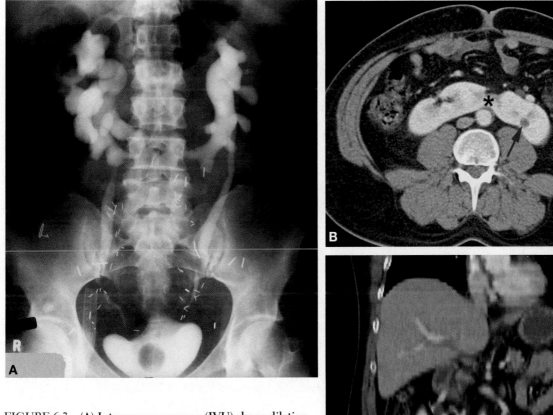

FIGURE 6-3   (A) Intravenous urogram (IVU) shows dilation
of the urinary collecting system bilaterally. Notice the
alteration of orientation of both renal poles. A pair of kidneys
orientated in this manner should suggest the diagnosis.
(B) CT axial image shows the contrast-enhanced isthmus (*).
Notice the small renal cyst on the left (*arrow*). (C) Coronal
reconstructed image shows the kidneys oriented with their
bottoms pointing medially (*arrows*). (A–C: Daffner RH.
Clinical Radiology: The Essentials. 3rd ed. Philadelphia, PA:
Lippincott Williams & Wilkins; 2007.)

assessed for the formation of cysts. Cysts in the liver
will be found in as many as 50% of patients with polycystic disease (Fig. 6-8). Also associated with this disorder are brain aneurysms and diverticula of the colon.
In the early stages of the disease, the cysts multiply and
enlarge, causing enlarged kidneys. In the end stages,
the kidneys are small and scarred, preventing normal
function.

Polycystic renal disease affects both infants and
adults. While the disease is much more common in
adults, *infantile polycystic disease* is more serious and
progresses rapidly. Characterized by dilated collecting tubules and smooth renal borders bilaterally, this
classification can be further delineated into newborn
and childhood types. *Newborn infantile polycystic*

disease (Fig. 6-9) develops in utero and results in *oligohydramnios* and *nephromegaly*. Unfortunately, most
infants with this disease are still born or die within
days of birth. *Childhood infantile polycystic disease*
(Fig. 6-10) occurs between the ages of 3 and 5 years. As
in newborn types, the disease is eventually fatal. *Hepa-
tosplenomegaly*, *portal hypertension*, and esophageal
varices are associated conditions of childhood PKD.

The adult version of polycystic renal disease still
falls under the category of congenital pathology
because the patient carries the genetic factors that
cause multiple cysts to grow in the parenchyma, only
at a later age. *Adult polycystic renal disease* begins
early in life with the formation of multiple tiny cysts
in the cortex. The formation of these cysts progress

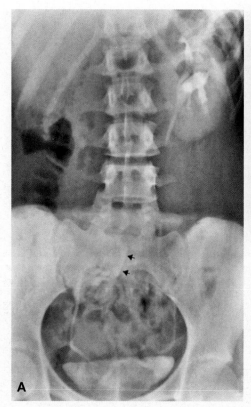

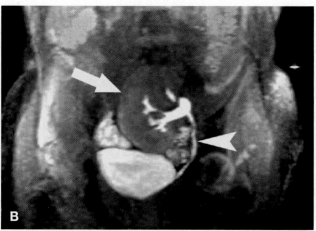

FIGURE 6-4   (A) Ectopic kidney located near the sacrum. The *arrows* point to the collecting system. (B) Another patient with a pelvic kidney (*arrow*). In this patient, the kidney is sitting completely in the pelvic cavity. The *arrowhead* points to the congenitally short ureter that is attached directly to the bladder immediately below the kidney. (A: Eisenberg RL. *Clinical Imaging: An Atlas of Differential Diagnosis*. 5th ed. Philadelphia, PA: Lippincott Williams & Wilkins; 2010. B: Leyendecker JR, Brown JJ. *Practical Guide to Abdominal and Pelvic MRI*. Philadelphia, PA: Lippincott Williams & Wilkins; 2004.)

so slowly that manifestation of the disease does not present until the patient is approximately 30 years old (Fig. 6-11A, B). As the cysts continue to grow and multiply, the nephrons located within the cortex are

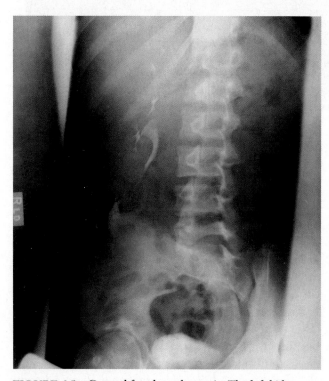

FIGURE 6-5   Crossed fused renal ectopia. The left kidney is rotated and fused with the lower, medial aspect of the right kidney.

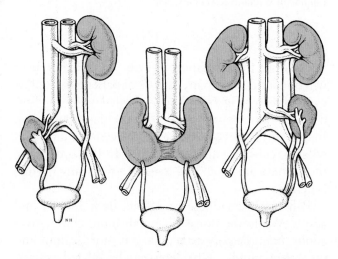

FIGURE 6-6   These drawings depict the different congenital anomalies that may occur in the urinary system. (A) Ectopic pelvic kidney. (B) Horseshoe kidney. (C) Supernumerary kidney (bifid). (Neil O. Hardy, Westpoint, CT.)

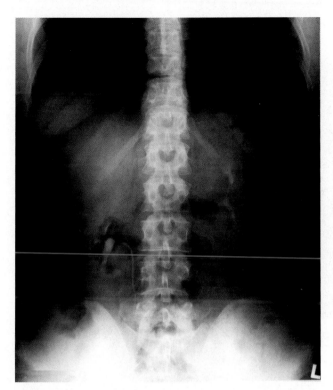

FIGURE 6-7   Nephroptosis or "floating" kidney. The kidney was in the normal position while the patient was supine. However, when the patient stood up for the upright position, post void, the right kidney fell almost 4 inches. *Note:* The technologist that took this image apparently did not follow the Tech Tip!

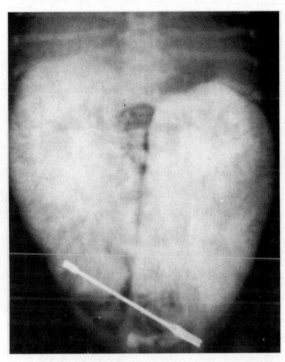

FIGURE 6-9   An IVU of a 2-day-old girl with autosomal recessive polycystic kidney disease shows the sunray appearance of the contrast material and the enormous renal size. (From Kelalis PP, King LR, Belman AB, eds. *Clinical Pediatric Urology*. Vol. 2. Philadelphia, PA: WB Saunders; 1976:686, with permission.)

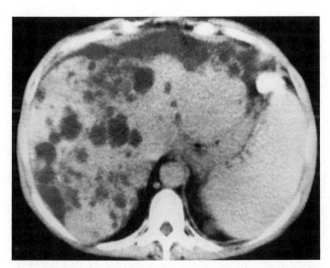

FIGURE 6-8   Innumerable lucent lesions of various sizes in a markedly enlarged liver in a patient who has severe polycystic kidney disease. (Eisenberg RL. *Clinical Imaging: An Atlas of Differential Diagnosis*. 5th ed. Philadelphia, PA: Lippincott Williams & Wilkins; 2010.)

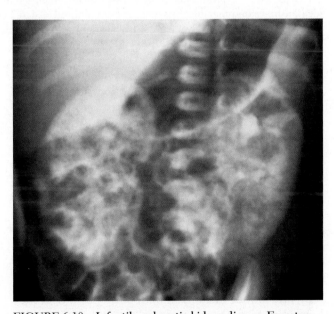

FIGURE 6-10   Infantile polycystic kidney disease. Excretory urogram in a young boy with large, palpable abdominal masses demonstrates renal enlargement with characteristic streaky densities leading to the calyceal tips. There is only minimal distortion of the calyces. (Eisenberg RL. *Clinical Imaging: An Atlas of Differential Diagnosis*. 5th ed. Philadelphia, PA: Lippincott Williams & Wilkins; 2010.)

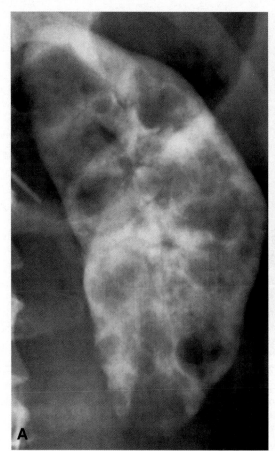

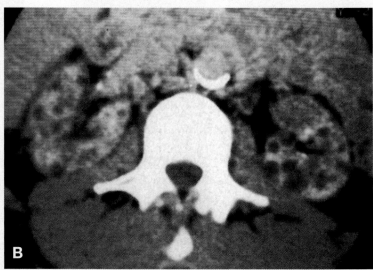

FIGURE 6-11   (A) Adult polycystic kidney disease. Nephrogram phase from selective arteriography of the left kidney demonstrates innumerable cysts ranging from pinhead size to 2 cm. (B) Adult polycystic disease. A CT scan of this patient shows bilateral renal involvement (A: Eisenberg RL. *Clinical Imaging: An Atlas of Differential Diagnosis*. 5th ed. Philadelphia, PA: Lippincott Williams & Wilkins; 2010.)

compromised and unable to function appropriately (Fig. 6-12). As more nephrons are destroyed, the kidney is unable to filter waste, reabsorb vital supplements, and regulate the balance of fluids, electrolytes, and pH in the blood. Hypertension, renal insufficiency, and uremia are all manifestations of adult polycystic disease. Hypertension caused by PKD is often difficult to control. This co-existing condition creates a decrease in the amount of blood flow through the kidney that must be filtered causing the uremia.

As the cysts continue to grow and compress the cortex, they will push outward on the capsule of the kidney. The kidney loses its smooth border as it becomes lumpy and lobulated due to the pressure from the inside cysts. This will also increase the length of the kidney as the cysts grow and extend the capsule to its limit. Patients diagnosed with this condition may live for extended periods of time or may die in a short time, depending on the degree of nephron involvement.

The cause of death is renal failure. Patients without systemic disease or autoimmune disease may be good candidates for kidney transplantation to prolong their lives.

There are various modalities that will demonstrate PKD such as computed tomography (CT), magnetic resonance imaging (MRI), and ultrasonography. For the diagnostic radiographer, the IVU will be the most common procedure performed. In the early stages, the kidneys will appear larger than normal with lobulated borders, elongated renal pelvis, and distortion of the calyces. The normal filling time will be longer as the nephrons are compromised and unable to process the contrast as well as a normal kidney. The "nephron blush" may not occur for more than 3 to 5 minutes or longer, depending on the severity of the disease.

Renal agenesis (Fig. 6-13) is an uncommon congenital anomaly that occurs unilaterally. It is the total failure of a kidney to develop. *Hypoplasia* describes a

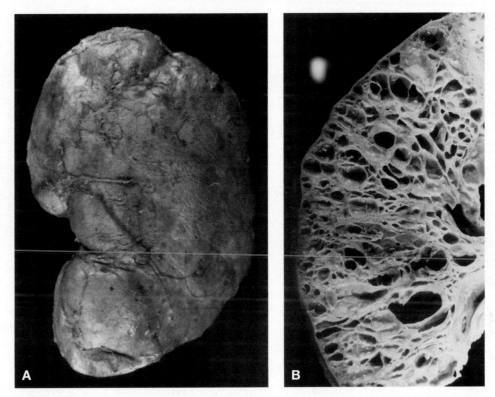

FIGURE 6-12   Polycystic kidney specimen. The left image shows the enlarged size. The right image shows how the cysts invade the cortex and can then disrupt the function of the nephrons.

kidney that is less developed than normal. Both agenesis and hypoplasia are usually associated with hyperplasia of the opposite kidney. **Renal hyperplasia** is an overdeveloped kidney that occurs when the opposite kidney is either absent or so underdeveloped that it is unable to perform the necessary function to maintain

body health. The normal kidney will enlarge as it works harder to take over the functions not performed by the opposing kidney.

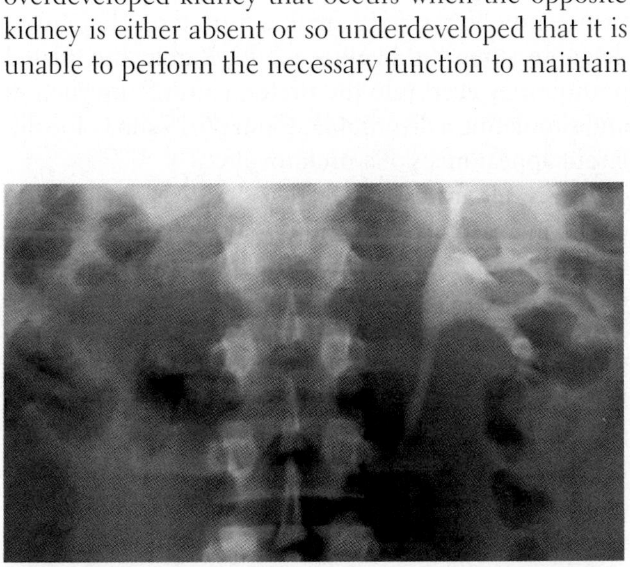

Inflammatory Processes

An inflammatory disease of the capillary loops of the renal glomeruli, located within the nephrons is known as **glomerulonephritis**. A more common term is **Bright disease**. This process may develop after an acute Streptococcal infection as a result of antigen–antibody complex being deposited in the glomerulus. It is the most common cause of underdeveloped kidneys (hypoplasia) in young adults. Bright disease is characterized by hypertension caused by the stimulation of the juxtaglomerular apparatus and edema of the face and ankles due to loss of protein. Symptoms include nausea, malaise, and arthralgia. Laboratory tests will indicate an increase in albumin, BUN, and creatinine levels. A chest X-ray may show pulmonary infiltrates (Fig. 6-14).

FIGURE 6-13   **Renal agenesis on the right. The left kidney is slightly enlarged.** (Eisenberg RL. *Clinical Imaging: An Atlas of Differential Diagnosis.* 5th ed. Philadelphia, PA: Lippincott Williams & Wilkins; 2010.)

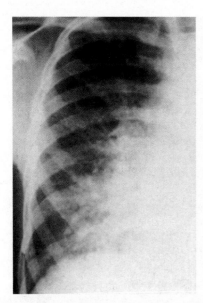

FIGURE 6-14   Very extensive interstitial edema producing pronounced reticulation through the lung and some underlying parenchymal haziness. Kerley A and B lines are present. This patient had acute glomerulonephritis. (Swischuk LE. *Emergency Radiology of the Acutely Ill or Injured Child*. 2nd ed. Philadelphia, PA: Lippincott Williams & Wilkins; 1986.)

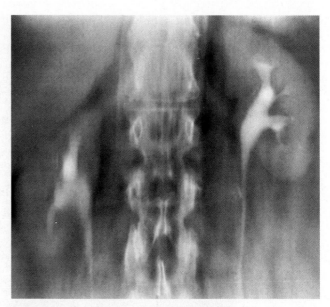

FIGURE 6-15   Chronic glomerulonephritis. Nephrotomogram shows bilateral small, smooth kidneys. The uniform reduction in parenchymal thickness is particularly apparent in the right kidney. Note that the pelvocaliceal system is well opacified and without the irregular contours and blunted calyces seen in chronic pyelonephritis. (Eisenberg RL. *Clinical Imaging: An Atlas of Differential Diagnosis*. 5th ed. Philadelphia, PA: Lippincott Williams & Wilkins; 2010.)

The majority of patients with Bright disease will recover spontaneously, but a small number of patients develop progressive renal failure, and death may be caused by uremia. In other cases, patients experience chronic inflammation. Chronic infection develops weeks or months after an episode of acute glomerulonephritis. It is associated with progressive hypertension and renal failure. Chronic glomerulonephritis leads to fibrosis that results in the shrinkage of the kidney. Because the fibrosis will affect the nephrons, there is loss of renal function with accompanying uremia. The kidneys initially appear larger due to the inflammation and the body's defense mechanism. After the fibrosis causes scarring and shrinkage, the kidneys will become small and dysfunctional (Figs. 6-15 and 6-16).

Diverticula, like those found in the bowel, can occur in the bladder (Fig. 6-17) or ureters, or both. These abnormal pouches appear in variable sizes and allow the urine to lie stagnant, resulting in stones or infection.

A cyst-like dilation of the ureter near its opening into the bladder is called a **ureterocele**. The radiographic sign "cobra head" is derived from the radiographic appearance on the IVU (Fig. 6-18). The ureter is the long body of a snake and the dilated flaring of the submucosal ureteric segment is reminiscent of the cobra snake as it flares its gills as a warning. If the image is

taken at the exact moment that contrast is excreted into the bladder, one can envision the tongue of the snake. As the bladder fills, the ureterocele is progressively diminished in size by the increasing pressure from urine and contrast. This makes a ureterocele hard to diagnose when the bladder is full. Rarely, the dilated portion may evert into the ureter, causing obstruction and simulating a diverticula. Figure 6-19 shows the different appearances of a ureterocele.

Prostatic hypertrophy describes prostate gland enlargement and subsequent obstruction of urinary output. Almost all men over 55 years of age experience some enlargement of the prostate gland. The early symptoms include reduced urine output but the feeling of a full bladder. The urethra passes through the prostate gland. As the gland enlarges it closes the lumen of the urethra, thus causing diminished urine output. The residual urine retained in the bladder tends to undergo decomposition and becomes infected. Cystitis (inflammation of the bladder) is a common complaint associated with hypertrophy of the prostate gland. As a result of increased pressure, the trabecular cords on the inner surface of the bladder pull on the wall. This causes the borders of the bladder

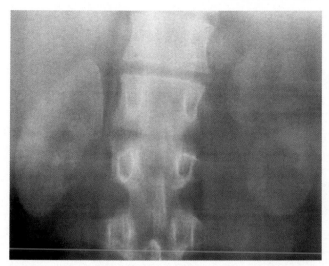

FIGURE 6-16 Patient with bilateral small smooth kidneys due to chronic glomerulonephritis. This patient does not have the contrast in the kidneys as does the patient in figure 6-15. However, there are fine calcifications located in the renal parenchymea. (Eisenberg RL. *Clinical Imaging: An Atlas of Differential Diagnosis.* 5th ed. Philadelphia, PA: Lippincott Williams & Wilkins; 2010.)

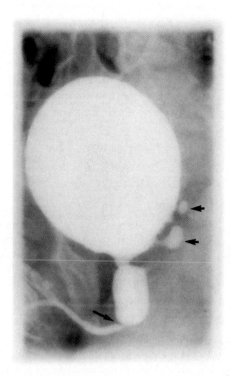

FIGURE 6-17 Cystourethrogram shows the valve (*long arrow*), dilated proximal urethral segment, and bladder diverticula (*short arrows*). (Daffner RH. *Clinical Radiology: The Essentials.* 3rd ed. Philadelphia, PA: Lippincott Williams & Wilkins; 2007.)

to assume a lumpy, irregular appearance. Additionally, the base of the bladder has a notched appearance as a result of the enlarged prostate pushing up into the bladder (Fig. 6-20).

Water in the nephrons of the kidney is the literal meaning of **hydronephrosis.** While technically there is no water in the nephrons, hydronephrosis is a result of some obstruction causing dilation of the renal pelvis, calyces, and ureter from backpressure of urine that cannot flow past the obstruction. In other words, hydronephrosis is the result of another process and is not a disease itself. One out of every 100 people has unilateral hydronephrosis. Bilateral hydronephrosis occurs when there is an obstruction in both ureters. This most commonly occurs in pregnancy where both ureters are compressed by the fetus (Fig. 6-21). In this case, the condition of hydronephrosis disappears when the baby is delivered.

The patient will suffer from hematuria, pyuria, flank pain, and fever. Diagnostic studies include an IVU, nuclear medicine, ultrasonography (Fig. 6-22), and CT and MRI. The radiographic images from an IVU will show enlargement above the obstruction with no anatomy demonstrated below. Calyces remain sharp, although enlarged (Fig. 6-23). If bilateral hydronephrosis is allowed to continue, the nephrons will eventually become damaged, leading to renal insufficiency or failure. Complications in

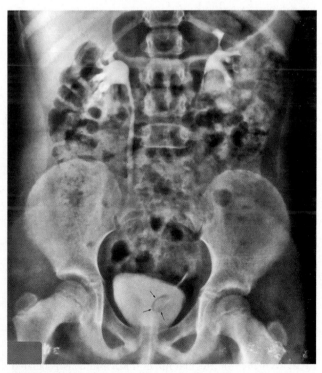

FIGURE 6-18 Simple ureterocele presenting as a "cobra head" filling defect in the bladder (*arrows*). The kidneys above are normal. (Daffner RH. *Clinical Radiology: The Essentials.* 3rd ed. Philadelphia, PA: Lippincott Williams & Wilkins; 2007.)

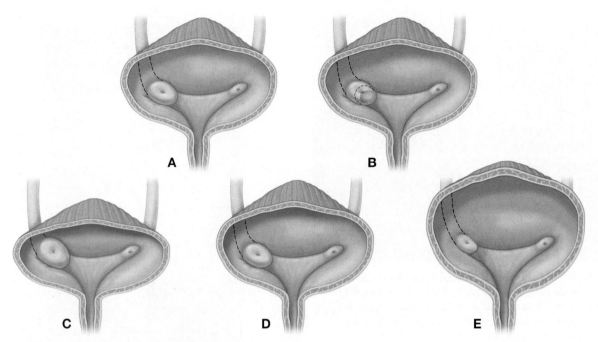

A   **B**

C   **D**   **E**

FIGURE 6-19   A ureterocele is a dilation of the submucosal ureteric segment. Rarely the dilated portion may slide up into the ureter, causing obstruction (A) and simulating a diverticulum (B). (C) A ureterocele in an empty bladder. As the bladder fills, the ureterocele becomes smaller (D) until it is difficult to identify (E).

unilateral hydronephrosis are rare as the normal kidney has the ability to take over the workload and compensate for the obstructed kidney. However, treatment such as a ureteral stent or a nephrostomy tube may be necessary. If an infection is the cause of the blockage, antibiotics are required to clear the infection.

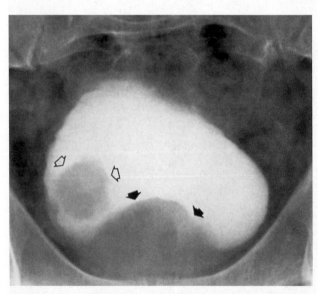

FIGURE 6-20   An irregular tumor (*open arrows*) is associated with a large filling defect (*closed arrows*), representing benign prostatic hypertrophy at the base of the bladder. (Eisenberg RL. *Clinical Imaging: An Atlas of Differential Diagnosis.* 5th ed. Philadelphia, PA: Lippincott Williams & Wilkins; 2010.)

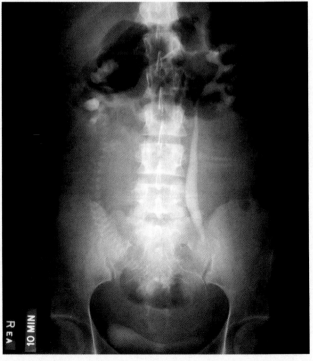

FIGURE 6-21   Hydronephrosis of both kidneys caused by a fetus obstructing the flow from the ureters to the bladder.

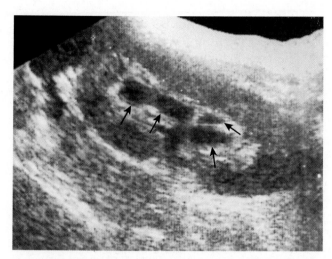

FIGURE 6-22 Hydronephrosis in a patient with moderate disease: the dilated calyces and pelvis appear as echo-free sacs (*arrows*) separated by septa of compressed tissue and vessels. (Eisenberg RL. *Clinical Imaging: An Atlas of Differential Diagnosis.* 5th ed. Philadelphia, PA: Lippincott Williams & Wilkins; 2010.)

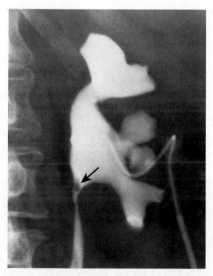

FIGURE 6-23 Hydronephrosis. Dilatation of the entire pelvocaliceal system proximal to an obstruction (*arrow*) at the ureteropelvic junction. (Eisenberg RL. *Clinical Imaging: An Atlas of Differential Diagnosis.* 5th ed. Philadelphia, PA: Lippincott Williams & Wilkins; 2010.)

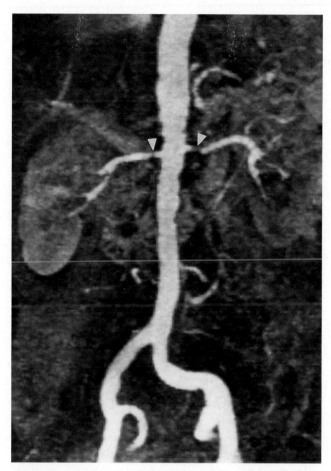

FIGURE 6-24 Renovascular hypertension. MR angiogram shows stenosis in both renal arteries (*arrowheads*). The left is more severely involved than the right, reflecting the changes in the renogram. No intravenous contrast was used for this examination. (Daffner RH. *Clinical Radiology: The Essentials.* 3rd ed. Philadelphia, PA: Lippincott Williams & Wilkins; 2007.)

Ninety-five percent of **hypertension** cases are idiopathic. The risk of hypertension is increased with the use of alcohol, smoking, and a sedentary lifestyle. Hypertension (high blood pressure) can be the result of a narrowing of either one or both of the renal arteries (Fig. 6-24). Renal artery stenosis causes the kidney to release rennin, an enzyme that causes vasoconstriction. Because of the vasoconstriction, the left ventricle of the heart has an increased workload to try to pump more blood to systemic circulation. This in turn leads to elevated blood pressure known as primary (essential) hypertension. Renal artery stenosis is present in 77% of hypertensive patients. Hypertension may also be the result of a preexisting condition such as Bright disease or pyelonephritis. This is known as secondary hypertension.

Hypertension is a serious process. The human heart beats about 100,000 times a day. As the heart works to pump the blood through the vessels, it causes the blood to hit the vessel wall. With increased blood pressure, the blood will hit the vessel walls harder, leading to damage. This can lead to strokes or heart attack. One in every four Americans has hypertension. This astounding number is believed to be so high because of the American lifestyle of a diet high in fat and cholesterol, little exercise, and high levels of stress. Many people do not even know they have hypertension, as there may be no symptoms. The only way to be sure is to routinely monitor the blood pressure.

Radiographically, a hypertensive kidney may appear so similar to a kidney with end-stage Bright disease that it may be difficult to tell the difference by imaging alone. Other names for hypertensive kidneys include arteriosclerotic kidney (because of the change in the blood vessels) and nephrosclerotic kidney (because of scarring within the kidney as it tries to repair itself). The kidney that is the source of hypertension is usually smaller in size and shows delayed excretion and over-concentration of the contrast media.

Pyelonephritis means inflammation of the kidney and renal pelvis. It is the most common single type of renal disease. Pyogenic bacteria, most commonly *Escherichia coli*, invade the renal tissue causing *acute pyelonephritis*. These bacteria may enter the kidney in a retrograde fashion from the bladder (reflux) or through the blood in about 20% of the cases. Pyelonephritis is about twice as common in women than in men because of the higher incidence of urinary tract infections (UTIs) in women. Patients characteristically experience flank pain, **bacteriuria**, **pyuria**, **dysuria**, **nocturia**, and increased frequency of urination. The infection causes the calyces to become enlarged, such as in hydronephrosis; however, the classic difference in radiographic images is the blunting of the calyces found in pyelonephritis (Fig. 6-25). The calyces remain sharp in hydronephrosis.

Chronic pyelonephritis is caused by chronic reflux of infected urine from the bladder into the renal pelvis. The eventual outcome of chronic pyelonephritis is decreased kidney size with destruction and scarring due to fibrosis of the renal tissue (Fig. 6-26).

Pyelonephritis is not an automatic indication for imaging of the urinary system. If the patient is a diabetic, has a history of urinary tract stones, has a poor response to antibiotics, or has frequent recurrences, then the clinician will request imaging procedures to help determine the etiology of the process. IVUs are normal in 75% of all cases, so they may not be the best primary diagnostic medium. The IVU will show diffuse involvement of the kidney. There may be delayed opacification of the collecting system. A CT will demonstrate generalized renal enlargement or focal swelling but with normal attenuation. The majority of sonography cases will demonstrate normal kidneys or perhaps a swollen kidney with decreased echogenicity.

Despite the difficulty in determining the cause of the pyelonephritis, it is important to treat the disease. With quick response to antibiotic treatment, the kidneys should heal with no scarring. When treatment is delayed during the first several years of affliction, the kidneys will be damaged so as to affect renal function causing hypertension and even end-stage renal disease (ESRD).

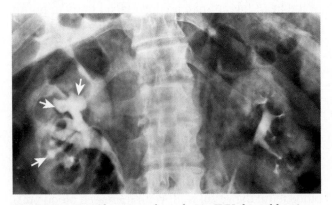

FIGURE 6-25   Chronic pyelonephritis. IVU shows blunting and clubbing of the calyces in the right kidney (*arrows*). The left kidney is normal. (Daffner RH. *Clinical Radiology: The Essentials*. 3rd ed. Philadelphia, PA: Lippincott Williams & Wilkins; 2007.)

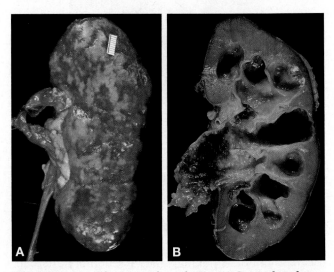

FIGURE 6-26   Chronic pyelonephritis. (A) Cortical surface contains many irregular depressed scars. (B) Marked dilation of calyces caused by inflammatory destruction of papillae, with atrophy and scarring of overlying cortex. (Rubin R, Strayer DS. *Rubin's Pathology: Clinicopathologic Foundations of Medicine*, 5th ed. Philadelphia, PA: Lippincott Williams & Wilkins; 2008.)

Vesicoureteral reflux (VUR) can be either congenital or acquired (known as secondary). The congenital cause is an incompetent ureteral valve that allows urine to flow back into the ureters and kidneys from the urinary bladder. This common condition occurs in 1 to 2 children out of every 100. Twice as many females as males and twice as many whites as blacks will have VUR. Reflux of urine will occur when the valve at the ureteral–vesicle junction (UVJ) is abnormal. Normally, the ureter will enter the bladder on the superior posterior aspect. This allows a good length of ureter to tunnel its way through the bladder wall entering the bladder. There will be a

"flap" of tissue from the bladder wall that covers the opening of the ureter after it enters the bladder. This flap (or valve) allows the flow of urine in one direction into the bladder. However, sometimes a ureter will enter the bladder too far laterally. In this case, the ureter is not long enough to tunnel through the bladder wall and have sufficient length to penetrate into the bladder cavity. Other causes of reflux include obstruction, abnormal bladder contractions, infrequent voiding, or constipation. A family history of VUR is often an indicator of problems in the children. If one child has VUR, the siblings should be checked.

Case Study

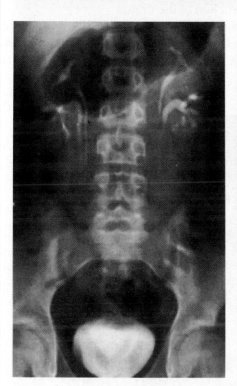 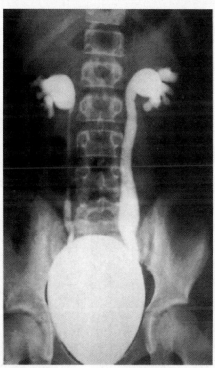

(Belman AB. The clinical significance of vesicoureteral reflux. *Pediatr Clin North Am* 1976;23:707.)

In this patient, a young girl, several conditions are present at once. An intravenous ureogram was performed and it shows complete, bilateral duplication of the collecting system. Looking the image on the left it can be seen that the lower calyces are blunted. Blunting of calyces is a sign of pyelonephritis. Now the question becomes, what caused the pyelonephritis? The image on the right is a cystogram done several days later. Reflux of urine is demonstrated into both the lower collecting systems. Because the urine that was flowing back into the kidneys now carried bacteria from the urethra, the renal tubules became infected and the cause of the pyelonephritis was determined.

An acquired cause of VUR is a UTI. It is known as secondary reflux because it is secondary to some other process. Fifty percent of infants and children with UTI have reflux. Not all patients with this condition experience symptoms however. It is estimated that 4 out of every 1,000 children have no symptoms yet have VUR. This is because the symptoms of UTI are not common in children. The main indication of an infection is trouble in urinating. Repeated UTIs should be cause to check for VUR as it may be the only symptom of the problem.

Children may need a renal ultrasound or voiding cystourethrography (VCUG) (see Case Study). It is important to diagnose and grade the condition early, before the infection causes scarring and loss of future growth potential. Scarring in the kidneys may cause elevated blood pressure later in life. Grade 1 has the least amount of involvement, while a grade 5 is the worst form of the condition. A grade 1 or 2 may resolve spontaneously as the patient ages. A grade 4 or 5, on the other hand, requires surgical intervention, usually in the form of a kidney transplant with removal of the scarred kidney.

Renal calculi are solid masses that consist of a collection of tiny crystals containing calcium, calcium salts, and oxalates. Oxalate is present in certain foods and is the most common substance to combine with calcium to form stones. Under most normal conditions, the minerals can form minute crystals that are passed out of the body along with the urine flow. Sometimes, however, the minerals clump together and cling to the tissue lining inside of the kidney. There they continue to grow as new crystals are added. As time passes, they harden. The urine shows elevated crystalline salts, pus, and blood upon examination and testing. Stones form in the urinary tract, usually in the renal pelvis, but they are sometimes found in the bladder. Calculi are usually asymptomatic and they begin to descend through the ureters (Fig. 6-27) or until they cause an obstruction. The hematuria and severe flank pain radiating to the groin or genitals are common manifestations. It is important to identify stones as renal failure can occur from an obstruction of the ureter.

Renal calculi are found in about 5% of the population. More have been found at autopsy to increase the incidence to 20%. There is a recurrence of renal

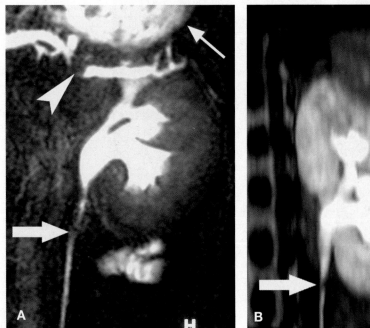

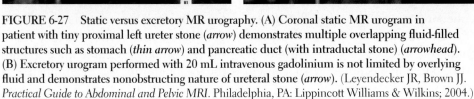

FIGURE 6-27   Static versus excretory MR urography. (A) Coronal static MR urogram in patient with tiny proximal left ureter stone (*arrow*) demonstrates multiple overlapping fluid-filled structures such as stomach (*thin arrow*) and pancreatic duct (with intraductal stone) (*arrowhead*). (B) Excretory urogram performed with 20 mL intravenous gadolinium is not limited by overlying fluid and demonstrates nonobstructing nature of ureteral stone (*arrow*). (Leyendecker JR, Brown JJ. *Practical Guide to Abdominal and Pelvic MRI*. Philadelphia, PA: Lippincott Williams & Wilkins; 2004.)

calculi in almost 50% of previous cases. Kidney stones are also common in premature infants due to the high concentration of their urine. As in gallstones, there are different types of renal stones. Calcium stones are the most common, particularly in men. *Uric* stones (Fig. 6-28) are also more common in men as they are associated with gout. Uric stones are radiolucent making them difficult to see on radiography except as a filling defect on contrast studies. *Struvite* stones (Fig. 6-29) are composed of magnesium ammonium phosphate that is found with UTIs. These stones are mainly found in women because of their increased incidence of UTIs. Because of their composition and connection to UTI, struvite stones are called "infection" stones. All types of stones can grow very large and may obstruct the kidney, ureter, or bladder.

If a stone begins formation in the renal pelvis and continues to grow there, it may take on the shape of the pelvicaliceal junction as it completely fills the renal pelvis. Known as a *staghorn calculus* because of its appearance as horns on a head of a deer, this condition will block the flow of all urine (Fig. 6-30). Struvite calculi represent 70% of staghorn calculus. *Nephrocalcinosis* describes numerous irregular spots of calcium contained in the renal parenchyma. There may be only a few scattered areas of calcium or there may be numerous densities throughout both kidneys

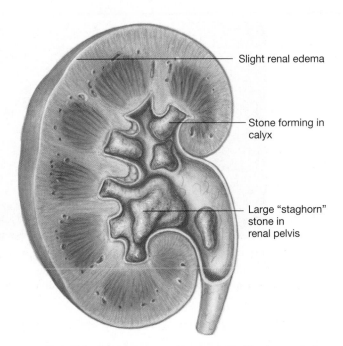

FIGURE 6-29   Struvite stones. (Asset provided by Anatomical Chart Co.)

(Fig. 6-31A, B). Those who are at risk for nephrocalcinosis are those who have increased alkali in the urine or who have chronic glomerulonephritis. Abdominal radiographs taken prior to injection of the contrast medium are an important part of an IVU, as contrast will hide some of the smaller calculi.

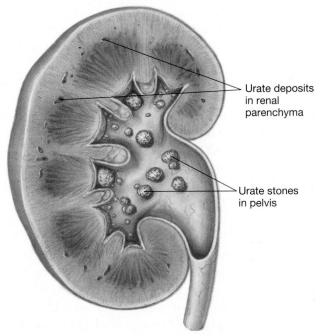

FIGURE 6-28   Uric acid stones. (Asset provided by Anatomical Chart Co.)

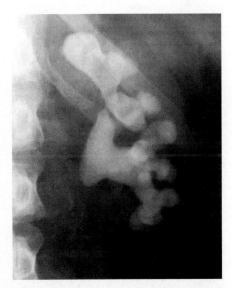

FIGURE 6-30   This 35-year-old woman was undergoing combined percutaneous nephrostolithotomy and extracorporeal shock wave lithotripsy (ESWL) for staghorn calculi. This is the scout image. (Harwood-Nuss A, Wolfson AB, Lyndon CH, et al. *The Clinical Practice of Emergency Medicine*. 3rd ed. Philadelphia, PA: Lippincott Williams & Wilkins; 2001.)

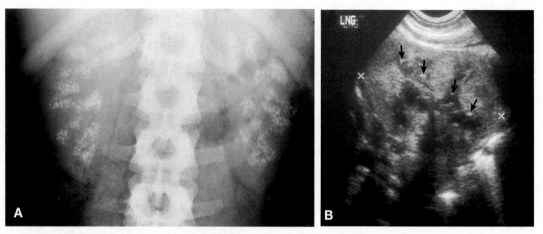

FIGURE 6-31   (A) Nephrocalcinosis. Radiograph shows fine deposition of calcium within the renal pyramids of both kidneys. (B) Ultrasound image shows multiple small calcifications (*arrows*) in the same patient from previous image. This is a reversible condition. (A and B: Daffner RH. *Clinical Radiology: The Essentials*. 3rd ed. Philadelphia, PA: Lippincott Williams & Wilkins; 2007.)

Although not as common as calculi in the kidney, stones do form in the urinary bladder. These can be single or multiple and can vary in size (Fig. 6-32). Bladder stones have a tendency to form from stagnant urine that is unable to be passed because of some urethral outlet obstruction or because of size. Since the stones are heavier than the urine, an upright position will demonstrate a filling defect at the base of the

FIGURE 6-32   **Multiple bladder stones of various sizes.** (Eisenberg RL. *Clinical Imaging: An Atlas of Differential Diagnosis*. 5th ed. Philadelphia, PA: Lippincott Williams & Wilkins; 2010.)

bladder and the post-void projection should show contrast outlining the stone.

Stones or obstruction may be seen on a kidney ultrasound, IVU, abdominal radiographs, retrograde pyelogram, abdominal CT, and abdominal/kidney MRI. Treatment goals include control of pain with analgesics and the prevention of further symptoms. Drinking enough fluid on a daily basis to increase urine output is highly desirable. Not all fluids are appropriate however. Coffee contains caffeine that will dehydrate the body and many sodas contain oxalates that combine with calcium to form crystallites. Water is the recommended fluid in the amounts of about 64 oz per day (8 glasses that are 8 oz each).

Renal failure is the condition where the kidneys fail to function properly through a decrease in the glomerular filtration rate (GFR). Renal failure can be broadly classified into two categories: acute or chronic. *Acute renal failure* (ARF) is the rapid, severe deterioration in kidney function caused by acute degeneration and necrosis of the renal tubules (known as **nephrosis**). Nephrosis rapidly leads to oliguria or anuria. Causes of nephrosis include ischemia or toxic injury, especially by alcohol. Other causes include obstruction of the renal artery, glomerulonephritis, pyelonephritis, and severe hypertension. Whatever the cause, it must be identified if the progress of failure is to be stopped. Water and potassium retention results in a life-threatening situation as the balance of fluid and electrolytes in the blood are disrupted. The patient will exhibit massive edema and uremia. Dialysis may be necessary to allow the underlying cause to be treated before the failure can be addressed. ARF is treatable, with long-term survival rates of 60%.

ARF can occur again, after chronic renal failure has been diagnosed. Known as acute-on-chronic renal failure, the purpose of treatment is to return the patient to their baseline renal function (prior to the onset of the newly diagnosed acute failure).

Chronic renal failure (CRF) is the slow, progressive, and irreversible loss of renal function. CRF is often caused by hypertension and diabetes. Because of the kidney's role in maintaining water balance and regulating acid–base balance and electrolyte levels, CRF causes major changes noted in all body systems. Hypertension, ventricular tachycardia, congestive heart failure, anemia, generalized edema, nephrocalcinosis, and clotting disorders are some of the manifestations of CRF. The patient experiences oliguria or anuria and exhibits signs of fluid overload. There is usually extensive scarring and fibrosis of the renal parenchyma resulting in decreased kidney size. With CRF, the patient undergoes regular dialysis on a permanent basis, unless a kidney transplant is undertaken. CRF is a common disease. The National Kidney Foundation reports that over 20 million Americans live with CRF, with approximately another 20 million at risk for the disease.

In renal failure, the kidneys cannot concentrate well, and large doses of contrast agents are necessary to visualize the cortex of the kidney. IVUs that are performed on patients in ARF demonstrate bilateral renal enlargement and prolonged nephrocortical blush (Fig. 6-33). Tomography is especially helpful in demonstrating the pelvic structures that are poorly visualized. The liver excretes the contrast agent when the kidneys fail, and occasionally opacification of the gallbladder is noted.

Because of the large amounts of contrast needed for an IVU, this procedure may be deemed detrimental to the patient's health. Renal failure lengthens the time necessary for excretion of contrast medium or prevents it all together. The longer the contrast media remains in the body, the more toxic it becomes. Therefore, sonography is one of the procedures that is most often requested to determine size of the kidney (Fig. 6-34).

Once kidney function decreases to less than 10%, they can no longer process wastes effectively to maintain life. The patient is now in end stage renal disease (ESRD). Only dialysis or a kidney transplant will prolong the patient's life. Dialysis is not a cure and may cause infection. Long-term dialysis has been linked to

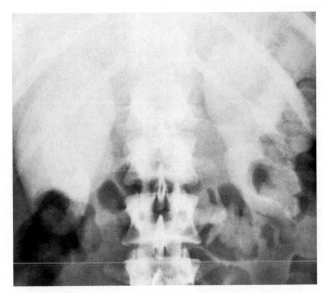

FIGURE 6-33   Acute renal failure (ARF). IVU image 20 minutes after the injection of contrast material shows bilateral persistent nephrograms with no calyceal filling. (Eisenberg RL. *Clinical Imaging: An Atlas of Differential Diagnosis*. 5th ed. Philadelphia, PA: Lippincott Williams & Wilkins; 2010.)

renal cancer. Transplants are a more permanent solution; however, the number of organs donated does not meet the medical demand. Over 67,000 Americans die each year of renal failure.

Neoplasms

Benign

A renal cyst is an acquired condition that usually occurs in the cortex of the lower pole of the kidney. Approximately 50% of the population over the age of 50 years have or have had a renal cyst. They generally are asymptomatic unless they are quiet large in which case pain or obstruction caused by pressure being excreted from the cyst may be present. Figures 6-35–6-37 readily show a simple renal cyst on CT, MRI, and ultrasonography. Radiographically, the cyst shows calyce spreading but does not demonstrate the irregular opacification after injection of a contrast agent that a tumor will.

Malignant

Benign tumors of the kidney are rare. The most common renal tumor in patients of any age is the **hypernephroma**. Other names for kidney cancer are **Grawitz**

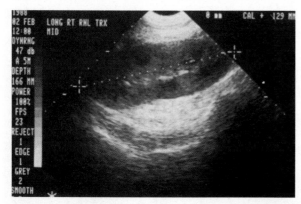

FIGURE 6-34 Ultrasonography is an excellent medium to measure the length of a kidney.

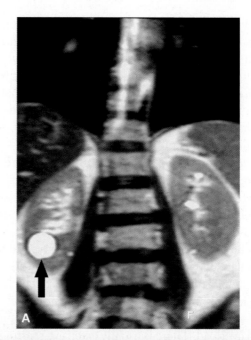

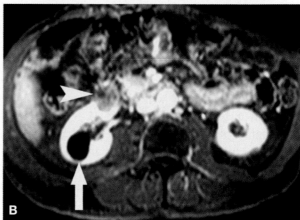

FIGURE 6-36 Simple renal cyst. Simple cyst in lower pole right kidney (*arrows*) demonstrates typical high signal intensity on T2-weighted coronal image (A) and lack of enhancement on axial postgadolinium, fat-suppressed T1-weighted image (B). Note the enhancing lesion (*arrowhead*) in anterior right kidney for comparison. (Leyendecker JR, Brown JJ. *Practical Guide to Abdominal and Pelvic MRI*. Philadelphia, PA: Lippincott Williams & Wilkins; 2004.)

tumor and **renal cell carcinoma**. It is an idiopathic process that has been linked to cigarette smoking, and certain genetic syndromes such as Von Hippel-Lindau syndrome (Fig. 6-38). It is also thought that long-term dialysis may also increase the risk of developing renal cell carcinoma. The tumor arises from the renal tubule cells and destroys the kidney while invading the blood vessels, particularly the renal vein and the IVC. This allows the spread of malignant cells to the lungs, liver, and the bones (Fig. 6-39). The main symptom is hematuria. The tumor has an increased incidence after the age of 40 years and is twice as common in

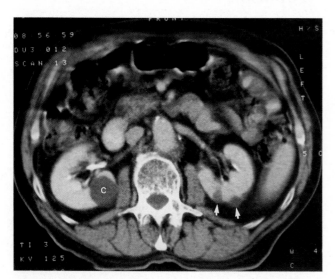

FIGURE 6-35 Computed tomography (CT) image shows a large cyst (C) in the posterior portion of the right kidney. Notice the two smaller cysts (*arrows*) on the left. (Daffner RH. *Clinical Radiology: The Essentials*. 3rd ed. Philadelphia, PA: Lippincott Williams & Wilkins; 2007.)

men. The radiograph shows a space-occupying lesion that distorts and displaces the collecting systems (Fig. 6-40). The tumor commonly shows an abnormal vasculature as seen during angiography (Fig. 6-41). Ultrasonography not only shows the composition of the tumor but also can demonstrate invasion of the renal vessels by the tumor (Fig. 6-42).

Nephroblastoma (Wilms tumor) is the most common malignant abdominal neoplasm occurring in

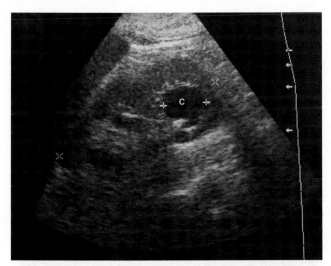

FIGURE 6-37   Longitudinal image shows the sonolucent cyst (C). Notice the increased echoes beneath the cyst (through transmission). (Daffner RH. *Clinical Radiology: The Essentials.* 3rd ed. Philadelphia, PA: Lippincott Williams & Wilkins; 2007.)

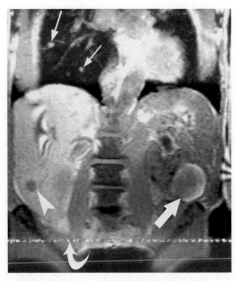

FIGURE 6-39   Metastatic renal cell carcinoma. Coronal gradient echo survey image demonstrates left renal cell carcinoma (*arrow*) with liver (*arrowhead*) and lung (*thin arrows*) metastases. This illustrates importance of careful scrutiny of entire image set when staging malignant tumors. Note the zipper artifact (*curved arrow*). (Leyendecker JR, Brown JJ. *Practical Guide to Abdominal and Pelvic MRI.* Philadelphia, PA: Lippincott Williams & Wilkins; 2004.)

A possible genetic cause has been suggested, as it is more common among siblings and twins. Most cases are noticed by symptoms of a palpable abdominal mass, blood in the urine, and fever. An IVU shows a large

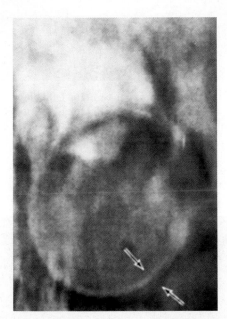

FIGURE 6-38   Renal cell carcinoma. Nephrotomogram demonstrates a lucent, well-demarcated renal mass with a thick wall (*arrows*). (Eisenberg RL. *Clinical Imaging: An Atlas of Differential Diagnosis.* 5th ed. Philadelphia, PA: Lippincott Williams & Wilkins; 2010.)

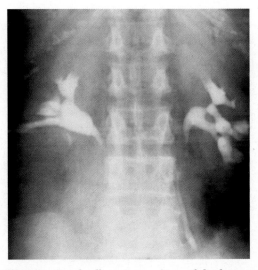

FIGURE 6-40   Renal cell carcinoma. Upward displacement of the right kidney and distortion of the collecting system by the large lower pole mass that cannot be seen on the X-ray. (Eisenberg RL. *Clinical Imaging: An Atlas of Differential Diagnosis.* 5th ed. Philadelphia, PA: Lippincott Williams & Wilkins; 2010.)

children. Only leukemia and brain tumors are more common in children. It is estimated that 1 out of every 10,000 children have a Wilms tumor. That is, 450 cases per year in the United States! The peak incidence is 3 years of age and the occurrence of the tumor after the age of 8 years is rare. The exact cause is unknown, but it is associated with birth defects of the urinary tract.

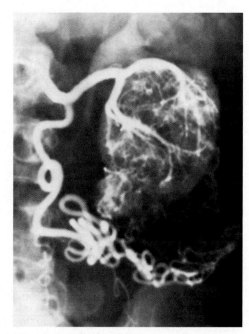

FIGURE 6-41   Renal cell carcinoma. Left renal arteriogram demonstrates a large hypervascular mass with striking enlargement of capsular vessels. (Eisenberg RL. *Clinical Imaging: An Atlas of Differential Diagnosis*. 5th ed. Philadelphia, PA: Lippincott Williams & Wilkins; 2010.)

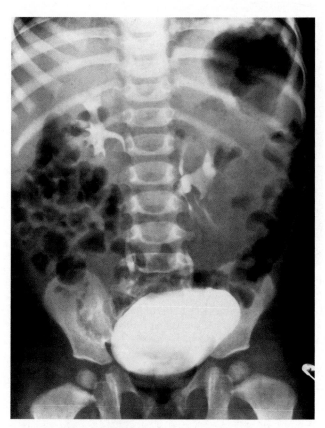

FIGURE 6-43   IVU shows a mass in the left kidney distorting the renal architecture, which was shown to be a nephroblastoma. (Daffner RH. *Clinical Radiology: The Essentials*. 3rd ed. Philadelphia, PA: Lippincott Williams & Wilkins; 2007.)

abdominal mass that displaces the kidney because of its location (Fig. 6-43). The use of abdominal CT will help stage the tumor and determine a prognosis (Fig. 6-44). Forty-three percent of patients with Wilms

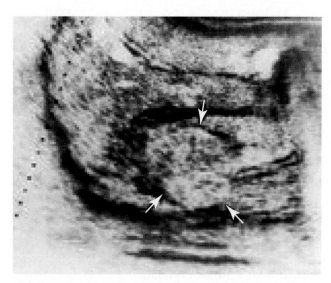

FIGURE 6-42   Renal cell carcinoma. Echo-filled solid mass (*arrows*) with no posterior enhancement. (Eisenberg RL. *Clinical Imaging: An Atlas of Differential Diagnosis*. 5th ed. Philadelphia, PA: Lippincott Williams & Wilkins; 2010.)

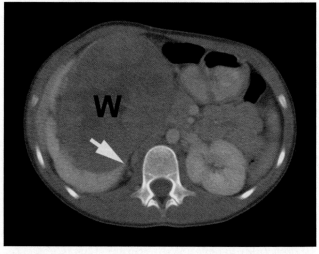

FIGURE 6-44   CT image shows the large right renal mass (W) of the Wilms tumor. Notice the "beak" sign at the junction of the tumor with normal kidney (*arrow*). (Daffner RH. *Clinical Radiology: The Essentials*. 3rd ed. Philadelphia, PA: Lippincott Williams & Wilkins; 2007.)

tumor are classified as stage I. In this stage, the kidney is intact and the tumor has not ruptured. If the tumor is completely removed and chemotherapy is initiated, 98% of patients have a 4-year survival rate. Stages II and III each involve 23% of the population. In these stages, the tumor involvement is more extensive and nephrectomy is indicated with radiation and chemotherapy. Prognosis is still high with a 4-year or more survival rate for 95% of the patients. The last two stages, stage IV and stage V, capture the remaining 15% of the patients with this disease. Stage IV shows metastases to the lung, liver, bone, or brain, and stage V requires bilateral renal involvement. The survival rate for both of these stages drops to approximately 76% surviving up to 4 years.

Nuclear medicine will demonstrate a nonfunctioning kidney by demonstrating the absence of the tracer accumulation in the kidney. Ultrasonography is done as a preoperative procedure to eliminate the possibility of IVC involvement with the tumor. Radiation therapy or chemotherapy may also be done preoperatively to shrink the tumor and decrease the risk to the patient.

Bladder carcinoma will usually begin in the epithelial tissue of the bladder. It occurs more often in men over the age of 50 years. The cause of this type of carcinoma has been related to excessive cigarette smoking, as the carcinogenic metabolites are excreted in the urine. There is also a high incidence of bladder cancer among workers in factories that manufacture aniline dyes. The tumor usually projects into the bladder in a papillary form, causing a filling defect on the bladder film of the ureogram (Fig. 6-45). However, because most tumors are small and located in the area of the trigone, detection by radiography is not as reliable a method as with CT, which can stage the tumor.

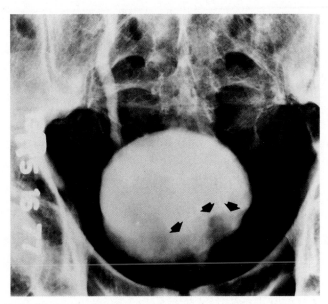

FIGURE 6-45   Bladder carcinoma (*arrowheads*) that has completely obstructed the left ureter. (Daffner RH. *Clinical Radiology: The Essentials*. 3rd ed. Philadelphia, PA: Lippincott Williams & Wilkins; 2007.)

Imaging Strategies

Extracorporeal Shock Wave Lithotripsy

Although extracorporeal shock wave lithotripsy (ESWL) is not an imaging modality, but rather a treatment procedure, the decision to include it in this section of the chapter was made due to its use of fluoroscopy and ultrasonography. ESWL was introduced in 1980 and has dramatically changed the way

renal stones were treated. For the past 30 years, it has remained the treatment of choice for renal and ureteral calculi. ESWL literally pulverizes a stone into smaller fragments by shock waves. The small fragments can now pass through the system and be excreted in the urine. This noninvasive procedure may even allow the patient to avoid surgery or an endoscopic procedure.

ESWL is an outpatient procedure that is usually performed with a mild sedative because the procedure may take about an hour to complete and the patient must lie reasonably still. It is generally painless and there is no need for general anesthesia.

Fluoroscopy and ultrasonography are used to localize the stone in the renal system. Fluoroscopy allows treatment to take place without interruption because of the ability to make continuous adjustments to pinpoint the shock wave placement on the stone. There are several drawbacks to the use of fluoroscopy. It uses radiation and it has limited, or no, ability to visualize the radiolucent stones unless contrast is injected.

Ultrasonography is able to locate both radiopaque and radiolucent stones. Also, it is not an ionizing modality so no radiation is involved. However, the kidneys often have overlapping bowel gas that hinders the ability of the sound waves to pass through and visualize the stone.

Newer generation lithotriptors are incorporating the use of ultrasonography and fluoroscopy in one unit. This is advantageous because each system is able to compensate for the limitation of the other.

Once the stones are located, energy is created by a shock wave generator called a lithotriptor, and sent across the skin through the visceral tissue and into the stone. First-generation lithotripsy units required the patient to be emerged in a water bath. Now, small water-filled cushions with a silicone membrane are placed on top of the patient's skin to provide an air-free contact. As many as 120 impulses per minute are used to break the stones into smaller pieces. To help with the stones passage after the treatment, a ureteral stent is sometimes put into place to allow for easier transit and passage through the ureter.

Ultrasonography

Ultrasonography becomes the method of choice for evaluating patients who are allergic to contrast media, have renal failure, have an elevated BUN level, or who are pregnant (during which time radiation should be avoided if at all possible). It can determine the source of abdominal pain, evaluate renal infection, identify congenital abnormalities, evaluate problems related to the prostate gland, and help in identifying injuries to the kidneys and bladder in an accident. Although sonography is helpful in imaging areas of the renal system, obesity can make this examination more difficult to perform and less accurate. Sonography plays a secondary role in the assessment of renal infection, abscess localization, evaluation of flank mass in children, and distinguishing cystic from solid components in renal masses. Doppler flow is useful for renal artery stenosis and thrombosis.

The kidneys are traditionally studied in both the transverse and longitudinal planes with the patient in the prone position. A complete study should also include scans with the patient in the decubitus position and supine position as well. Coronal sections correlate best with the kidney anatomy seen on IVUs.

Computed Tomography and Magnetic Resonance Imaging

Most renal abnormalities are best seen on **CT** after IV contrast has been administered. Studies done without contrast are best for demonstrating calcifications because the use of contrast would obstruct the visualization of the calculi. CT is useful in staging renal and bladder neoplasms or evaluating constricting ureteral lesions. CT is most useful in obese patients as adipose tissue enhances the renal boundaries. CT urography (CTU) has been recently designed to evaluate the entire urinary system by using thin slices to image the excretory phase.

Renal **MRI** helps to establish renal cell carcinoma and the extent to which this process has invaded the renal system. Because of the artifacts that occur on the CT scan near the IVC, MRI is most useful in assessing this area. MRI is also able to assess lesions and classify them as either cysts or cystic neoplasms. The best use of MRI is in patients with suspected renal artery stenosis. Since renovascular disease is one of the most common treatable causes of hypertension, it is a common indication for MRI.

Nuclear Medicine

Nuclear medicine scans of the renal system are used to image the function of the kidneys. It can be a screening tool, a diagnostic procedure, or a complimentary modality. Because of the sensitivity of the modality, it has become the modality of choice to study the function of the kidneys.

The **dynamic renal scan** (also known as a renogram) studies the function of the kidneys. The procedure studies the blood flow to the kidneys and how well each kidney is functioning for the production of urine. The procedure also shows if there are any obstructions in the output of urine. The radioisotope is injected and a series of scans will be taken over a period of about 30 minutes.

A **static renal scan** tells the physician about the size, shape, and location of the kidneys. It will also demonstrate any fibrous tissue on the kidney left from previous infections. Like the dynamic scan, an injection is given; however, this time, the patient may leave the department and return 3 hours later. The scan itself only requires about 30 minutes.

A third study, the **glomerular filtration (GFR) study** is not an actual scan but is a blood test done over a period of several hours. After an injection, the patient returns to the department in 2 hours. A blood sample is taken every hour for the next 3 hours. The blood itself is studied and tested for the amount of injected material that is still in the blood.

Interventional Radiography
Intravenous Urography

Intravenous urography (IVU) is a radiographic procedure for the entire urinary system. Although CT and sonography are used more frequently than an IVU in the imaging of the urinary system, it is still essential to understand how an IVU progresses and the impact of the contrast on the patient's system. An IVU is performed to determine the presence and location of an obstruction, the cause of abnormal laboratory results, the presence of arterial hypertension, and the location of a mass. For example, if the right kidney is displaced down and laterally, there could be a duodenal, pancreatic, or adrenal mass. In the male patient, a superiorly displaced bladder may indicate a prostate tumor. The contrast agents used, such as Conray or Isovue, are normally excreted and help to determine glomerular filtration. It takes about 15 minutes for an intravenously injected contrast medium to reach its greatest level of concentration in the renal collecting system. Fluid restriction in order to produce some dehydration improves the concentration of the contrast. The first portion of the excretory system to be shown by an IVU is the calyces. The post-void image also gives information, as it shows any reflux of urine from the bladder back into the ureters.

An IVU is performed in various manners in each imaging department. However, the following general information will apply to most facilities. After an injection into the venous system, the contrast will appear in the collecting system of the kidneys. The first radiographic image is usually taken 5 minutes after injection to identify the nephrocortical blush and the appearance of the collecting system. At 10 minutes postinjection, a KUB may be performed to see bladder filling, and then obliques are done to see the length of the ureter without superimposition of the vertebrae.

Variations of these times could include an image taken immediately postinjection. Known as a *nephrogram*, this first radiograph shows the blush of the renal cortex. If the contrast is injected under pressure as a bolus, a *hypertensive IVU* for high blood pressure may be underway. In hypertensive patients, there is decreased urinary flow and more concentration of contrast material on the affected side. Images taken at 1-minute intervals for 5 minutes will show the disproportionate concentration of contrast on the affected side.

T E C H   T I P

The technologist must be alert to the patient and any reactions following the injection of contrast in the advent that an allergic reaction is about to happen. It is essential to know the location and the contents of the "crash cart" in case it is needed.

Percutaneous Antegrade Pyelography and Percutaneous Nephrostomy

Percutaneous antegrade pyelography can study renal emptying after nephrostomy. Performed by direct puncture of the renal pelvis through the posterior lateral aspect of the patient, a catheter is placed into the renal pelvis and contrast material is injected directly into the kidney. The catheter can be left in place for therapy purposes. **Percutaneous nephrostomy** is performed when urinary drainage is difficult due to supravesical urinary tract obstruction or urinary diversion in patients with fistulas, leaks, or traumatic/iatrogenic ureteral dissections. Nephrostomy tubes have the advantage of allowing medication to be administered for the treatment of infections, to allow the drainage of infectious material and for the dissolution of stones through irrigation.

Retrograde Studies
Retrograde Urethrography

In order to study the length of the male urethra, patients are often moved to the surgery suite for mild sedation. The urinary meatus is opened to allow the tip of a syringe to be positioned into the urethra. Contrast is injected directly into the urethra to visualize the anatomical aspects. This procedure does not allow the study of the bladder as a voiding cystogram would.

Retrograde Pyelography

The study is also performed under mild sedation in the surgery area for cystoscopy. The patient is placed in a modified lithotomy position so that the ureterocystoscope can be inserted into the ureter with the tip placed as near the renal pelvis as possible. Contrast medium is injected into the renal pelvis and images are taken. Retrograde studies cannot study the function of any area that is assessed.

Cystography

Cystography is a study of the bladder. A catheter is inserted through the urethra into the bladder and contrast media is instilled into the bladder. When the bladder is full, the catheter is removed and radiographic images are taken. If the images are also taken as the patient voids, the term cystourethrography is used since now the urethra can be studied in addition to the bladder. This procedure is used to determine the cause of infections, locations of tumors or stones, and to check for reflux into the ureters (see the figure in Case Study).

Pediatric Voiding Cystourethrogram

Also known as a voiding cystourethrography (VCUG), this procedure allows the visualization of the bladder and lower urinary tract (urethra). As explained earlier in the section "Cystography," a catheter is inserted into the bladder and contrast is instilled into the bladder. Once the bladder is full, the catheter is removed and the patient is required to void while fluoroscopic images are taken to visualize the anatomy and function of the bladder and lower urinary tract. Abnormalities in the flow of urine through the tract are seen during the voiding phase of the procedure.

RECAP

The nephron, found in the renal cortex, is the functioning unit of the kidney. If the nephron is compromised by disease, the kidney's function will be impacted. If a kidney's function falls to less than 10% of its ability, it is considered to be in failure.

Pathology

- Congenital
  - Bifid: double collecting system; can be multiples of any part of the urinary system
    - Incidental finding on the image and it is of little consequence in most cases
  - Horseshoe kidney: lower poles unite causing the renal pelvis to become more horizontal leading to the formation of renal calculi.
  - Ectopia
    - Crossed (where the lower kidney is on the opposite side) or
    - Located in another location, such as in the pelvis
    - Congenitally short ureter will differentiate ectopia from a floating kidney (nephroptosis)
    - In most cases, ectopic kidneys pose no problems
  - Polycystic renal disease
    - Two types: infantile and childhood
    - Symptoms include high blood pressure, masses in the kidney or abdomen, and abdominal tenderness over the liver
    - Complications include high blood pressure, anemia, recurrent urinary tract and kidney infection, kidney stones, and mild to severe kidney failure
  - Renal agenesis: uncommon absence of one kidney
    - Associated with hyperplasia of remaining kidney
    - Inflammatory processes
  - Glomerulonephritis (aka Bright disease) is caused by strep infection
    - Signs/symptoms include hypertension, edema of face and ankles, and arthralgia
    - Complications are possible progressive renal failure leading to uremia or chronic inflammation of the kidneys leading to fibrosis
  - Weakening of the ureteral or bladder wall causes diverticula
    - Asymptomatic
    - Complications are usually in the form of calculi due to stagnant urine collecting in the pouch of the "tick"

- Best seen on a retrograde urogram or intravenous urogram (IVU)
○ Ureterocele is a cyst-like dilation of the ureter
  - Radiographic sign is "cobra head"; the size becomes smaller as urine pressure increases in the bladder
○ Prostatic hypertrophy is enlargement of prostate gland
  - Most men over age 55 years experience some problem
  - The base of the bladder can have an indentation from the gland pushing up
○ Hydronephrosis
  - Enlargement of the collecting system caused by any obstruction to the ureter
  - Signs and symptoms are hematuria, pyuria, and fever
  - Radiographic images from an IVU will show enlargement of the system above obstruction with sharply defined calyces
○ Hypertension
  - Caused be narrowing of the renal artery (primary) or an infectious process such as glomerulonephritis or pyelonephritis (secondary)
  - Symptoms are usually in the form of elevated blood pressure
○ Pyelonephritis is inflammation of the kidney and renal pelvis
  - Caused by *E. coli* that causes bacteriuria, pyuria, dysuria, and flank pain
○ Vesicoureteral reflux (VUR)
  - Caused by an incompetent ureteral valve
  - Children with VUR and urinary tract infection (UTI) need to be diagnosed early to avoid loss of growth
○ Renal calculi are solid masses of calcium and oxalates
  - Grow in the urinary tract of the kidney but may form in the bladder
  - Usually asymptomatic until descending then cause pain and hematuria
  - Calcium stone most common
  - If the stone fills the renal pelvis, it is called a staghorn calculus
  - Nephrocalcinosis is numerous calcifications within the renal parenchyma

○ Renal failure
  - Two forms: acute and chronic
  - Nephrosis occurs leading to oliguria
  - Patient has edema and uremia
  - Dialysis may be necessary
  - IVU is difficult because the nephrons cannot concentrate the contrast media well
○ Cysts
  - Benign and occur in the cortex
  - Asymptomatic
  - Seen on CT or ultrasonography better than radiography
  - Neoplasms
○ Hypernephroma is also called a Grawitz tumor
  - Arises from the renal tubule cells
  - Destroys the kidney and invades the blood vessels
○ Nephroblastoma is also known as a Wilms tumor
  - Most common in children
  - It metastasizes quickly
  - Prognosis is poor if not treated early
○ Bladder carcinoma
  - Found more often in males aged over 50 years who have a history of excessive smoking or in factory workers where aniline dye is manufactured
  - Causes a filling defect in the bladder
  - CT is the best modality for diagnosing

Imaging Modalities

- While CT, MRI, and ultrasound can all study the size, shape, and location of the organs, they cannot study their function
  ○ Nuclear medicine scans study renal function but do not assess the structure
  ○ Antegrade studies and retrograde studies can show anatomy but not the function
  ○ IVUs will demonstrate not only structure but also function
    - IVU cannot quantify the amount of glomerular filtration like a nuclear medicine study can

CLINICAL AND RADIOGRAPHIC CHARACTERISTICS OF COMMON PATHOLOGIES

Pathologic Condition	Causal Factors to Include Age, if Relevant	Manifestations	Radiographic Appearance
Horseshoe kidney	Congenital	Kidney stones	Lower poles fused across the midline

PKD
  Newborn
  Childhood
  Adult
	Congenital
	—
	Seen at 3–5 y
	Seen after 30 y
		Oligohydramnios
		Nephromegaly
		Hepatosplenomegaly, portal hypertension
		Hypertension, renal insufficiency, uremia
			Large, lobulated kidneys with elongated renal pelvis, distorted calyces

Glomerulonephritis	Strep infection Young adults	Hypertension, edema, nausea, arthralgia	Large kidneys early, with small kidneys later

Diverticula
  Ureterocele
	Weak wall
	Weak distal ureter
		Stones and infection	Outpouchings
			  Cobra head

Hydronephrosis	Obstruction of renal pelvis or ureter	Hematuria, pyuria, fever	Enlarged, well-defined calyces, dilation proximal to obstruction
Hypertension	Narrowing of renal arteries	High blood pressure	Small kidney, delayed excretion, hyperconcentration of contrast agent
Pyelonephritis	Pyogenic bacteria	Flank pain, bacteriuria	Blunted calyces, decreased kidney size

Calculi
  Staghorn
  Nephrocalcinosis
	Clusters of calcium	Hematuria, flank pain	Calcifications
			Large stone fills renal pelvis
			Multiple calcifications in cortex

Renal failure
  Acute
  Chronic
	Ischemia, toxic injury	Massive edema
		Hypertension, CHF
			Bilateral enlargement, prolonged blush
			Sonography recommended

Renal cyst	<50 y	Asymptomatic	Calyceal spreading
Hypernephroma	<40 y	Hematuria	Space-occupying lesion
Nephroblastoma	>5 y	Firm, palpable abdominal mass	Large abdominal mass, displaces kidney
Bladder cancer	Males <50 y Excessive smoking	Asymptomatic	Filling defect, CT recommended

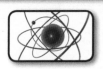

CRITICAL THINKING DISCUSSION QUESTIONS

1. Describe a hypertensive intravenous urogram.

2. Define cystography. Indicate why each is done and how it is performed. What examination can be combined with cystography and what will this demonstrate?

3. Describe each of the following procedures. What will each demonstrate?
   a. Retrograde urethrography
   b. Retrograde pyelography
   c. Percutaneous antegrade pyelography

4. Name two nuclear medicine studies of the kidneys. Why is each of them performed? Why is nuclear medicine necessary for renal imaging?

5. Describe extracorporeal shock wave lithotripsy (ESWL). Include in the description what it is, why it is performed, and how it is performed. What other procedures are performed with it?

6. When is ultrasonography used to image the renal system and why is this modality useful to the study of urinary disease?

7. Define horseshoe kidney. Describe its radiographic appearance. What condition is common with this condition? Why?

8. Describe polycystic kidney disease. What are the complications of this disease? What do the images demonstrate?

9. Describe glomerulonephritis. What causes it? How may death be caused? Why does this cause small kidneys? Which imaging modality is best to demonstrate this?

10. Compare and contrast acute and chronic renal failure (what each is, what they cause, what causes them, what the manifestations are of each). Explain why intravenous urography is detrimental to the patient of renal failure. If it is performed, how is the contrast material excreted? What other organ can be seen if this occurs? Why? What imaging modality is best suited for a patient of renal failure? What can this procedure demonstrate?

11. Compare and contrast a Wilms tumor and a Grawitz tumor by addressing the following: what is the definition; what are the alternative names; what causes it; who is more likely to have it; and where does it actually occur?

12. Describe where bladder cancer occurs and how this relates to the use of CT. What will the radiographic appearance be?

The Reproductive System

Goals

1. To review the basic anatomy of both the male and the female systems

   OBJECTIVE: Identify anatomic structures on diagrams and radiographic images of the reproductive system

2. To become acquainted with the physiology of the reproductive system

   OBJECTIVE: Describe the physiology of the male and the female reproductive systems

3. To become familiar with the radiographic manifestations of all the common congenital and acquired disorders of both the male and the female reproductive systems

   OBJECTIVE: Describe the various pathologic conditions affecting the female reproductive system and their radiographic manifestations

   OBJECTIVE: Describe the various pathologic conditions affecting the male reproductive system and their radiographic manifestations

Key Terms

Adenomyosis
Chocolate cysts
Corpus luteum
Cryptorchidism
Dermoid
Dysmenorrhea
Endometriosis
Epididymitis
Fibroadenoma
Gynecomastia
Hydrocele
Leiomyoma
Menopause
Menstrual cycle
Nulligravida
Nullipara
Orchiectomy
Orchiopexy
Ovulation
Pelvic inflammatory disease (PID)
Polycystic ovarian disease
Prostatic calculi
Prostatic hyperplasia

● Goals *continued*

4. To determine the special modalities and procedures that will demonstrate the pathologies of both systems

   OBJECTIVE: Describe the special radiographic examinations of the female reproductive system

   OBJECTIVE: Briefly explain mammography and its importance in women's health

● Key Terms *continued*

Pyosalpinx
Seminomas
Spermatocele
Spermatogenesis
Teratoma
Testicular torsion
Tubal ovarian abscess

184

The reproductive system of the female is studied by radiography more often than the reproductive system of the male. Subspecialties of radiography such as ultrasonography and nuclear medicine play an important role in demonstrating various pathologic conditions. Many pathologic conditions are quite common and present symptoms that should be familiar to the technologist. The external genitalia of the female are collectively termed the vulva and include the mons pubis, labia major and minor, clitoris, vaginal orifice, and Bartholin glands. The male external genitalia consist of the scrotum and the penis. Although these areas are considered to be a portion of the reproductive system (accessory organs in the urinary system in the male), the external genitalia will not be discussed further.

TECH TIP

Ultrasonography is now the major method of choice for demonstrating the reproductive organs of both the female and male patients because there is no radiation involved.

Anatomy

Female Reproductive Organs

The female reproductive organs are a uterus, a vagina, a pair of ovaries, and a pair of fallopian tubes. The breasts are accessory organs.

The uterus is a thick-walled, hollow, pear-shaped organ that lies in the pelvic cavity between the bladder and the rectum. The upper portion of the uterus, the body, also known as the corpus, has a rounded swelling, just above and between the entry points of the uterine tubes, called the fundus. The lower, narrower portion of the uterus is the cervix. The opening from the cervix of the uterus into the cervical canal is called the internal os, and the opening from the cervical canal into the vagina is called the external os.

The uterine wall is composed of three layers. The internal lining is a specialized epithelial mucous membrane called endometrium. The middle layer, the myometrium, is formed of three layers of smooth muscle, extending diagonally, crosswise, and lengthwise. The external layer is formed of serous membrane, called perimetrium, which covers only a portion of the body of the uterus.

The uterus normally sits in the pelvis at a forward angle, with the fundus of the uterus toward the abdominal wall. There should be an almost 90° angle between the vaginal canal and the body of the uterus. This position is known as anteverted. Additionally, the uterus can be slightly anteflexed and not be considered in a deviated position. When the bladder is filled, the anteflexion becomes less pronounced. Normally the uterus is located in the midline of the pelvic cavity; however, the uterus may extend to the right or left side of the patient's midline. A uterus that is deviated to the left may be termed livo-rotated, while a uterus that is deviated to the right of the patient's midline may be termed dextro-rotated.

The vagina is a flattened dilatable canal that enters the cervix at right angles when in a normal position. The vagina forms a cuff around the cervix known as the fornix.

The ovaries lie in the ovarian fossa behind the broad ligament on either sides of the uterus. They lie at an angle between the external iliac vein in front and the ureter behind. Each ovary lies beneath the suspended end of a uterine tube but does not come into contact with the tube.

There are two uterine (fallopian) tubes. The proximal ends of the tubes open into the uterus at the isthmus. This opening is known as the uterine ostium. The distal ends, the infundibulum, are funnel-shaped with fringed, finger-like processes called fimbriae. The fimbriated ends are over but not attached to or touching the ovaries. The opening at this end is known as the abdominal ostium. The ampulla is the largest portion immediately adjacent to the infundibulum. Figure 7-1A, B shows the coronal and sagittal sections of the female reproductive organs.

The female breasts are lobulated, glandular structures on the anterior lateral surface of the thorax. Their development is controlled by hormones secreted by the ovaries. The breast is cone-shaped, with the base

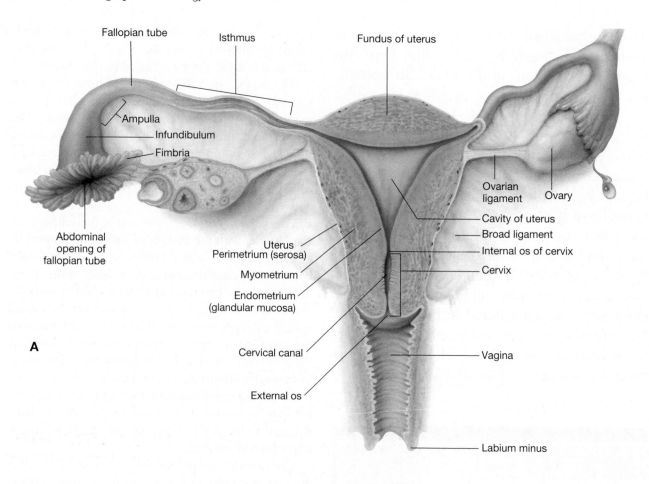

Fallopian tube

Isthmus

Fundus of uterus

Ampulla

Infundibulum

Fimbria

Abdominal opening of fallopian tube

Uterus Perimetrium (serosa)

Myometrium

Endometrium (glandular mucosa)

Cervical canal

External os

Ovarian ligament

Ovary

Cavity of uterus

Broad ligament

Internal os of cervix

Cervix

Vagina

Labium minus

A

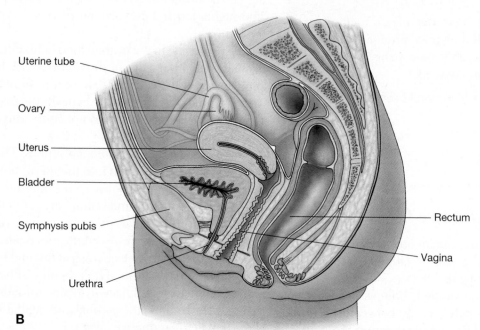

Uterine tube

Ovary

Uterus

Bladder

Symphysis pubis

Urethra

Rectum

Vagina

B

FIGURE 7-1   (A) This coronal section shows the interior aspect of the uterus and the relationship of the ovaries to the fallopian tubes. (B) This lateral view shows the relationship of the fundus of the uterus to the cervix as well as the bladder and uterus. (A: Asset provided by Anatomical Chart Co.; B: Daffner RH. *Clinical Radiology: The Essentials.* 3rd ed. Philadelphia, PA: Lippincott Williams & Wilkins; 2007.)

against the chest wall, and tapers down to the nipple, which is surrounded by a circular pigmented area called the areola. Breast tissue is composed of adipose and connective tissue consisting of lobules and milk ducts. Each breast consists of 15 to 20 lobes that are divided into 20 or 40 lobules, which contain the milk-producing acini cells. These lobules are the basic structural unit of the breast. Within the lobules are the lactiferous ducts, which unite to drain to the nipple.

The layer of subcutaneous fibrous tissue provides support for the breast. Cooper ligaments extend from the connective tissue layer, through the breast, and attach to the underlying muscle fascia, providing further support for the breast. The muscles forming the floor of the breast are the greater and smaller pectorals, the anterior serratus, the latissimus dorsi, the subscapular, the external oblique, and the straight abdominal muscles.

The glandular and connective tissues are water-dense, firm, homogeneous breast that show little tissue differentiation. During pregnancy and lactation, the breasts become very dense and opaque. After pregnancy, the breasts undergo involution and fatty infiltration. Involution is the process of the lobules decreasing in size as well as number. The space left is filled with fat. The tissue regenerates for each pregnancy to a point, but with each succeeding pregnancy, the breast tissue becomes fattier. Menopausal women have almost no density in their breast because the entire organ is made up of fat.

Male Reproductive Organs

The male reproductive organs are the testes, epididymides, vas deferens, ejaculatory ducts, seminal vesicles, prostate gland, and Cowper glands.

The testes are a pair of egg-shaped glands normally located in a sac-like structure that hangs from the perineal areas known as the scrotum. The scrotum, which is divided into two sacs internally, also contains one epididymis and the inferior part of a spermatic cord. Each testicle is enclosed in a fibrous white capsule and is divided into compartments, each of which contains a seminiferous tube that joins into a cluster from which several ducts appear and enter the head of the epididymis. It is in the seminiferous tubules that sperm are formed.

The epididymis is a tightly coiled, tube-like structure about 20 feet long. It lies along the posterior border of the testis. The epididymis stores sperm before

ejaculation. The vas deferens is a tube that is the continuation of the epididymis. It extends from the epididymis up through the inguinal canal, where it is encased by the spermatic cord, into the abdominal cavity and down the posterior side of the bladder where it connects with the seminal vesicle duct and forms the ejaculatory duct. The ejaculatory ducts pass through the prostate gland and extend to the urethra.

The seminal vesicles are two twisted pouches lying along the bladder's lower posterior surface and in front of the rectum. They secrete a portion of the liquid part of semen. The prostate gland is composed of smooth muscle and glandular tissue. It surrounds the neck of the bladder and the urethra. The prostate gland secretes a thin, alkaline substance that makes up the majority of the seminal fluid (Fig. 7-2).

Cowper glands (bulbourethral glands) lie on either side of the urethra below the prostate gland. These glands secrete an alkaline fluid similar to that produced by the prostate gland that protects the sperm from the acid present in the vagina.

Physiology and Function

Female

The ovaries are responsible for the production of ova and the secretion of the female hormones estrogen and progesterone. Estrogen is responsible for growth and maintenance of the reproductive organs and secondary sex characteristics. Progesterone and estrogen prepare the endometrium for pregnancy and the breasts for milk production.

Females are born with approximately 200,000 potential ova-containing follicles in each ovary. Menarche usually begins between the ages of 11 and 15. Once each month, around the first day of menstruation, the follicular cells start to secrete estrogen. In most cycles, only one follicle matures and migrates to the surface of the ovary, where it ruptures and expels the mature ovum into the pelvic cavity. The expulsion of the mature follicle is known as **ovulation**.

The remaining cells of the ruptured follicle enlarge. With the deposit of lutein, the follicle becomes known as the **corpus luteum** and continues to grow for 7 to 8 days. The corpus luteum secretes progesterone in increasing amounts. If fertilization of the ovum has not occurred, the size and secretions of the corpus luteum

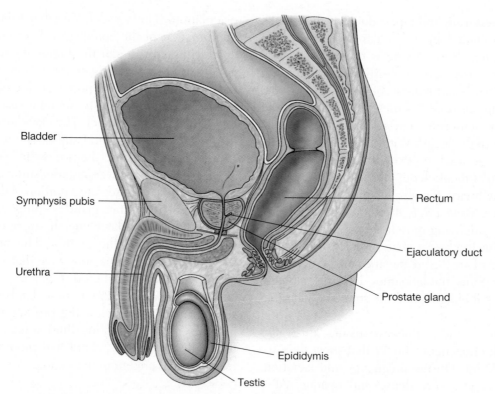

Bladder

Symphysis pubis

Urethra

Rectum

Ejaculatory duct

Prostate gland

Epididymis

Testis

FIGURE 7-2   Sagittal section of the male pelvic cavity. (Dean D, Herbener TE. *Cross-Sectional Human Anatomy*. Baltimore, MD: Lippincott Williams & Wilkins; 2000.)

gradually diminish until the nonfunctional structure is reduced and eventually disappears. If fertilization does occur, the corpus luteum remains intact throughout the pregnancy.

The cyclic changes in the ovaries are controlled by a variety of substances secreted by the anterior pituitary gland. Growth of the primitive Graafian follicles and ova and the secretion of estrogen are controlled by the follicle-stimulating hormone, whereas follicular rupture, expulsion of its ripe ovum, and the secretion of progesterone are under the control of the luteinizing hormone.

The **menstrual cycle** refers to the changes in the endometrium of the uterus that occur in women throughout the childbearing years. Each cycle lasts about 28 days and is divided into three phases: proliferative, secretory, and menstrual.

The *proliferative phase* occurs between the end of the menses and ovulation. The *secretory phase* occurs between ovulation and the onset of menses. The length of this phase is fairly constant and usually lasts 14 days. The *menstrual phase* of the cycle is when the actual flow of blood, mucus, and endometrium from the uterus begins and ends. This usually lasts about 4 to 6 days, until the low level of progesterone causes

the pituitary gland to again secrete follicle-stimulating hormone and a new menstrual cycle begins.

The reproductive years of a woman terminate with the cessation of the menstrual cycle. This is known as **menopause** and usually occurs in the late 40s or early 50s, but may be later.

Male

The major function of the male reproductive system is the formation of sperm, known as **spermatogenesis**. In addition to sperm cell production, the testes secrete the male hormone testosterone, which is responsible for adult male sexual behavior. Testosterone also helps regulate metabolism by promoting growth of skeletal muscles and is thus responsible for the greater male muscular development and strength. The final maturation of sperm occurs in the epididymis. The sperm spend from 1 to 3 weeks in the epididymis before they become motile and capable of fertilizing an ovum. From the epididymis, sperm are conveyed into the vas deferens where they may remain up to 1 month without loss of fertility. An alkaline fluid is secreted by the vas deferens to maintain viability of the sperm.

Male fertility is related not only to the number of sperm ejaculated but also to their size, shape, and motility. It is hypothesized that sterility results when the sperm count falls below about 50 million sperm per milliliter of semen. Unlike those for a woman, the reproductive years for a man never end. He is able to fertilize an ovum throughout his life.

Pathology

Female

Congenital Anomalies

Congenital anomalies of the female reproductive organs usually are in the form of duplications. There are various positions of the uterus that are not considered normal yet are of little consequence.

As was stated earlier, the normal position of the uterus is a slight anteflexion, which means the fundus is anterior to the cervix. It is also anteverted in that the fundus is away from the rectum (see Fig. 7-1B). If the uterine fundus is tipped backward so that there no longer exists a 90° angle between the vagina, cervix, and uterine body, and the fundus is now posterior to the cervix, the condition is known as retroversion. If there is backward flexion and the uterine body is now pointing down toward the rectum, the uterus is said to be retroflexed. Both of these anomalies are quite common and present no significant problems. The fundus of the uterus may also be flexed forward more than it should be. This position is known as acute anteflexion. The meanings of these terms are described in Display 7-1.

Figures 7-3 through 7-5- show these abnormal positions of the uterus.

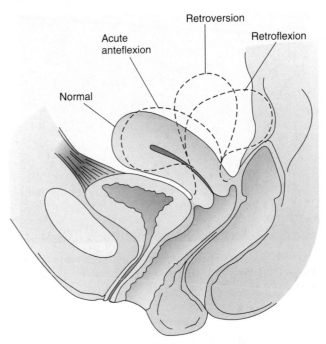

FIGURE 7-3   The dotted lines show the following abnormal positions of the uterus: retroverted; severely anteflexed; retroflexed. (Porth CM. *Pathophysiology Concepts of Altered Health States.* 7th ed. Philadelphia, PA: Lippincott Williams & Wilkins; 2005.)

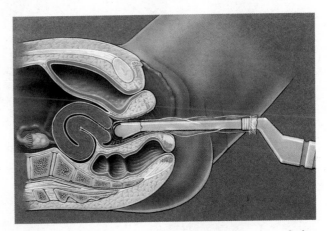

FIGURE 7-4   Schematic of transvaginal sonography with the probe adjacent to the cervix in a retroflexed uterus. (Drawing by Paul Gross, MS.)

The uterus is made from paired ducts called Müllerian ducts that fuse from the lower end. The lower end fuses to become the uterus and the two top ends of the ducts each become a fallopian tube. Congenital anomalies result from varying degrees of failure of fusion of the Müllerian ducts (Fig. 7-6). Many of these malformations can be detected by radiographic studies such as hysterosalpingography.

DISPLAY 7-1 POSITION ANOMALIES

Distinction	More Common	Less Common
Position tipped	"Anteverted": tipped forward	"Retroverted": tipped backward
Position of fundus	"Anteflexed": Fundus is pointing forward relative to the cervix	"Retroflexed": Fundus is pointing backward

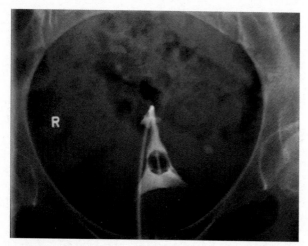

FIGURE 7-5   Hysterosalpingogram showing a retroverted uterus. Note the uterus is positioned completely upside down.

In rare occasions, the Müllerian ducts do not form in utero. When this happens, there can be no uterus. This condition is known as **uterine aplasia**. If only one duct forms, there can be no fusion. One duct remains as one half of an elongated uterus and only one fallopian tube. This is known as a **unicornuate uterus** (Fig. 7-7). However, a normal vagina is present and successful pregnancy can occur. In most patients, the kidney is missing on the same side as the missing half of the uterus.

A rare condition known as **didelphic uterus** occurs when there is nonfusion of the two Müllerian ducts. The result is complete duplication (Figs. 7-8 and 7-9). There are two cervixes and two uterine bodies (Fig. 7-10) but the normal number of fallopian tubes. In most patients, the vagina is septate, causing a double

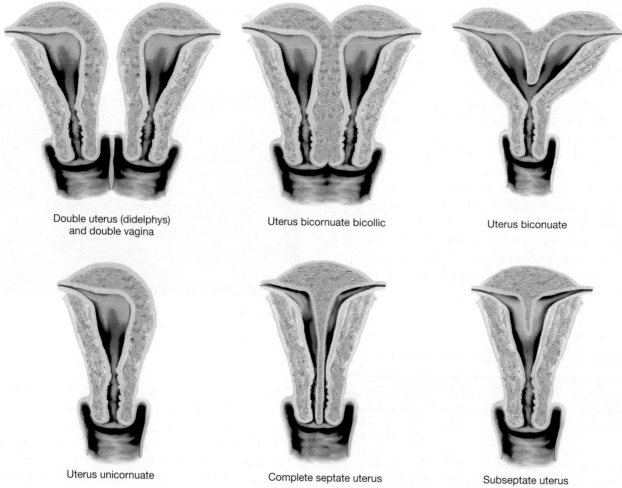

Double uterus (didelphys)
and double vagina

Uterus bicornuate bicollic

Uterus biconuate

Uterus unicornuate

Complete septate uterus

Subseptate uterus

FIGURE 7-6   **Uterine anomalies.** (Baggish MS, Valled RF, Guedj H. *Hysteroscopy: Visual Perspectives of Uterine Anatomy, Physiology and Pathology*. Philadelphia, PA: Lippincott Williams & Wilkins; 2007.)

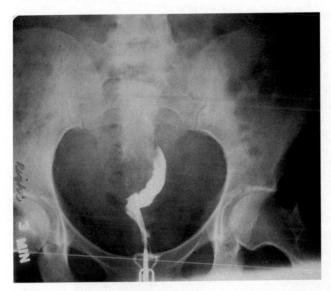

FIGURE 7-7   Unicornuate uterus.

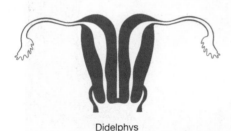

Didelphys

FIGURE 7-8   Didelphic uterus. There are two complete vaginas, cervices, and uterine bodies. (LifeART image, copyright © 2013. Lippincott Williams & Wilkins. All rights reserved.)

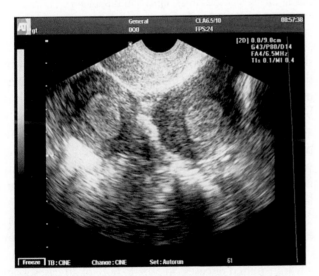

FIGURE 7-9   Two-dimensional transvaginal sonographic image of a didelphic uterus. Both endometrial cavities are clearly visible. (Baggish MS, Valled RF, Guedj H. *Hysteroscopy: Visual Perspectives of Uterine Anatomy, Physiology and Pathology.* Philadelphia, PA: Lippincott Williams & Wilkins; 2007.)

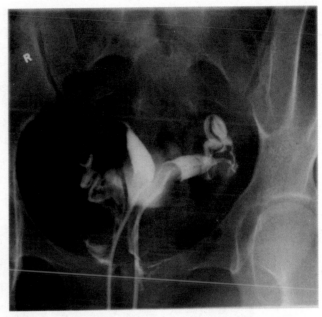

FIGURE 7-10   Hysterosalpingogram showing two complete vaginas, cervices, and uterine bodies.

vagina. In such cases, the two uterine bodies are often of different sizes.

A **bicornuate bicollic uterus** (Figs. 7-11 and 7-12) occurs when the ducts fuse to the level of the cervix, creating one vagina, two cervixes, and two uterine bodies. A very common duplication anomaly is called a **bicornuate uterus**, which occurs when the ducts fuse to the level of the body so that there are two fundi. A bicornuate uterus is important in pregnancy in that twin gestational sacs could implant in each horn of the fundus. It is possible for a mass to form in one horn with a pregnancy in the other (Fig. 7-13).

If the nonfusion of the Müllerian ducts begins at the level of the fundus, the condition is known as an **arcuate uterus** (Figs. 7-14 and 7-15). This is the most common anomaly and produces only minimal external contour deformity.

In the **septate uterus**, a septum extends through the normal uterine body to reach the cervix, dividing the uterus into two complete compartments (Fig. 7-16).

A **subseptate uterus** has a partial septum dividing the body only. The septum does not extend to the cervix. For some unexplained reason, twins occur in women with this condition three times more often than women with a normal uterus. Pregnancy may still occur in many women despite these anomalies. The incidence of complications during pregnancy is considerably increased, however. Complications include

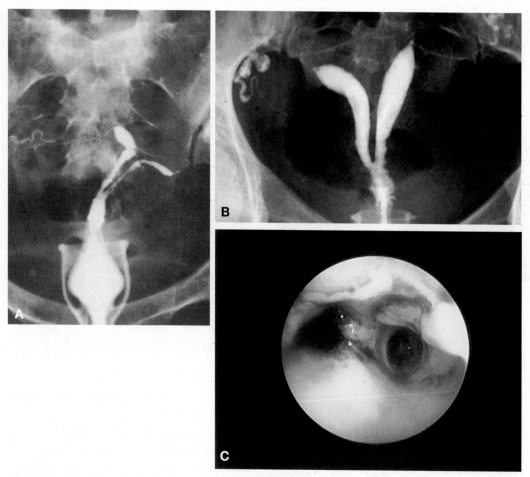

FIGURE 7-11   Hysterosalpingogram of a bicornuate bicollic uterus. (A) Hysteroscopy demonstrated a long central adhesion reaching the fundus. (B) New radiologic view of a complete septum. (C) Hysteroscopic view of the septum taken just at the internal os. (Baggish MS, Valled RF, Guedj H. *Hysteroscopy: Visual Perspectives of Uterine Anatomy, Physiology and Pathology*. Philadelphia, PA: Lippincott Williams & Wilkins; 2007.)

abortion, premature delivery, hemorrhages, retained placenta, and breech presentation.

Inflammatory Processes

Endometriosis is defined as the growth of endometrial tissue outside the uterus, usually on the ovary, fallopian tube, broad ligament, pouch of Douglas, or retrovaginal septum. This condition is more common in women who have never been pregnant (**nulligravida**) and are over the age of 30. When the endometrium sloughs off during the monthly cycle, some of the blood and mucus refluxes into the pelvis and attaches to the aforementioned ectopic areas.

Even though the endometrial tissue lies outside the uterus, it still responds to hormonal changes and undergoes a proliferative and secretory phase along with

sloughing a subsequent bleeding. Old blood turns brown; therefore, the pockets of endometrial tissue are known as **chocolate cysts**. The blood that escapes each month is brown in color. Sterility may occur if the tubes are badly affected. Symptoms of endometriosis include severe pain with the period (**dysmenorrhea**) and a dull aching pain during the remainder of the month. **Adenomyosis** is the ingrowth of endometrium into the uterine musculature. This condition may coexist with endometriosis.

Pelvic inflammatory disease (PID) is an inflammation of the female upper genital tract including the fallopian tubes. It is one of the most serious complications of sexually transmitted diseases. In 50% to 60% of all cases, bacteria that are the result of gonorrhea cause PID. Infection may occur by other routes such as an intrauterine contraceptive device and nonsterile abortions or deliveries. *Acute PID* causes slight uterine enlargement. In the

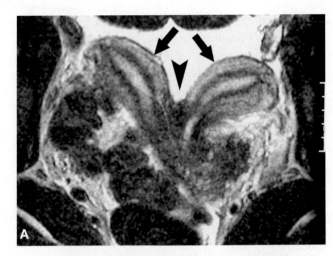

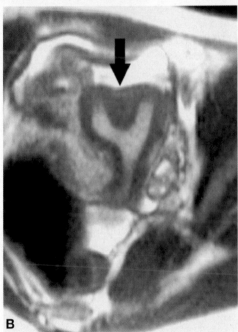

FIGURE 7-12   (A) is a bicornuate bicollic uterus. Note the large separation between the uterine horns (arrows) and a cleft in the fundus (arrowhead). (B) A subseptate uterus. Note the lack of fundal cleft (arrow) at the site of the thick septum. (Leyendecker JR, Brown JJ. *Practical Guide to Abdominal and Pelvic MRI.* Philadelphia, PA: Lippincott Williams & Wilkins; 2004.)

early stages, the pelvic sidewall structures can still be identified. Because the fallopian tubes open into the pelvic cavity, infection may spread to the ovaries and adjacent structures if the infundibulum is not closed by scar tissue. As the disease progresses, the adnexa become thicker and begins to merge with the sidewall. More than 25% of women with advanced PID have at least one complication, which can include ectopic pregnancy, infertility, and/or chronic abdominal pain.

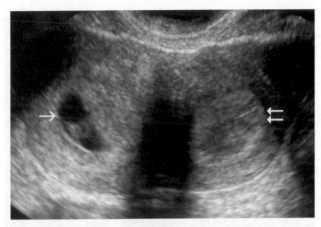

FIGURE 7-13   Bicornuate uterus. Sonographic transverse view clearly shows the two separate horns of the fundi in which one horn has a pregnancy. The gestational sac is in the right horn and the left horn shows decidual changes.

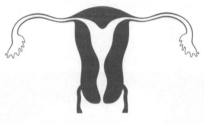

Arcuate

FIGURE 7-14   Schematic representation of an arcuate uterus. (LifeART image, copyright ©2013. Lippincott Williams & Wilkins. All rights reserved.)

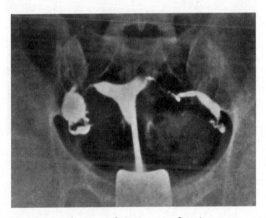

FIGURE 7-15   A hysterosalpingogram showing an arcuate uterus. (Beckmann CRB, Ling FW, et al. *Obstetrics and Gynecology.* 5th ed. Philadelphia, PA: Lippincott Williams & Wilkins; 2006.)

If left untreated, a **pyosalpinx** (pus in the tube) will develop. This will eventually lead to a **tubal ovarian abscess** (TOA) (Fig. 7-17). If a TOA or a pyosalpinx ruptures, peritonitis may ensue, which can be

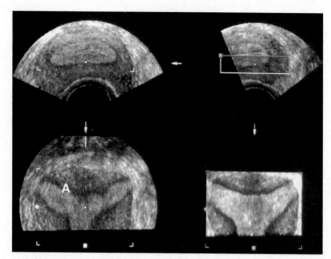

FIGURE 7-16   Three-dimensional sonographic examination of a septate uterus. *Top row (left to right)* demonstrates the transverse and longitudinal planes, respectively. *Bottom row, left* is a coronal section showing the fundus being divided into two compartments. *Bottom row, right* is a composite performed to enhance diagnostic accuracy to assure septate versus bicollic uterus.

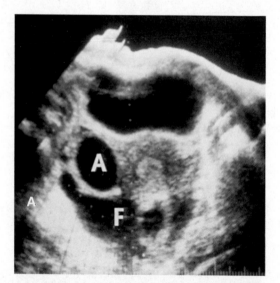

FIGURE 7-17   Tubal ovarian abscess (TOA) (A). There is fluid (F) in the cul-de-sac posterior to the abscess. (Eisenberg RL. *An Atlas of Differential Diagnosis.* 4th ed. Philadelphia, PA: Lippincott Williams & Wilkins; 2003.)

localized in the right upper quadrant under the liver. Free fluid in the cul-de-sac is usually seen with PID.

Ultrasonography should be the first diagnostic imaging procedure performed when PID is suspected. Transvaginal sonography allows detailed visualization of the uterus and the adnexa, including the ovaries. Magnetic resonance imaging (MRI) serves as

an excellent imaging modality in cases in which the sonographic findings are equivocal. Occasionally, computed tomography (CT) scanning may be used; however, the radiation exposure is high and must be considered before utilizing CT over ultrasonography.

In *chronic PID*, all the signs of acute PID are gone and the uterus has sharp borders. The adnexa may demonstrate nonspecific thickening because of continued scarring (Fig. 7-18). PID is a common cause of ectopic pregnancy. The fertilized ovum is unable to pass through the scarred, narrow tubes and therefore becomes implanted at this point. Ultrasound is used to determine the location of the ectopic pregnancy before it ruptures.

Neoplasms
Benign

Leiomyomas, also known as fibroids, leiomyomata, or myomata, are composed of connective tissue and muscle fiber. While the more common term "fibroid" is used to define benign tumors of the uterus, this term has been determined to be not technically correct and its use should be discouraged. They are the overgrowth of the normal muscular wall of the uterus. Leiomyomas are very common after the age of 35 years. Since they thrive on estrogen, postmenopausal women do not grow new tumors. If a neoplasm exists before menopause, it will atrophy as the estrogen levels drop after menopause.

Leiomyomas are the most common benign tumor of the uterus. There are three types: submucosal, intramural, and subserous (Fig. 7-19).

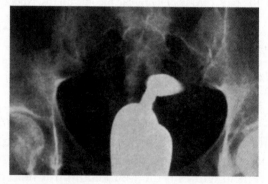

FIGURE 7-18   Hysterosalpingogram showing complete blockage of both fallopian tubes due to pelvic inflammatory disease (PID). The uterus is overdistended with contrast medium. (Beckmann CRB, Ling FW, et al. *Obstetrics and Gynecology.* 5th ed. Philadelphia, PA: Lippincott Williams & Wilkins; 2006.)

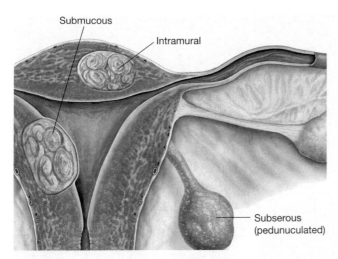

FIGURE 7-19   The various types of leiomyomas.

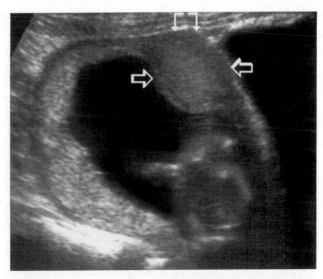

FIGURE 7-20   This submucosal leiomyoma is seen between the *arrows* growing off the anterior wall of the uterus.

The *submucous* types are the least common and grow off the endometrium into the uterine cavity (Fig. 7-20). The most common type is known as *intramural* and grows within the myometrium. The *subserous* type is mostly pedunculated and grows off the perimetrium into the pelvic cavity. Many times, myomas will calcify with time (Fig. 7-21). It can be present with pregnancy and can cause an abortion or an abruption placenta. They can prevent a normal vaginal delivery if they are located near the cervix. Myomas can also cause the premature rupture of the membranes.

Teratomas, also known as **dermoids**, are benign "cysts" of the ovary that contain skin, hair, teeth, and fatty elements that derive from ectodermal tissue. About one-half contain calcifications usually in the form of teeth, but may include the wall of the cyst (Fig. 7-22). These are of no clinical significance unless they grow so large that they compress adjacent structures. Teratomas account for about 15% of all benign ovarian masses.

Single cystic lesions of the ovaries are rarely significant and are usually a follicular cyst or a corpus luteum cyst. Multiple cystic areas may be an indication of endometriosis. **Polycystic ovaries** are enlarged ovaries consisting of many small cysts. This manifestation may be associated with Stein-Leventhal syndrome, which is characterized by facial hair, excess weight, amenorrhea, and infertility.

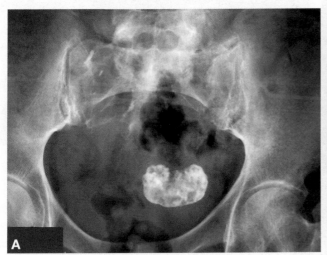

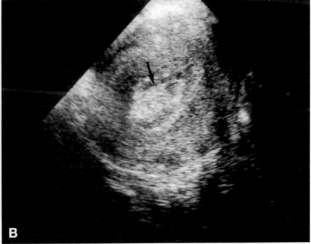

FIGURE 7-21   Pelvic radiograph (A) shows a calcified mass that often looks like popcorn. (B) The ultrasound image demonstrates the echogenic mass of the calcified leiomyoma seen at the *arrow*. (Daffner RH. *Clinical Radiology: The Essentials.* 3rd ed. Philadelphia, PA: Lippincott Williams & Wilkins; 2007.)

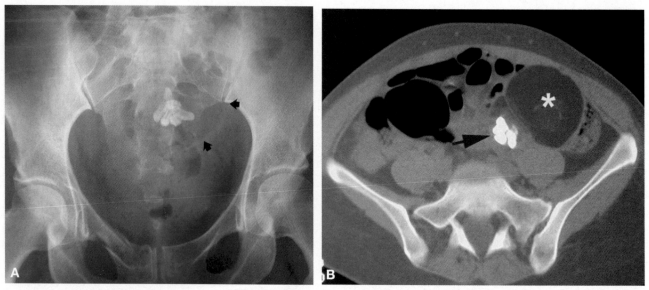

FIGURE 7-22   (A) The AP view shows calcification (malformed teeth) along the mid to left side of the pelvis. (B) A CT image shows the calcifications (*arrow*) and also some fatty components of the tumor (*). (Daffner RH. *Clinical Radiology: The Essentials.* 3rd ed. Philadelphia, PA: Lippincott Williams & Wilkins; 2007.)

Case Study

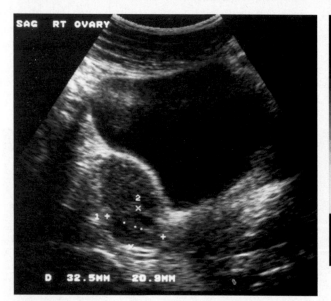

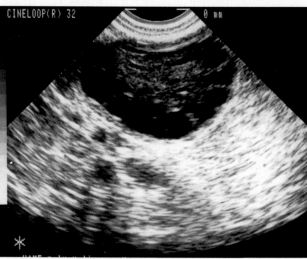

The image on the left shows the relationship of the ovary to the midsection of the body of the uterus. Notice how small the ovary is when it is normal. Polycystic ovarian disease shows a much enlarged ovary that is filled with multiple cysts (the dark, radiolucent areas) as seen on the image on the right. When polycystic ovarian disease is present, it is wise to check the patient's renal area, as the kidneys are often involved and will contain multiple cysts.

Fibrocystic disease of the breast is a common benign condition occurring in about 20% of women who are premenopausal. Fibrocystic disease is a general term that encompasses a variety of changes that occur. The most obvious changes are fibrous and cystic dilation of the ducts. It is usually bilateral with cysts of various sizes distributed throughout the breasts. The breast will also contain an increased amount of fibrous tissue (Fig. 7-23). A more important change is hyperplasia of the ducts. This change is thought to be a precursor to cancer. If hyperplasia is present with fibrosis and cystic dilation, the term proliferative fibrocystic disease is used.

A fibroadenoma is the most common benign breast tumor (Figs. 7-24 and 7-25). It generally appears as a smooth, well-circumscribed mass with no invasion of surrounding tissue. The masses may be moved around within the breast as they have no attachments to the overlying skin or underlying tissue. Ultrasonography permits differentiation of a solid fibroadenoma from a fluid-filled cyst. Mammography may demonstrate these masses. Fibroadenomas are easily removed and carry no threat of developing into cancer.

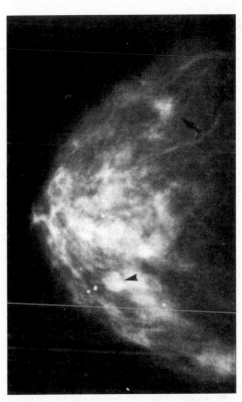

FIGURE 7-24   In this cephalocaudal film-screen mammogram, a small scirrhous carcinoma (*arrow*) is seen with a well-marginated fibroadenoma (*arrowhead*). (Beckmann CRB, Ling FW, et al. *Obstetrics and Gynecology.* 5th ed. Philadelphia, PA: Lippincott Williams & Wilkins; 2006.)

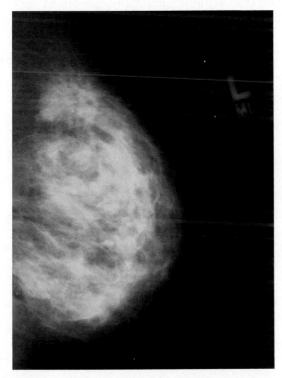

FIGURE 7-23   Fibrocystic disease. Dense breasts have multiple fibrous areas. The round radiopaque marker at the top of the breast indicates where the patient felt a mass.

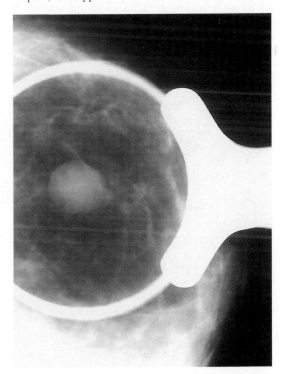

FIGURE 7-25   The use of compression and spot imaging of the suspected area will clearly define the smooth borders of the fibroadenoma.

Malignant

Adenocarcinoma of the endometrium accounts for 90% of all uterine malignant neoplasms. It is the most common invasive gynecologic malignancy (excluding breast cancer). Approximately 40,100 new cases were expected in 2008 with approximately 7,400 deaths.

There are two classifications. Type I occurs most often in the pre- and perimenopausal women. Type II occurs in older, postmenopausal women who have never borne a viable baby (nullipara). Prolonged estrogen stimulation has been associated with increased frequency of endometrial carcinoma; therefore, women on hormone replacement therapy are at an increased risk for endometrial cancer. Clinical symptoms include bleeding, hypermenorrhea, or postmenopausal bleeding. The tumor may project into the uterine cavity (Fig. 7-26) or it may infiltrate the wall of the uterus.

An intravenous urogram (IVU) will show the bladder wall depressed by an enlarged uterus. Ultrasonography (Fig. 7-27), CT, and MRI are all modalities that differentiate endometrium from myometrium, thus accurately locating the tumor. Hysterectomy combined with radiation therapy gives an overall survival rate of approximately 80%. This high cure rate is attributed to early detection (bleeding in postmenopausal women is abnormal) and containment of the cancer within the body of the uterus.

Cystadenocarcinoma is ovarian cancer. Although this neoplasm is less common than other malignancies, it is important because it is relatively asymptomatic until the disease has progressed to a stage at which chances for a cure are slim (Fig. 7-28).

Cervical cancer arises from epithelial tissue around the neck of the uterus (Fig. 7-29). It is caused by certain types of human papillomavirus (HPV). Researchers have identified certain types of HPV that are transmitted through sexual contact as the cause of nearly all cervical cancers. When a female has been infected by certain types of HPV and the virus does not go away on its own, abnormal cells can develop in the lining of the cervix. If not discovered early and treated, these abnormal cells can become cervical precancers and then cancer.

In the United States, there are 30% more cases of cervical cancer in African Americans as compared to Whites, and 41% more cases in Hispanics than Whites. Asians/Islanders and Whites are almost equal in numbers with 8 in 100,000 women contracting the virus and being diagnosed with cervical cancer. The Center for Disease Control and Prevention reported 12,280 new cases of cervical cancer being identified in 2007. In 2006, an HPV vaccine was introduced. It is hoped that as more women are vaccinated against this virus, the number of cases will decline.

The IVU demonstrates hydronephrosis in one-third of the patients. In fact, the most common cause of death

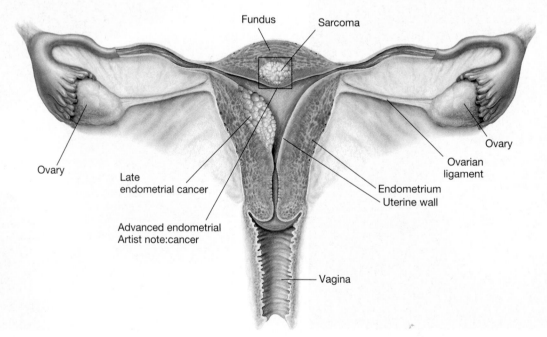

FIGURE 7-26 This drawing shows how endometrial cancer will project into the body of the uterus. (Asset provided by Anatomical Chart Co.)

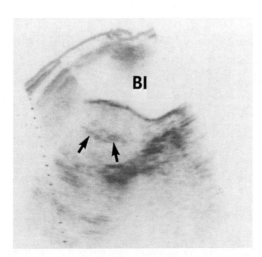

FIGURE 7-27   Longitudinal sonogram shows the uterus to be enlarged and bulbous. There are clusters of high-amplitude echoes (*arrows*) in the region of the central cavity echo. Bl, bladder. This was proven to be an endometrial carcinoma. (Eisenberg RL. *Clinical Imaging: An Atlas of Differential Diagnosis.* 5th ed. Philadelphia, PA: Lippincott Williams & Wilkins; 2010.)

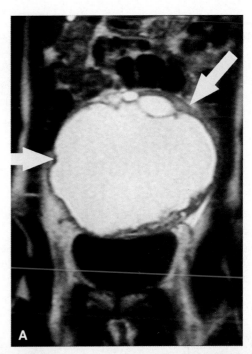

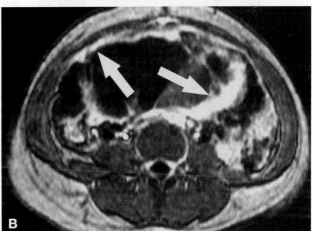

FIGURE 7-28   Ovarian carcinoma. (A) Coronal T2-weighted image demonstrates large complex cystic mass (*arrows*) with thick irregular walls occupying pelvis and lower abdomen. (B) Following gadolinium administration, mass demonstrates thick enhancing walls and septations (*arrows*) consistent with malignant process. Mucinous cystadenocarcinoma diagnosed at surgery. (Leyendecker JR, Brown JJ. *Practical Guide to Abdominal and Pelvic MRI*. Philadelphia, PA: Lippincott Williams & Wilkins; 2004.)

in patients with carcinoma of the cervix is impaired renal function caused by ureteral obstruction. Again, as with endometrial carcinoma, CT, MRI (Fig. 7-30), and ultrasonography are accurate in locating the tumor cells and determining any invasion of other organs. Cervical cancer is preventable and curable if detected early. Important strategies to reduce the risk of cervical cancer include screening with the Papanicolaou and, for some women, HPV tests, as well as prevention of HPV infection with the HPV vaccine.

Breast cancer is the most common malignancy among women. It has the highest mortality rate of any malignant neoplasm in women. If a woman lives to her mid-80s, her overall risk of getting breast cancer is roughly one in eight. Factors that increase the risk of breast cancer include the age at which a woman has her first full-term pregnancy. Women who delay childbirth tend to have a higher relative risk compared with women who had a first pregnancy at age of 17 years. Other risk factors include early menarche. Those who begin menses at the age of 12 or younger are at a higher risk. Age is another factor with the risk increasing with age.

Almost all breast cancers are seen mammographically as a tumor mass, clustered calcifications, or both. Either feature, when clearly demonstrated, is so suspicious of malignancy as to require prompt biopsy, whether the lesion is palpable or not. Secondary changes of breast carcinoma include skin thickening around the areola and nipple retraction.

The typical malignant tumor mass is poorly defined, has irregular margins, and demonstrates numerous fine linear strands or spicules radiating out from the mass (Fig. 7-31). This appearance is characteristic but not diagnostic of malignancy and is in stark contrast to the typical mammographic picture of a benign mass,

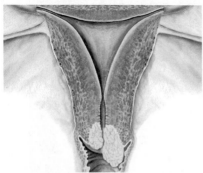
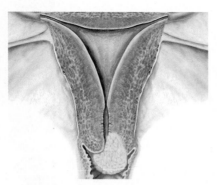
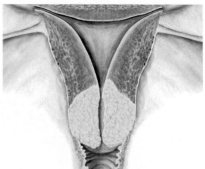

Carcinoma confined to the cervix.

Carcinoma confined to the cervix, "cauliflower" lesion.

Bulky endocervical barrel-shaped lesion.

FIGURE 7-29 Three images of cervical carcinoma. The *left image* is confined to the cervix, the *middle image* is a cauliflower lesion, and the *right image* shows an endocervical barrel-shaped lesion.

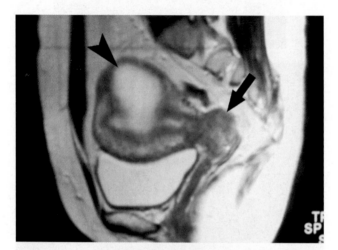

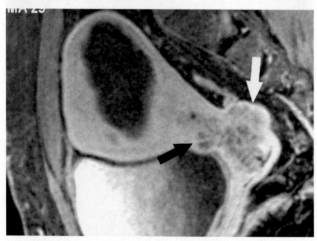

FIGURE 7-30 The MRI on *top* shows a cervical mass (*arrow*) and a cystic leiomyoma (*arrowhead*). The *bottom* image demonstrates the margins of the mass at the *arrows*. (Leyendecker JR, Brown JJ. *Practical Guide to Abdominal and Pelvic MRI.* Philadelphia, PA: Lippincott Williams & Wilkins; 2004.)

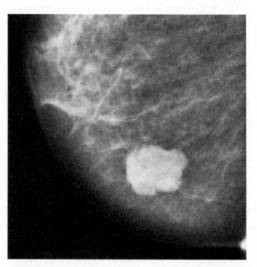

FIGURE 7-31 This large mass demonstrates the irregular borders so indicative of carcinoma of the breast. (Reprinted with permission from Mitchell GW. *The Female Breast and Its Disorders.* 1st ed. Baltimore, MD: Williams & Wilkins; 1990:140.)

which has well-defined smooth margins and a round, oval, or gently lobulated contour.

Clustered calcifications in breast cancer are typically numerous, very small, and localized to one segment of the breast. They demonstrate a wide variety of shapes, including fine linear, curvilinear, and branching forms.

Although relatively infrequent, breast cancer also can develop in men. It accounts for only 1% of all breast cancers. Male breast cancer is a disease of the elderly and has a somewhat worse prognosis than female breast carcinoma.

Male

Congenital Anomalies

The testes normally descend from the intra-abdominal area through the inguinal canal into the scrotum near the end of the gestational period. After birth, both testes should be palpable in the scrotum. If one or both are not felt, it must be determined if the testes are absent or ectopic. **Cryptorchidism** is the condition of undescended testes. About 3% of full-term and 30% of premature infant boys are born with at least one undescended testis, making cryptorchidism the most common birth defect of male genitalia.

Ultrasonography is used as a screening mechanism to determine the location of an undescended testicle in the inguinal canal, the pelvis, or the abdomen. If ultrasonography fails to locate the testicle, the patient will be referred to CT or MRI. Undescended testes are associated with reduced fertility, testicular torsion, and a higher rate of malignancy. In fact, malignance is approximately 40 times higher in males with cryptorchidism. The testicle must be brought down and surgically fixed in the scrotum by a procedure called **orchiopexy**, or it must be removed (**orchiectomy**). Orchiectomy is performed on those patients who are diagnosed after the onset of puberty.

Inflammatory Processes

Prostatic hyperplasia is enlargement of the prostate gland. This benign condition is very common in men over the age of 50 years and is related to decreased hormone secretions. As the prostate gland enlarges, it pushes on the bladder, which results in an inability to completely empty the bladder. This leads to obstructions, bilateral ureteral dilation, and hydronephrosis. As the urine stagnates in the bladder, urinary tract infections and even pyelonephritis are complications that must be dealt with.

The intravenous urogram (IVU) demonstrates the elevation and smooth impression on the floor of the bladder by the prostate (Fig. 7-32). The elevation of the bladder also causes the elevation of the insertion of the ureters on the trigone. The characteristic J-shape, or "fish hook," appearance of the distal ureters will be demonstrated. Symptoms of obstruction are relieved by a surgical procedure known as transurethral resection of the prostate (TURP).

MRI is an excellent imaging tool because there is no radiation involved in this sensitive area (Fig. 7-33).

Prostatic calculi are small, multiple calcifications found in the prostate gland. Males over the age of

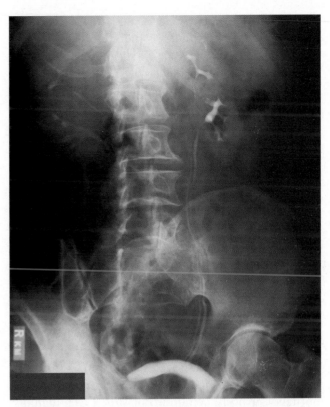

FIGURE 7-32 Because of the enlarged prostate gland, the contrast medium does not fill the base of the bladder on this image demonstrating prostatic hyperplasia.

50 years are prone to this common condition. The calculi, if dense enough, are visible on plain abdominal radiographs. They are of no clinical significance.

Testicular torsion occurs when the testicle twists over on its pedicle. If this happens, there is a compromise of

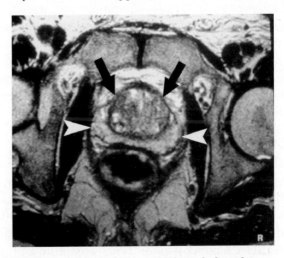

FIGURE 7-33 High-resolution MRI through the pelvis shows the round borders of an enlarged prostate (*arrows*). The peripheral zone of the prostate is marked by the arrowheads. (Leyendecker JR, Brown JJ. *Practical Guide to Abdominal and Pelvic MRI.* Philadelphia, PA: Lippincott Williams & Wilkins; 2004.)

the vascularity of the testicle. A sudden onset of severe scrotal pain and swelling are the clinical symptoms. Doppler ultrasound will make a diagnosis through the absence of the sound of blood flow.

Epididymitis is inflammation of the epididymis and also leads to swelling of the scrotum accompanied by pain and erythema. Orchitis (inflammation of the testes) may be associated with epididymitis. Doppler ultrasonography is used to demonstrate the intratesticular arterial blood flow to distinguish between torsion and epididymitis. Arterial perfusion is decreased or absent in testicular torsion, whereas in epididymitis the blood flow is increased.

Nuclear medicine may also be used to differentiate between the two problems. Similar to ultrasonography, nuclear medicine shows decreased isotope uptake in the affected side in torsion due to decreased blood flow, and increased uptake in the testicle involved in epididymitis.

Enlargement of the male breast is known as **gynecomastia**. This proliferation of ducts and connective tissue is the result of estrogen stimulation. A variety of stimuli can cause males to secrete more estrogen than normal. Cirrhosis, certain neoplasms, TCH, digitalis, and Klinefelter syndrome are all possible causative agents. Aging, with decreased androgen production, is the usual cause of bilateral gynecomastia.

Neoplasms

Benign

Masses in the testes may be the result of trauma or inflammation, but most commonly are neoplasm. Males between the ages of 25 and 40 years are most often afflicted. Benign masses include hydroceles and spermatoceles. A **hydrocele** is a collection of fluid in the testis or along the spermatic cord. A **spermatocele** is a cystic dilation of the epididymis. Both of these conditions are easily demonstrated by ultrasonography.

Malignant

Malignant tumors of the testes are more common than the benign variety. The two major types are seminomas and teratomas. **Seminomas** arise from the seminiferous tubules. These tumors are extremely radiosensitive and the prognosis is excellent. **Teratomas**, on the other hand, have a poor prognosis. They arise from a primitive germ cell and consist of a variety of structures. Both of these tumors are highly malignant and tend to spread by the lymphatics and the blood to the area of the renal hilum. CT scan best demonstrates testicular

tumors, as this modality will also detect metastasis to the lung, liver, or bone.

Lung cancer is the most common malignancy in men. However, **adenocarcinoma** of the prostate gland is a close second. About 200,000 new cases are diagnosed each year in the United States alone with 1 in 10 men being affected. The tumor is rare before the age of 50 years, but as men age, the risk increases. Seventy percent of the cases occur in men aged 65 years or more. Prostate cancer occurs 2.4 times more often in African Americans than in Whites. A family history and obesity are also tied into the high risk group. Figure 7-34 shows the different stages of prostate cancer.

The intravenous urography examination again demonstrates an elevated bladder. However, unlike hyperplasia of the prostate, which makes a smooth border, carcinoma makes an irregular impression on the bladder floor because of the irregular, lobulated borders of the tumor. It is important to determine carcinoma of the prostate early, as it spreads to the rectum directly. It metastasizes to the bone in 75% of all cases. With early detection, 99% of patients can live for 5 or more years.

Ultrasonography, with the use of a transrectal probe, has proved useful in detecting carcinoma of the prostate gland particularly for growth and biopsy guidance. MRI can delineate the prostate and surrounding organs to accurately stage any pelvic neoplasms (Fig. 7-35).

Imaging Strategies

Mammography

TECH TIP

Mammographers must pass a separate examination at the ARRT level. In addition, many states also require a state mammography license in addition to the national certification. Because mammography requires specialized equipment and quality control, the mammography team must be dedicated to continued education that is geared toward increasing quality images to improve patient survival rates.

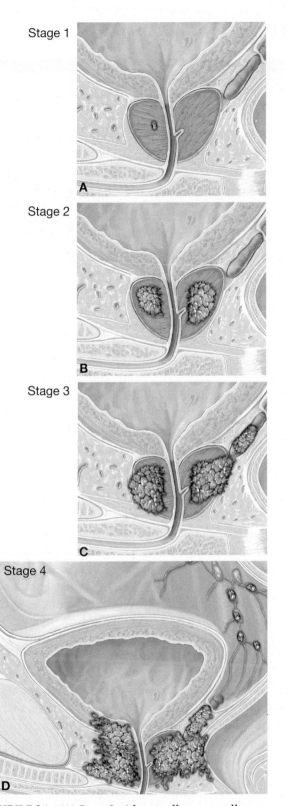

Stage 1

Stage 2

Stage 3

Stage 4

FIGURE 7-34   (A) Stage I with a small cancer cell seen on
the left of the image; (B) stage II shows the cancer growing
but still contained with the prostate gland; (C) stage III
indicates that cancer cells have started to invade the seminal
vesicle. (D) In stage IV, the cancer has spread into the lymph
nodes.

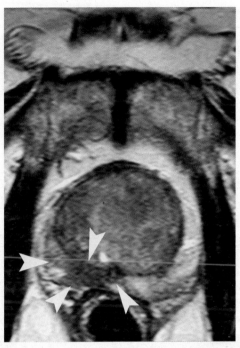

FIGURE 7-35   MRI demonstrating a low-signal area
indicated by the *arrowheads*. This was identified as prostate
carcinoma. (Leyendecker JR, Brown JJ. *Practical Guide to
Abdominal and Pelvic MRI.* Philadelphia, PA: Lippincott
Williams & Wilkins; 2004.)

This radiologic procedure of the breast can show
the size of a mass, reveal calcifications, and demonstrate nipple inversion. However, the most
important function of mammography is the early
detection and diagnosis of breast cancer. There is
a 90% to 98% chance of long-term survival if cancer is detected and treated in its early stages. To
ensure early diagnosis, the American Cancer Soci-
ety advises women between the ages of 35 and 40
to have a baseline mammogram (Fig. 7-36A, B).
Guidelines call for women aged 50 years and older
to have yearly mammography; however, decisions
for radiographic examination any sooner than these
recommendations should be a personal decision
between the patient and her physician. All patients
with any clinical history such as discharge, nipple
retraction, skin thickening, palpable masses, or
a family history of breast cancer should undergo
mammography.

It has been demonstrated that radiation exposure
to the breast can induce breast cancer and that this
risk is dose dependent. Although radiation health
professionals consider any radiation dose to be a

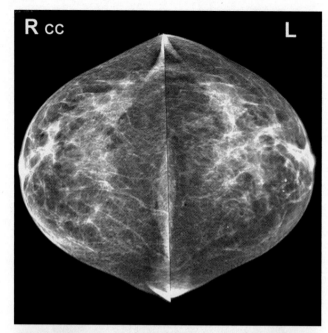

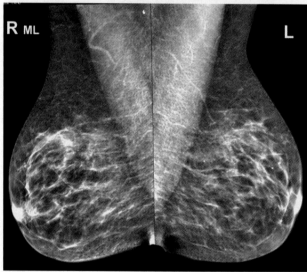

FIGURE 7-36   Routine digital mammogram showing
normal results on a 63-year-old woman. (A) Right and left
craniocaudal (CC) view. (B) Right and left mediolateral
(ML) view. Notice the exquisite details the digital image
provides. (Daffner RH. *Clinical Radiology: The Essentials.*
3rd ed. Philadelphia, PA: Lippincott Williams & Wilkins;
2007.)

nonthreshold dose (no safe dose), a maximum of 0.01
Gy has been set as the safe limit of radiation exposure
in mammography. The absorption of 0.01 Gy of radiation by the breast raises the chance of cancer from 8%
to 8.08%. Normally, only 0.003 to 0.008 Gy are given
at the skin surface, which is well under the 0.01 Gy
safety mark.

Hysterosalpingography

> ### TECH TIP
>
> Hysterosalpingography is performed with the use
> of fluoroscopy. This modality has the ability to
> produce a large radiation dose to the reproduc-
> tive organs. Judicial use of radiation must be
> considered.

Hysterosalpingography is a procedure that may be diagnostic as well as therapeutic. Diagnostic indications for
hysterosalpingography include abnormal bleeding or
spotting between menstrual periods, patency of tubes,
anomalies, habitual spontaneous abortions, amenorrhea, dysmenorrhea, and a lost intrauterine contraceptive device. Therapeutic indications include restoring
patency to the tubes, stretching adhesions, dilation of the
tubes, or straightening of the tubes. Contraindications of
hysterosalpingography include pregnancy, pelvic inflammatory disease, vaginal or cervical infection, or menses.

Two types of contrast media are used for hysterosalpingography: water soluble and oily, each with their
advantages and disadvantages. A water-soluble medium
may either be in the form of Salpix or Sinografin. This
contrast medium is absorbed quickly and leaves no
residue. The disadvantage to water-soluble mediums is
the great deal of pain they produce. Ethiodol is an oily
contrast medium that is very opaque and causes little
or no pain. Unfortunately, the oil persists in the body.

Besides considering the above advantages and disadvantages when choosing a contrast medium, the
radiographer should also keep in mind the time it takes
the body to rid itself of the contrast material. It should
be either excreted or absorbed rapidly. The contrast
medium must also be dense and viscous enough to
coat the uterus and not be diluted too easily with the
uterine fluids. Finally, it should be nonreactive.

Only about 4 mL is required to fill the uterus.
Another 4 mL is used to fill the tubes. If no pathology
is present contrast will spill into the pelvic cavity
proving patency of the fallopian tubes. Carbon dioxide
may also be used in addition to the positive contrast
medium. About 100 mL is necessary and will be
absorbed in approximately 25 to 30 minutes.

The patient assumes the lithotomy position and
the cervix is exposed with a speculum. A cannula is

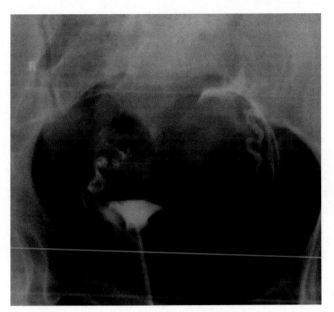

FIGURE 7-37   Normal hysterosalpingogram.

placed into the cervical os and is held in place by a tenaculum. The speculum is then removed over the cannula. Contrast material is slowly injected under fluoroscopic guidance. A rubber plug is fixed to the cannula and fits tightly against the external os of the cervix to prevent backflow of the contrast material. Overhead radiographs are usually taken in several projections (Fig. 7-37).

Ultrasonography

TECH TIP

Ultrasound does not use ionizing radiation and as such, it is now the modality of choice for examinations of the reproductive organs. Ultrasonography requires additional education. With the examinations of the reproductive system, the sonographer must be professional in order to put the patient at ease.

Ultrasound can be performed to visualize both the female and the male reproductive organs. With the improved resolution of diagnostic ultrasonographic instrumentation, almost all radiographic procedures of the reproductive system have been replaced with ultra-sound. When combined with clinical and laboratory features, the ultrasonographic findings help to limit the diagnostic possibilities. In obstetrics, ultrasonography is useful in evaluating normal fetal development and positioning and a variety of obstetric complications. Of these applications, those complications arising in the first trimester of pregnancy are by far the most important. No other imaging modality is able to compete with the value of ultrasonography in this respect.

Female pelvic ultrasound is done either transabdominally or transvaginally. Transvaginal ultrasound has a much smaller field of view, making it difficult to become oriented to the anatomy on the images. With transabdominal images, the "slices" are either in the longitudinal or cross-sectional plane. In the longitudinal images, the bladder, uterus, cervix, and vagina can be easily identified. Refer to the figure on the left of the case study presented earlier to view a normal ultrasound of the female bladder and uterus.

In the male, ultrasonography has been used to evaluate testicular masses and prostatic nodules. Doppler ultrasonography and color flow ultrasonography are excellent means of demonstrating blood flow to the testes. In cases of torsion of the testicle, there will be blockage or decreased blood flow, thus the Doppler will not demonstrate much, if any, flow. In cases of infection, such as in epididymitis, there will be increased blood flow to the area and Doppler will demonstrate such.

Computed Tomography and Magnetic Resonance Imaging

CT is useful in demonstrating the lymph nodes of the pelvis and the invasion of surrounding areas by a tumor. It is particularly advantageous for differentiation of pathology from the bowel. The immediate postoperative patient tolerates examination by CT better than that of ultrasonography. However, CT utilizes a large amount of radiation that is directed to the area of the gonads. Unless the patient is beyond childbearing years or the benefit outweighs the risk, CT is not advised.

MRI provides additional information over ultrasonography and aids in the clinical decision-making for patients being evaluated for other procedures. MRI is highly accurate in the determination of the presence of leiomyomas, their size, and location. While ultrasonography remains the modality of choice for the assessment of reproductive organ disorders, pelvic MRI provides clinically relevant information beyond the scope of ultrasound.

Nuclear Medicine

Nuclear medicine has a limited role in the assessment of disorders of the reproductive system. Sentinel node scans are performed after biopsies by injecting radioisotope in the area. Scans are then done to see if there is any uptake of the isotope in the lymph nodes. Bone scans are performed in patients with breast cancer and prostate cancer to determine if metastasis has occurred.

RECAP

Anatomy and Physiology

- Female
  - Single uterus is made when the Müllerian ducts fuse together
    - Three layers: endometrium, which is the lining; myometrium, which is the actual muscle wall; perimetrium, which is the outer lining
  - Each uterine tube (aka fallopian tube) is the top half of one of the Müllerian ducts
  - Uterus can be to the left (livo-rotated) or to the right (dextro-rotated)
  - Fimbriated ends of the uterine tube help sweep the ovum from the ovary into the uterine tube
  - Ovary is attached to the uterine body laterally by the broad ligament
  - The woman is born with all her eggs (approximately 200,000)
    - Each ovary will rupture an ovum (mature egg) every other month
    - Each ovary will secrete hormones: estrogen and progesterone
- Male
  - Testicles are formed in the abdomen and descend to the scrotum shortly after birth
    - Testicles secrete the hormone: testosterone
  - Epididymis is coiled on top and posterior of each testicle
    - It stores the sperm
  - Prostate gland
    - Surrounds the ejaculatory duct
    - Surrounds the urethra

Congenital Pathologies

- Female
  - Agenesis: missing uterus
  - Arcuate: small indentation on the top of the fundus
  - Bicornuate bicollic: one vagina, two cervixes, two uterine bodies
  - Bicornuate: common anomaly with two fundi
  - Didelphic: complete duplication
  - Unicornuate: one half of a uterus and one fallopian tube
  - Septate: septum in the uterine body extending the length of the body
  - Subseptate: partial septum dividing the body
  - Retroverted: fundus of the uterus is posterior to the cervix
- Male
  - Cryptorchidism
    - Undescended testicle
    - Worrisome for malignancy

Inflammatory Processes

- Female
  - Endometriosis: growth of endometrial tissue outside the uterus
    - Associated with chocolate cysts and adenomyosis
  - PID can be either acute or chronic; it is a common cause of ectopic pregnancy
  - Three types of leiomyomas
    - Submucous: projecting into the body of the uterus
    - Intramural: within the muscle wall
    - Subserous: projecting off the perimetrium and into the pelvic cavity
- Male
  - Epididymitis and testicular torsion
    - Tested by ultrasonography and nuclear medicine
    - Rely on blood flow to the area to make the diagnosis

Neoplasms

- Female
  - Benign neoplasms of the breast
    - Fibrocystic disease
    - Fibroadenomas
  - Malignant neoplasms
    - Endometrial carcinoma (90% of uterine malignancies)
    - Cervical carcinoma
    - Cystadenocarcinoma is ovarian cancer
    - Breast cancer
      - Most common malignancy in women
      - Highest mortality rate
      - Overall risk of having breast cancer is one in eight
      - Risk increases with age, family history, and a first pregnancy occurring late in life
- Male
  - Malignant neoplasms
    - Prostate cancer
      - Need early diagnosis before metastasis occurs to the bones

Imaging Strategies

- Mammography
  - Most important diagnostic tool for the early diagnosis of breast cancer
  - There is little risk of inducing cancer using modern equipment
- Hysterosalpingography
  - Diagnose and treat
  - Infection is a contraindication
- Ultrasonography
  - Imaging modality of choice for reproductive system imaging
  - With the use of transrectal transducers a close-up look at the uterus or prostate is possible
- CT and MRI
  - Complementary modalities that add information to that achieved by ultrasonography
  - Useful in staging of malignant neoplasms
  - Leiomyomas can be readily assessed
  - Surgical intervention can be planned after either of these modalities
- Nuclear medicine
  - Limited role in the assessment of the reproductive system
  - Sentinel node scans are performed after biopsies
    - Scans performed for uptake in the lymph nodes
  - Bone scans
    - To see if there is metastasis from breast cancer and prostate cancer

CLINICAL AND RADIOGRAPHIC CHARACTERISTICS OF COMMON PATHOLOGIES

Pathologic Condition	Age (if Known) Causal Factors	Manifestations	Radiographic Appearance
Endometriosis	Over 30 y and nulligravida	Dysmenorrhea, aching remainder of the month	Ultrasonography
Pelvic inflammatory disease	50–60% by gonorrhea	Pelvic pain, foul-smelling discharge	Ultrasonography
Leiomyoma	Over 30 y and nulligravid, estrogen stimulated	Asymptomatic	Ultrasonography
Teratoma		Asymptomatic	Calcifications (teeth)
Fibrocystic breasts	Premenopausal	Asymptomatic	Fibrosis bilaterally seen on mammography
Fibroadenoma		Asymptomatic, movable mass	Smooth, well-circumscribed mass

(continued)

CLINICAL AND RADIOGRAPHIC CHARACTERISTICS OF COMMON PATHOLOGIES *(continued)*

Pathologic Condition	Age (if Known) Causal Factors	Manifestations	Radiographic Appearance
Endometrial carcinoma	Postmenopausal, nullipara, estrogen stimulation	Bleeding, hypermenorrhea	Depression on bladder wall by uterine mass seen on IVU
Cervical carcinoma	High degree of sexual activity, chronic irritation, infection	Bleeding, pain	Hydronephrosis, ultrasonography or CT suggested
Breast carcinoma	Postmenopausal, delayed childbirth	Nipple retraction, skin thickening, nipple discharge	Tumor mass, clustered calcifications, irregular margins
Prostatic hyperplasia	Over 50 y, decreased hormones, enlarged prostate	Retention of urine	Hydronephrosis, ureteral dilation, "fish hook" sign
Prostatic calculi	Over 50 y	Asymptomatic	Small multiple calcium deposits near base of bladder
Prostatic carcinoma	Over 50 y	Retention of urine	Irregular impression on bladder floor
Cryptorchidism	Infant male	Nonpalpable testis in scrotum	Ultrasonography suggested
Hydrocele, spermatocele	25–40 y, trauma, inflammation	Swelling of the scrotum	Ultrasonography suggested

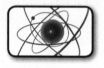

CRITICAL THINKING DISCUSSION QUESTIONS

1. Hysterosalpingography is both diagnostic and therapeutic. Explain how the procedure can do both.

2. Contrast media for hysterosalpingography can present problems. What are they?

3. Explain mammography and its importance in women's health.

4. Define and describe endometriosis. How is adenomyosis related?

5. Describe what happens to the adnexa with PID.

6. An IVU may detect adenocarcinoma of the endometrium or of the cervix. What would these processes look like on an IVU and what is a better diagnostic tool?

7. Define cryptorchidism. What diagnostic procedure is performed to determine the location of the organs? Why is it important to correct this condition?

8. What two procedures are performed to differentiate between torsion and epididymitis? What will each condition demonstrate?

9. What are complications of prostatic hyperplasia? What will the intravenous urography demonstrate with this condition?

10. Describe the process by which ultrasonography is useful in detecting carcinoma of the prostate gland. What other organs can be visualized by the use of this modality in this manner?

8

The Circulatory System

● Goals

1. To review the basic anatomy and physiology of the circulatory and lymph systems

   OBJECTIVE: Describe the internal anatomy of the heart and the basic anatomy of the lymph system

   OBJECTIVE: Describe the physiology of the circulatory and lymph systems

2. To understand cardiovascular disease and its two main components: diseases of the heart and diseases of the blood vessels

   OBJECTIVE: Describe the various pathologic conditions affecting the heart and blood vessels

3. To become familiar with the radiographic manifestations of all the common congenital and acquired disorders of the circulatory system

   OBJECTIVE: Explain how the different pathologic processes will manifest on radiographic images

4. To interpret which modalities are best suited for the different pathologic processes

   OBJECTIVE: List the different imaging modalities and which pathologies are best seen

● Key Terms

Anastomosis
Aneurysm
Arteriosclerosis
Atherosclerosis
Cardiac dilation
Cardiac heterotaxia
Cardiomegaly
Cardiovascular disease
Coarctation
Congestive heart failure
Dextrocardia
Dyspnea
Endocarditis
Hypertensive heart disease
Incompetent
Insufficient
Myocardial infarction
Pericardial effusion
Rheumatic heart disease
Septal defects
Shunts
Situs inversus
Stenosis
Thrombus
Valvular disease

Although the circulatory system may not seem to be as important to radiographers who have not specialized in modalities such as angiography and sonography, it is still important to understand the basic anatomy and conditions that will be visualized on a radiographic image. The radiographer that continues on in education for nuclear medicine and computed tomography (CT) or magnetic resonance imaging (MRI) will need to know the anatomy, physiology, and pathologies of the circulatory system in great detail to determine what images should be obtained to demonstrate the pathologic process.

Because the circulatory system runs parallel to the lymph system, the anatomy and physiology and function will be described in this chapter. However, because pathology of the lymph system is beyond the scope of radiographers, it will not be discussed. It is important to remember that malignant cells metastasize more commonly through the lymph system than in any other method.

Anatomy

Circulatory System

The circulatory system is made up of the heart, arteries, arterioles, capillaries, venules, and veins. The heart, a muscular organ, lies in the middle mediastinum with two thirds of it to the left of the midline. It is shaped like a closed fist or inverted cone. The apex of the heart is the rounded tip that is pointed down, to the left, and anterior. The base is the large end that points up, to the right, and posterior. The heart has four chambers: the right and left atria are found at the base, and the right and left ventricles found near the apex. Each of these chambers is separated by a septum. The interarterial septum is between the two atria, and the interventricular septum is located between the two ventricles.

The heart has 11 openings. Those openings are the right and left arterioventricular openings, the pulmonary opening, the aortic opening, the superior vena cava and inferior vena cava openings, two left and two

right pulmonary vein openings, and the coronary sinus opening. Some of the openings have valves within them to prevent retrograde blood flow. There are four that should be known by all radiographers. The left arterioventricular valve, also known as the mitral or bicuspid valve, is located in the opening between the left atrium and ventricle and has two cusps (flaps). The right arterioventricular valve, or tricuspid valve, has three flaps and is found between the right atrium and ventricle. The aortic semilunar valve, located between the left ventricle and the aorta, has three cusps as does the pulmonary valve, which is found at the pulmonary opening between the right ventricle and the pulmonary trunk. There are other valves in a few of the remaining openings, but they are not listed here because of their nonfunctional status.

The wall of the heart is made of three separate layers. The endocardium is the lining, the myocardium is the middle muscular layer, and the epicardium is the outer covering. The epicardium is actually the visceral layer of a membrane known as the pericardium. There is another layer to the pericardium called the parietal layer. This is what makes up the sac in which the heart is located. Figure 8-1 shows the chambers

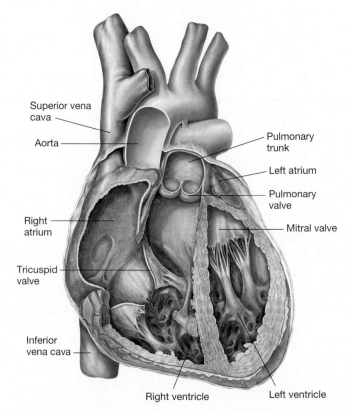

FIGURE 8-1   Cross-sectional anatomy of the heart.

and the valves of the heart. Also seen are the layers of the wall of the heart.

The thick-walled tubes that carry blood away from the heart are the arteries. Arteries are named either for their location or according to the direction of blood flow in them. The major trunk arteries are the aorta, which is to the left of the midline and sends blood from the heart to the body tissues, and the pulmonary artery, which arises from the right ventricle of the heart and supplies the lungs with blood. The various arteries end with short narrow vessels that are found in all tissues supplied by blood. These are called arterioles. From arterioles, the vessels become simple endothelial tubes known as capillaries. These are the minute structures that form the transition from artery to vein. From the capillary system, the vessels again become larger to form the venules, which are the counter part to the arterioles. Venules converge to form veins, which bring blood back to the heart. Figure 8-2 shows the blood flow from arteries through all phases to veins. The major trunk veins are the superior and inferior venae cavae, which drain the upper and lower body, respectively, and the four pulmonary veins that drain the lungs. Both venae cavae terminate in the right atrium, and all four pulmonary veins empty into the left atrium.

Lymphatic System

The lymph system is considered along with the circulatory system because it comprises lymph and tissue fluid obtained from blood. The lymph organs consist of the spleen, the thymus, and the tonsils and adenoids. The largest is the spleen, which is located in the left upper quadrant of the abdomen between the stomach and the diaphragm.

The spleen is a highly vascular organ that is composed of splenic pulp encapsulated by connective and muscular tissues. White splenic pulp is made up of lymphatic nodules and diffuse lymphatic tissue that cover the arteries of the spleen. Red splenic pulp is made up of lymphatic tissue that is permeated with sinusoids and flooded with blood. A blood-forming organ early in life, the spleen is a site for the storage of red corpuscles. It is an important part of the defense system as it has a plethora of blood-filtering macrophages.

The thymus is located in the superior mediastinum, extending upward into the lower portion of the neck, almost to the level of the thyroid. The thymus is relatively large in infants (Fig. 8-3) and continues to grow until puberty. After that, the gland atrophies so that by old age the gland has almost disappeared.

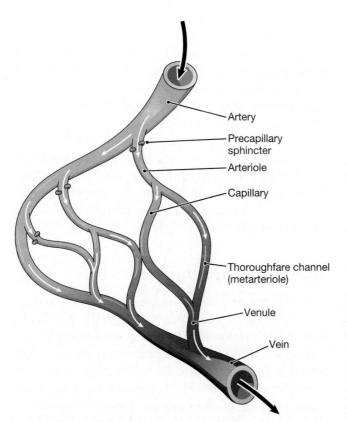

FIGURE 8-2   Blood flow from arteries to arterioles, to capillaries, to venules to veins. (Cohen BJ, Taylor JJ. *Memmler's the Human Body in Health and Disease.* 10th ed. Baltimore, MD: Wolters Kluwer Health; 2005.)

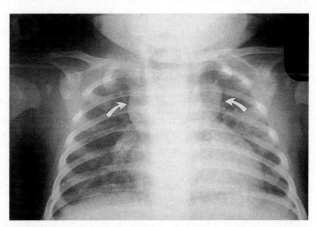

FIGURE 8-3   Enlarged thymus gland which is normal in babies and small children. (Terry R. Yochum, Lindsay J. Rowe, Yochum And Rowe's Essentials of Skeletal Radiology, Third Edition. Philadelphia: Lippincott Williams & Wilkins, 2004.)

The tonsils and adenoids are small, round masses of lymphoid tissue. They are covered with a mucous membrane. The tonsils are located at the back of the throat (palatine tonsils) and at the base of the tongue (lingual tonsils). The adenoids are actually the pharyngeal tonsils and are located at the back of the roof of the pharynx.

The lymphatic vessels begin as lymphatic capillaries and form a vast network. Every tissue supplied by blood vessels (with the exception of the placenta and brain) has lymphatic vessels. As the capillaries join other lymph vessels, they become progressively larger. These are known as lymphatics. Resembling the venous circulation, the lymphatics are the collecting vessels of the lymph system. They send the lymph fluid through round or oval bodies located in the path of the lymphatics. These bodies are the lymph nodes and are found grouped together by the area of the body being drained.

As the lymphatics collect lymph from the body, they empty into the right lymphatic duct (that eventually drains into the right subclavian vein) and the thoracic duct. As the major vessel of the lymphatic system, the thoracic duct drains lymph from the rest of the body and empties into the left subclavian vein.

Physiology and Function

The function of the circulatory (cardiovascular) system is to transport blood. To do this, two separate systems are required. The *pulmonary system* carries blood from the heart to the lungs and back to the heart. The systemic system takes blood from the heart to the body and back to the heart. The trip through the liver to become detoxified is the *portal system*. The circulation through the heart is the *cardiac system*. Both the portal and cardiac systems are parts of the systemic circulation. Figure 8-4 shows the blood flow through the heart and blood vessels for both pulmonary system (right side of the heart) and the systemic system (the left side of the heart).

Pulmonary Circulation

Unoxygenated blood flows through the superior and inferior venae cavae and dumps into the right atrium. By passing through the tricuspid valve, blood flows into the right ventricle. As can be seen in Figure 8-4, the pulmonary trunk originates off the right ventricle

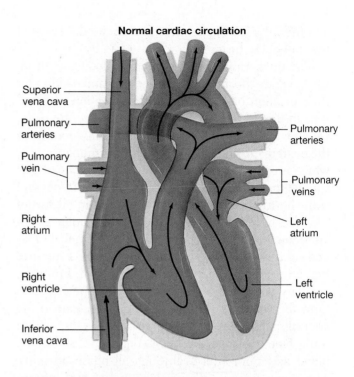

FIGURE 8-4   Normal blood flow through the vessels and the heart. (Asset provided by Anatomical Chart Co.)

and divides into two main branches, the right and left pulmonary arteries. Blood must be pumped through the pulmonary valve into the main pulmonary artery and into the right and left pulmonary arteries. These arteries send blood into the respective lungs, with 60% of the blood being sent to the right side and 40% of the blood going to the left side. After entering the lungs, the blood receives oxygen in the capillaries that surround the alveoli and returns to the heart through the right and left pulmonary veins into the left atrium. At this point, systemic circulation begins.

Systemic Circulation

The left atrium receives oxygenated blood from the pulmonary veins and sends it through the mitral valve into the left ventricle. The ascending aorta originates off the left ventricle, passes posterior to the main pulmonary artery and anterior to the right pulmonary vein. Superior to this, the aortic arch has three major branches. The brachiocephalic artery is also known as the innominate artery. The left common carotid and the left subclavian artery are the other two branches. The right common carotid artery does not originate off the aortic arch but rather is a branch of the innominate artery. Figure 8-5 shows these branches.

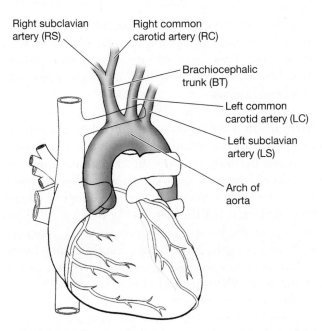

Right subclavian artery (RS)

Right common carotid artery (RC)

Brachiocephalic trunk (BT)

Left common carotid artery (LC)

Left subclavian artery (LS)

Arch of aorta

FIGURE 8-5 Common pattern of branches of the arch of the aorta (present in approximately 65% of people). The largest branch (BT) arises from the beginning of the arch and divides into two branches (RS and RC). The next artery (LC) arises from the superior part of the arch. The third branch (LS) arises from the arch approximately 1 cm distal to the left common carotid. (Moore KL, Dalley AF. *Clinically Oriented Anatomy.* 4th ed. Baltimore, MD: Lippincott Williams & Wilkins; 1999.)

The left ventricle pumps blood through the aortic valve into the ascending aorta to the arch. At this point, a portion of the blood flows through the three major branches of the arch to supply the upper body with oxygenated blood. The remaining portion of the blood flows through the descending aorta to reach the lower body. At about the level of L4, the abdominal aorta bifurcates into the right and left common iliac arteries. Each common iliac artery descends and divides into the internal and external iliac arteries. Branches from these arteries supply the pelvic organs and muscles. Within the capillaries of each structure of the body, blood releases it vital oxygen and then drains from the body part into either the superior or inferior vena cava. These two veins return venous blood back to the right atrium of the heart, thus completing the systemic circulation.

Portal Circulation

Blood in the vessels of the abdominal digestive organs must go through portal circulation. Blood from veins in the visceral walls and the visceral organs, including the gallbladder, pancreas, spleen, stomach, and

intestines, is carried to the liver by the portal vein. Nutrients that are carried to the liver are stored, after conversion, for later use by body tissues. The hepatic veins carry the blood from the liver to the inferior vena cava, which drains the blood into the right atrium. The blood is now ready for pulmonary circulation.

Lymphatic System

The lymphatic system as a whole has a major role in immunity. It moves lymph fluid in a closed circuit with the cardiovascular system. Lymphocytes and antibodies are produced; fat and fat-soluble substances from the intestinal tract are absorbed; phagocytosis is initiated as appropriate; and blood is manufactured when other sources are compromised.

The chief functions of the spleen are the formation of lymphocytes, monocytes, and plasma cells (hematopoiesis); phagocytosis; and the storage of red blood corpuscles. Although the spleen is an extremely useful organ, it can be removed without detrimental effects. The lymphatic tissue of the thymus gland helps to produce lymphocytes (T-cells and B-cells) that work to destroy foreign organisms. The tonsils filter out bacteria and other foreign matter and play a role in the formation of lymphocytes. The lymph vessels collect protein and water, which are continually filtered out of the blood. Lymph nodes filter out bacteria, particles, or other foreign bodies from the blood.

Pathology

Terminology

Cardiovascular disease is a broad, umbrella term that encompasses a collection of diseases and conditions. Its two main components are diseases of the heart and diseases of the blood vessels. Everything from aneurysms and heart attacks to varicose veins are types of cardiovascular diseases. A look at the diseases that a radiographer will most often encounter is described.

Lipids that are deposited in the arteries cause plaque. The gradual buildup of fatty deposits (mainly cholesterol) on the inner lining of an artery wall is termed **atherosclerosis**. Atherosclerosis progressively narrows the artery, decreasing the blood flow. The process of atherosclerosis begins at an early age. Significant disease may be present in some patients before the age of

20 years. **Arteriosclerosis** is the hardening of the wall of the arteries due to the plaque formation and calcification (Fig. 8-6). Several other conditions may arise from plaque buildup. The arteries may become narrow. This narrowing is known as **stenosis**. A change in the wall of blood vessels such as the irregularity caused by arteriosclerosis is the major cause of an intravascular clot known as a **thrombus**.

A thrombus is a blood clot that has attached itself to the inner wall of an artery or vein. A thrombus may disintegrate spontaneously or it may require medical treatment. Two other factors lead to the development of intravascular thrombosis. Clots tend to form where blood flow is slow. Thrombi especially occur in areas of stasis in patients who are inactive or immobilized, such as after major abdominal surgery. If a thrombus remains within the lumen of the vessel, it may occlude the flow of blood, cutting off oxygen that is vital to tissues. The thrombus may break off from the vessel wall and travel to the lungs or heart. Death may result when a thrombus completely occludes a major coronary vessel or a vessel to the brain or lungs.

If one of the coronary arteries becomes completely blocked, that part of the heart muscle will die, resulting in **myocardial infarction**. The major site of involvement is the left ventricle, although some infarcts extend into the right ventricle. Symptoms of myocardial infarctions are variable. Many patients have no symptoms prior to their first myocardial infarction, although a few may experience angina.

Isolated inflammation of the heart wall can occur. **Myocarditis** refers to inflammation of the myocardium, and **pericarditis** is inflammation of the pericardium.

When the muscle fibers stretch, causing the heart to enlarge, the process is known as **cardiac dilation**. When the heart remains enlarged because of a disease process, the term **cardiomegaly** (Fig. 8-7) is used. Shortness of breath, known as **dyspnea**, is often associated with cardiomegaly, as the heart compresses lung tissue.

Various terms are used for malposition of the organs of the body. **Dextrocardia** occurs when the heart is displaced to the right side of the body (known as dextroposition). If the heart is reversed so that it is a mirror image of a normal heart, this is known as **cardiac heterotaxia**. When all the organs of the body are reversed from normal and on the opposite side of the body, the condition is known as **situs inversus**.

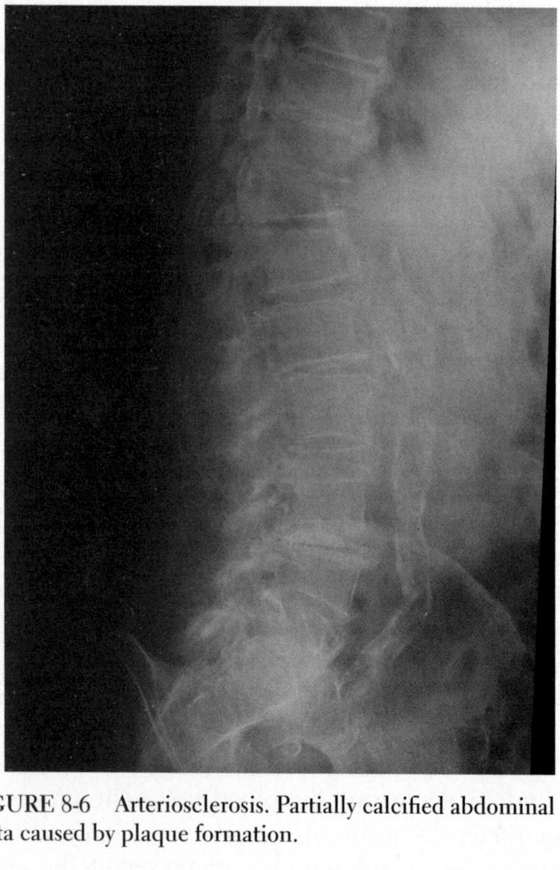

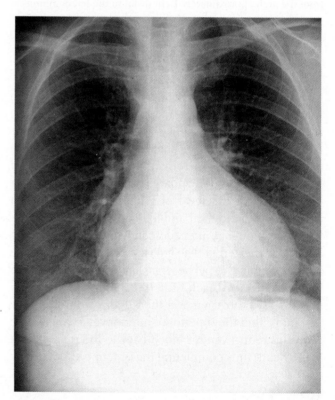

FIGURE 8-7 Massive cardiomegaly in a 45-year-old woman with immunoglobulin light chain (AL) amyloidosis. (Koopman WJ, Moreland LW. *Arthritis and Allied Conditions: A Textbook of Rheumatology.* 15th ed. Philadelphia, PA: Lippincott Williams & Wilkins; 2005.)

FIGURE 8-6 Arteriosclerosis. Partially calcified abdominal aorta caused by plaque formation.

Case Study

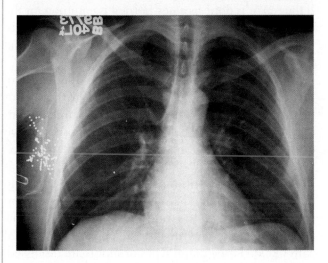

This 21-year-old patient was brought into the emergency department approximately 1 AM. A chest radiograph was ordered. The technologist marked the image with his initials, the date, the fact that it was an upright image and a 40L next to the upright arrow. The radiologist read this out as a gun shot wound (GSW) to the right axillary area. It was discovered the following morning that the report was incorrect. The patient had been shot on the left side. Yet that is the opposite side of the heart's apex. Looking closely at the heart and the diaphragm it can be seen that there is air in the stomach below the heart. If the patient was truly shot on the left side (as was confirmed by visual inspection of the patient in the operating suite) then this patient has the condition known as situs inversus.

When the valves of the heart are affected by some pathologic condition such as thickening or shrinking due to infection, the term **valvular disease** is used. Valvular disease refers to valves that will not operate normally. The valve may be **incompetent**, wherein the valve is normally formed but will not completely close the orifice, which allows retrograde blood flow. A valve that is considered **insufficient** is one that will not operate properly because it is deformed.

Congenital Anomalies

Congenital heart disease is a broad term and includes a wide range of diseases and conditions. These diseases can affect the formation of the heart muscle or its chamber or valves. Some congenital heart defects may be apparent right at the time of birth, while others may not be detected until later in life. Only the most common congenital defects are described here. Although the radiographer should be familiar with the various conditions that can be seen on a chest radiograph, it is not the intent here to cover areas that are rarely seen, or that only a physician can determine from advanced years of study.

Coarctation of the aorta is severe narrowing of the aorta (Fig. 8-8) that causes the left ventricle of the heart to suffer an increase in workload in order to push blood through a narrow passageway. The seriousness of the defect depends on the location of the constriction. If the narrowing is severe enough or complete, anastomotic vessels develop in an attempt to compensate

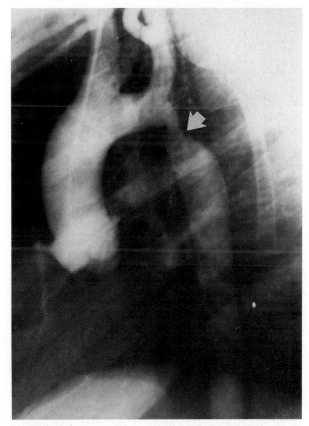

FIGURE 8-8 Angiogram shows the area of coarctation (**arrow**). (Daffner RH. *Clinical Radiology: The Essentials.* 3rd ed. Philadelphia, PA: Lippincott Williams & Wilkins; 2007.)

for the inadequate blood supply to the lower portion of the body. This results in hypertension in the upper extremities and hypotension in the lower extremities.

There are two varieties of coarctation of the aorta: localized and tubular. The most common is the *localized type* (formerly known as adult). This occurs four times more often in males than in females and is rarely seen in African Americans. In an adult, severe hypertension proximal to the coarctation results in dilation of the aortic arch. Rib-notching is an important radiographic sign of coarctation of the aorta (Fig. 8-9). The sign refers to sharply defined bony erosions along the lower margins of the ribs caused by the development of anastomotic vessels that enlarge under their increased volume and cause pressure erosions on the ribs.

Tubular coarctation is hypoplasia of a long segment of aortic arch after the origin of the innominate artery. Cardiac anomalies with tubular coarctation are common, whereas they are not common with a localized type coarctation. Depending on how quickly the ductus closes between the aorta and pulmonary trunk, the

newborn will develop congestive heart failure (CHF) by the second or third week of life due to overload of the left ventricle.

Coarctation can be removed by surgery or by balloon dilation done in the cardiac catheterization lab. If the repair is done as a newborn, it is common for the coarctation to return. As an adult, with equal pressure in the upper and lower extremities, it is unlikely that the aorta will become obstructed again.

Congenital heart abnormalities are the result of inborn defects caused by failure of the heart or major blood vessels near the heart to develop normally during the growth period before birth. The most common types of congenital abnormalities are those in which holes in the heart wall occur. These are known as **shunts** and allow pulmonary and systemic blood to mix. Blood is shunted from the systemic circulation (high pressure) to the pulmonary circulation (low pressure). This causes the lungs to become overloaded with blood. Three major types of shunts are discussed.

Septal defects are small openings in the septum of the heart. Openings in the septum between the two atria are known as *atrial septal defects* (ASDs) and are the most common congenital defect of the heart (Fig. 8-10).

In a large defect, a large amount of oxygen-rich blood leaks from the left side back to the right side and then back to the lungs. This is a left-to-right shunt because the pressure is higher in the left atrium

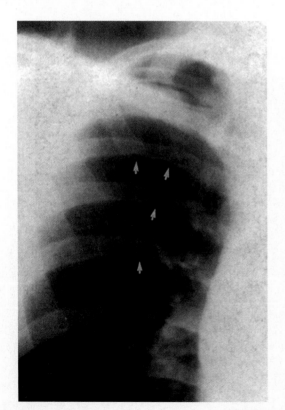

FIGURE 8-9   Close-up from the posteroanterior examination of a 24-year-old man with coarctation of the aorta. The sclerotic margin along the superior border of the scalloped inferior erosions (*arrows*) characterizes rib-notching. (Topol EJ, Califf RM, Isner J, et al. *Textbook of Cardiovascular Medicine.* 3rd ed. Philadelphia, PA: Lippincott Williams & Wilkins; 2006.)

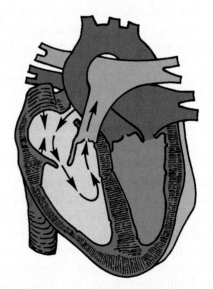

FIGURE 8-10   Atrial septal defect (ASD). (LifeART image, copyright ©2013. Lippincott Williams & Wilkins. All rights reserved.)

than it is in the right atrium. Pulmonary blood flow is increased because of this type of shunt. In addition to overloading the pulmonary bed, the right ventricle experiences an overload. This produces a radiographic appearance of enlargement of the right ventricle and right atrium.

If the defect occurs between the two ventricles, it is known as a *ventricular septal defect* (VSD; Fig. 8-11). This defect is more serious than an ASD because there is a greater pressure difference between the two ventricles than between the two atria. VSDs vary in size and may occur in the membranous or muscular portion of the ventricular septum. Owing to higher pressure in the left ventricle, a shunting of blood from the left to the right ventricle occurs during systole because of the higher pressure in the ventricle during that phase. If pulmonary vascular resistance produces pulmonary hypertension, the shunt of blood is then reversed from the right to the left ventricle, resulting in cyanosis. Some blood flows from the left ventricle to the right ventricle (left-to-right shunt), forcing both ventricles to pump the same blood more than once. The radiographic image shows enlargement of the left side of the heart. In small openings, there is no strain on the heart, and patients are usually asymptomatic except for a heart murmur in the first weeks of life. If the septal opening is large, symptoms can be severe.

Breathing is rapid; growth is retarded, and the infant has feeding difficulties.

Small defects often close in childhood. However, if the opening is large, closing the hole before the age of 2 years is necessary to prevent future problems. The defect can be surgically corrected by sewing a patch over the hole. Repairing a VSD restores the blood circulation to normal and the long-term outlook is good.

The third major type of left-to-right shunt is a *patent arterial duct*, which exists when the arterial duct in a newborn fails to close after birth (Fig. 8-12). Failure of closing of arterial duct is quite common in premature infants, but is somewhat rare in full-term babies. The arterial duct is a vessel that extends from the bifurcation of the pulmonary artery to join the aorta just distal to the left subclavian artery. It serves to shunt blood from the pulmonary artery into the systemic circulation during intrauterine life. If it does not close soon after birth, blood will continue to flow through the duct during systole and diastole. Oxygenated blood is

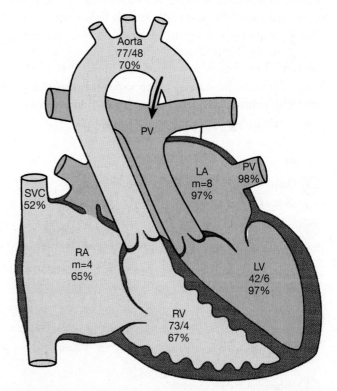

FIGURE 8-12   The patent ductus arteriosus shunts blood into the pulmonary circuit, and the foramen ovale shunts an equal amount out of the pulmonary circuit. **LA,** left atrium; **LV,** left ventricle; **PV,** pulmonary vein; **RA,** right atrium; **RV,** right ventricle; **SVC,** superior vena cava. (Mullins CE, Mayer DC. *Congenital Heart Disease: A Diagrammatic Atlas.* New York: Alan R Liss, 1988, with permission.)

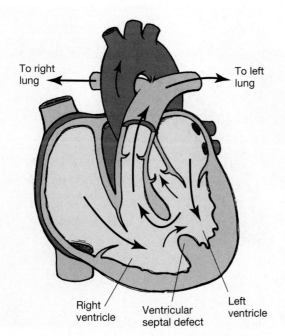

FIGURE 8-11   **A ventricular septal defect (VSD) is an abnormal opening between the right and left ventricle.**

continuously shunted from the aorta to the pulmonary artery and back to the lungs instead of going through the aorta to the body. The heart will be overworked in an attempt to balance the supply with the demand for oxygen. Since the heart depends on the lungs for its supply of oxygen, the lungs become overworked in their effort to keep pace with oxygen demands and breathing becomes dyspneic on light exertion, with resultant fatigue. Chest radiographs demonstrate enlargement of the left atrium and left ventricle and increased vascular congestion. A large opening will cause the child to tire quickly, grow slowly, and be more susceptible to things like pneumonia. If the opening does not close within a few weeks of birth, it must be surgically tied off.

Tetralogy of **Fallot** occurs when four conditions exist simultaneously. There must be pulmonary stenosis, a VSD, right ventricle hypertrophy (thickening), and displacement of the aorta to the right (or overriding of the aorta above the VSD) (Fig. 8-13). This combination of defects causes the blood to be unoxygenated, as it does not flow through the pulmonary system. Pulmonary stenosis is a narrowing of the pulmonic valve and the muscular region below the valve. This decreases the amount of blood that is trying to flow from the right ventricle into the pulmonary circulation. Thus, there is a decreased blood flow to the lungs. This in turn causes an elevation of pressure in the right ventricle and hypertrophy of that chamber

as it overworks to pump the blood through the narrow pulmonary valve.

The VSD allows unoxygenated blood in the right ventricle to mix with oxygenated blood in the left ventricle (known as a right-to-left shunt). This allows blood to travel up through the displaced aorta, which opens directly into both the right and left ventricles. Because the aorta is carrying both unoxygenated and oxygen-rich blood, the amount of oxygen the aorta carries to the body tissues is decreased. This gives rise to extreme cyanosis and is a common cause of "blue baby."

When the right ventricle enlarges, it causes the apex of the heart to become displaced upward and laterally. This is the classic radiographic appearance known as "Coeur en sabot." It resembles the curved-toe portion of a wooden shoe (Fig. 8-14). Clinical manifestations include clubbing of fingers and toes, systolic murmurs, and retardation of growth.

Complete repair tends to be done early in life but usually after the age of 1 year. If the infant is extremely small and cyanotic, a temporary operation may be done first to provide adequate blood flow to the lungs. This allows the baby to grow big enough to have a full repair. The temporary repair consists of a shunt being built between the aorta and pulmonary artery. This shunt is removed when a complete repair is undertaken. Unfortunately, it is being proven that 20 to 30 years after the repair,

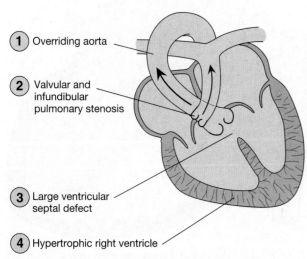

FIGURE 8-13   Classic anatomic features of tetralogy of Fallot. (1) Overriding aorta (dextroposition of the aorta); (2) obstruction to right ventricular outflow (infundibular or valvular pulmonic stenosis); (3) VSD; (4) right ventricular hypertrophy. (Blackbourne LH. *Advanced Surgical Recall.* 2nd ed. Baltimore, MD: Lippincott Williams & Wilkins; 2004.)

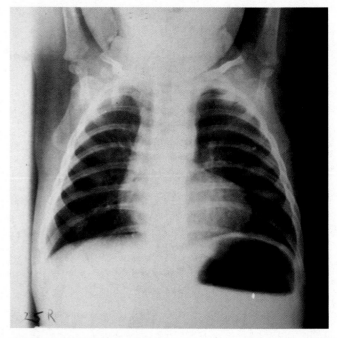

FIGURE 8-14   Classic appearance of "Coeur en sabot" resulting from tetralogy of Fallot.

pulmonary regurgitation is common. Because the valves that were put into the pulmonary main trunk have a point in which it will wear out, there is a need for valve replacement. MRI is extremely useful in determining the time for the replacement. MRI will be ordered to watch the valve and determine the optimal time for replacement before the actual failure of the valve.

Display 8-1 shows the different types of congenital heart defects.

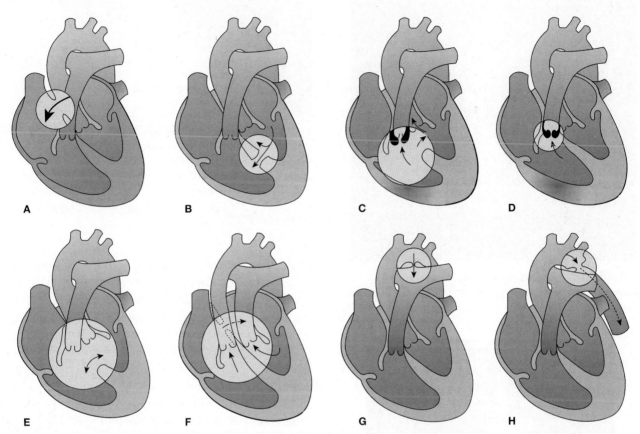

DISPLAY 8-1   Congenital heart defects. (A) Atrial septal defect: blood is shunted from left to right. (B) Ventricular septal defect: blood is usually shunted from left to right. (C) Tetralogy of Fallot: this involves a ventricular septal defect, dextroposition of the aorta, right ventricular outflow obstruction, and right ventricular hypertrophy. Blood is shunted from right to left. (D) Pulmonary stenosis, with decreased pulmonary blood flow and right ventricular hypertrophy. (E) Endocardial cushion defects: blood flows between the chambers of the heart. (F) Transposition of the great vessels: the pulmonary artery is attached to the left side of the heart and the aorta to the right side. (G) Patent ductus arteriosus: the high-pressure blood of the aorta is shunted back to the pulmonary artery. (H) Postductal coarctation of the aorta. (Porth CM. *Pathophysiology Concepts of Altered Health States.* 7th ed. Philadelphia, PA: Lippincott Williams & Wilkins; 2005.)

Inflammatory and Degenerative Processes

An **aneurysm** is a major process that will affect the adult aorta. An aneurysm is a dilatation of an artery (usually the aorta) and is caused by atherosclerosis in almost 80% of the cases. Trauma is normally the cause of the remaining cases; however, diseases such as syphilis, Marfan syndrome (congenital), and high blood pressure are also known to be a causative factor in an aneurysm.

A true aneurysm is a permanent dilation of all the layers of a weakened but intact vessel wall. Aneurysms are found to be one of three types. A *saccular* aneurysm (Fig. 8-15) is a localized outpouching of one side of the vessel wall, usually located in the cerebral arteries but it may be in the distal abdominal aorta.

A *fusiform* aneurysm is a uniform dilatation of the entire portion of the artery (Fig. 8-16). Such aneurysms are usually found in the distal abdominal aorta. The third type is known as a *dissecting* aneurysm (Fig. 8-17). This occurs when a hemorrhage occurs between the layers of the wall of the artery. Approximately 75% of these aneurysms are found in the arch.

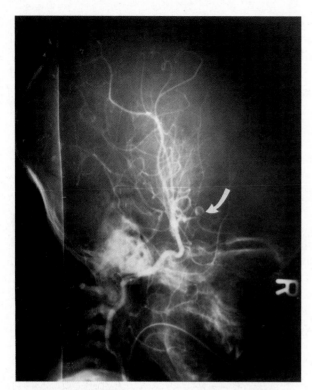

FIGURE 8-15   Cerebral angiography shows a saccular aneurysm (*curved arrow*) of the anterior communicating artery in an infant.

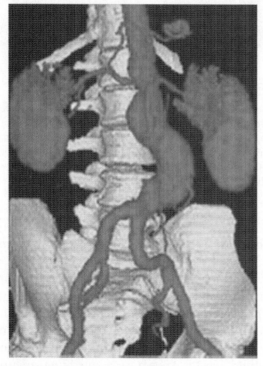

FIGURE 8-16   Three-dimensional CT shows an enlarged abdominal aorta inferior to the renal arteries. This represents a fusiform aneurysm. (Baim DS. *Grossman's Cardiac Catheterization, Angiography, and Intervention.* 7th ed. Philadelphia, PA: Lippincott Williams & Wilkins; 2006.)

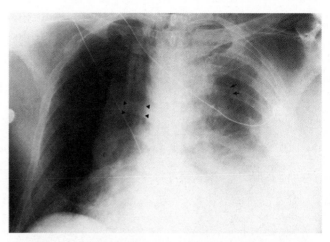

FIGURE 8-17   Chest radiograph of a 65-year-old woman with an aortic arch dissecting aneurysm. The *arrowheads* point to the misplaced trachea, the *arrow* points to an indistinct aortic knob. There is also massive left pleural effusion. (-Nuss, Wolfson AB, Lyndon CH, et al. *The Clinical Practice of Emergency Medicine.* 3rd ed. Philadelphia, PA: Lippincott Williams & Wilkins; 2001.)

Dissecting aneurysms can take on the appearance of a fusiform type as the dissection causes progressive widening of the aortic shadow. Any time when an aneurysm is found in the abdominal aorta, it is known as the triple A (AAA) for abdominal aortic aneurysm.

In addition to the listed types of aneurysms, there is a false aneurysm. This is a pulsating hematoma and must be distinguished as such. Ultrasonography of the abdominal aorta will determine if the palpable mass is truly an aneurysm or a hematoma. Display 8-2 shows the anatomical structures of each type of aneurysm as compared to the normal artery.

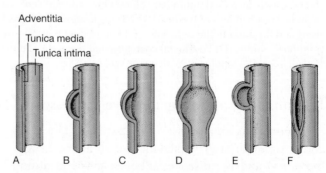

DISPLAY 8-2   Arterial aneurysm: (A) normal artery; (B) false aneurysm—the clot is outside the arterial wall; (C) true aneurysm with one, two, or all three layers of the wall involved; (D) fusiform aneurysm; (E) saccular aneurysm; (F) dissecting aneurysm—the layers of the arterial wall have been split. (Smeltzer SC, Bare BG. *Brunner & Suddarth's Textbook of Medical-Surgical Nursing.* 9th ed. Philadelphia, PA: Lippincott Williams & Wilkins; 2000.)

The danger of an aneurysm is its tendency to increase in size and to rupture, leading to massive hemorrhage that may be fatal if it involves a critical organ such as the brain. About 15,000 people in the United States die each year from ruptured aortic aneurysms. It is the 10th leading cause of deaths in men over the age of 50 years. It is recommended that men over 65 years of age who have ever smoked (even if they quit years ago) should be checked for abdominal aneurysms.

Angiography is the modality of choice to diagnose aneurysms. When a dissecting aneurysm is present, arteriography is used to define the site of extravasation and the extent of the dissection (Fig. 8-18). Ultrasonography is also used, especially if the injection of contrast medium under pressure is determined to be detrimental to the patient. However, if the aneurysm is located within the thoracic cavity, CT may be used if aortography is not indicated.

Surgery is generally recommended as treatment, unless the diameter of the aorta is small (less than 4.5 cm). The timing and indications for surgery differ depending on the type of aneurysm. Some people are candidates for endovascular stent repair (described below under imaging modalities).

Atherosclerosis is the major cause of vascular disease. It is characterized by irregularly distributed fat deposits in medium- and large-sized arteries. Atherosclerosis will begin when the lining of the artery becomes damaged through some process such as smoking. Plaque, which is low-density lipoproteins, will slowly accumulate at the site of damage. Arteries become narrowed from the plaque buildup. As stated earlier, the plaque can eventually occlude the arteries completely. Plaque formation and stenosis often involve the coronary arteries, causing arteriosclerotic heart disease.

TECH TIP

Even though the terms atherosclerosis and arteriosclerosis are often used interchangeably, these are two separate processes. The knowledgeable technologist will be able to see the difference on a radiographic image. Remember that lipids (cholesterol) building up in the artery is atherosclerosis. When those plaques become calcified and harden the wall of the vessel, it is now arteriosclerosis.

Arteriosclerotic heart disease is also known as cardiovascular disease (Fig. 8-19A, B). It remains the leading cause of deaths in the United States despite declining mortality rates since the 1960s. In 1992, more than two out of every five deaths were the result of major cardiovascular disease. Coronary artery bypass grafting remains among the most frequently performed surgical procedures and will continue to remain so because of hypertension.

Hypertension accelerates the development of atherosclerotic plaques, so it is often found in conjunction with arteriosclerotic heart disease. If enough plaque finally accumulates, the myocardium is damaged. Continual plaque buildup results in a myocardial infarction. Mild cardiomegaly as well as calcification in the coronary arteries can be seen on the radiographic image.

CHF results when the heart cannot supply enough blood at a sufficient rate to meet the metabolic requirements of tissues. It can be considered a symptom of impairment of the pumping action of the heart that is caused by an underlying disease. This can be caused by damage from a heart attack, cardiovascular disease, hypertension, or infection to the heart muscle and damage to the valves.

CHF can be divided into categories depending on the underlying heart condition present. It may affect

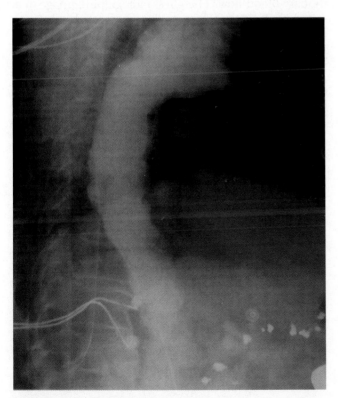

FIGURE 8-18 Angiography of a dissecting aneurysm of the aortic arch.

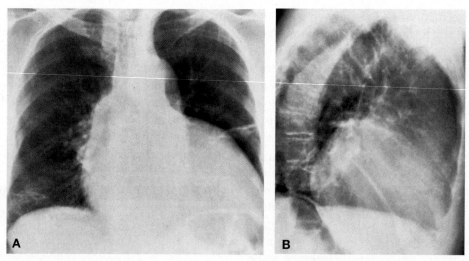

FIGURE 8-19   Arteriosclerotic heart disease. (A) Frontal and (B) lateral views of the chest show marked enlargement of the left ventricle. There is also tortuosity of the aorta and bilateral streaks of fibrosis. (Eisenberg RL. *Clinical Imaging: An Atlas of Differential Diagnosis.* 5th ed. Philadelphia, PA: Lippincott Williams & Wilkins; 2010.)

either the right or left side of the heart. One side of the heart fails while the other side continues its normal output. When this occurs, there is increased pressure in the pulmonary or systemic veins, or both, resulting in "backing up" of blood. CHF is commonly accompanied by pleural effusion. Diffuse cardiomegaly is the classic radiographic sign of CHF.

When there is *left heart failure*, the left ventricle does not pump a volume of blood equal to that of the venous return in the right ventricle. As fluid builds up, a point is reached at which it has nowhere to go but the alveoli and bronchial tree of the lungs. This produces rales and pulmonary edema. As a result, breathing may become more difficult, and the patient tires easily. Left-sided heart failure is usually caused by hypertension, but can result from coronary heart disease or valvular disease. The radiographs show a congested hilar region of the lungs with increased vascular markings. Left heart failure may lead to right heart failure because increased pressure is transmitted through the pulmonary circulation to the right heart.

Right-sided heart failure (Fig. 8-20) causes dilation of the right ventricle and right atrium. The transmission of increased pressure can cause dilation of the superior vena cava, widening of the right superior mediastinum, and edema of the lower extremities. The enlargement of a congested liver may elevate the right hemidiaphragm. Right-sided heart failure can be caused by pulmonary valvular stenosis, emphysema, or pulmonary hypertension resulting from pulmonary emboli. Normally, in an

upright chest radiograph, the pulmonary vessels in the lower lung zones are larger than those in the apices. With severe pulmonary venous hypertension, there is a redistribution of flow so that vessels in the upper zones are larger than those in the lower lung zones. This change is referred to as "cephalization" of pulmonary blood flow. The chest radiographic image of a person with CHF shows a pulmonary vascular shift, an increase in heart size and, more importantly, "cephalization," which is the hallmark on the image (Fig. 8-21).

TECH TIP

Remembering the respiratory system in Chapter 3, the chest radiograph provides an incredible amount of information from something as simple as that examination is. However, thinking back to how chest imaging is performed, if there is any rotation, the heart can be made to look like there is ventricular enlargement. If the technique is not proper, it can hide subtleties such as Kerley B lines or cephalization of the pulmonary vessels. Another error that will create the appearance of CHF is not a deep enough inspiration on the image. A little care and time devoted to the positioning of the patient will provide the physician with the best diagnostic image and allow a correct diagnosis.

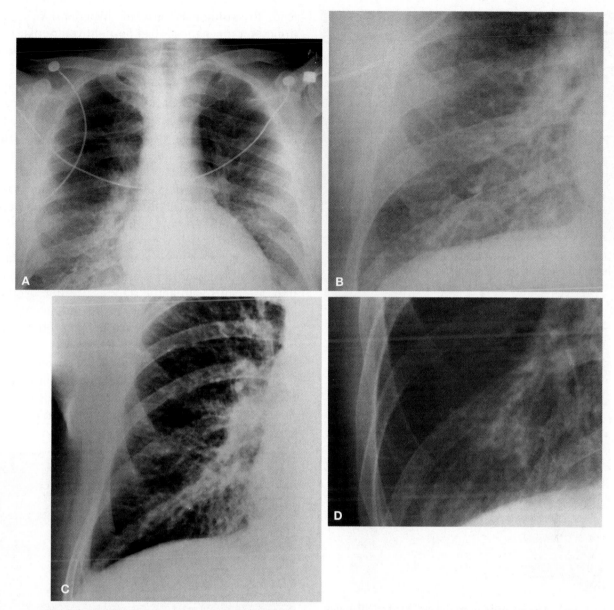

FIGURE 8-20   Kerley lines in patients with congestive right sided heart failure. (A) AP radiograph shows prominent interstitial markings in both bases with a fine interlacing pattern. (B) Detail view shows the linear horizontal Kerley B-lines in the periphery. (C) and (D) Detail views of two other patients show similar findings. (Daffner RH, *Clinical Radiology The Essentials*, 3rd ed. Philadelphia: Lippincott Williams & Wilkins, 2007.)

The most common cause of CHF in the older adult is **hypertensive heart disease**. As its name implies, hypertension is a major cause of this disease. High blood pressure, over a long period of time, causes narrowing of the systemic blood vessels. Because of this resistance, the left ventricle must work harder, causing dilation and enlargement of the ventricle (Fig. 8-22). There is often downward displacement of the apex of the heart. Failure of the left ventricle leads to increased pulmonary venous pressure and congestive failure. Radiographic signs and symptoms are the same as for CHF.

Hypertrophy of the separate chambers of the heart may help pinpoint other pathologic processes that are not yet obvious. **Right atrial enlargement** is recognized radiographically by enlargement of the cardiac shadow to the right of the thoracic spine in the frontal view. Malrotation of the patient, scoliosis, or mediastinal shift must be excluded before the appearance can

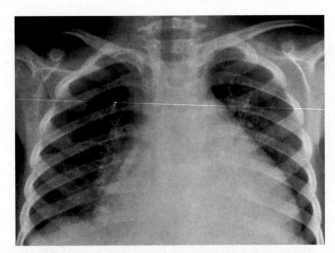

FIGURE 8-21   Congestive heart failure (CHF) with cephalization seen on the right upper apex. There is also increased heart size.

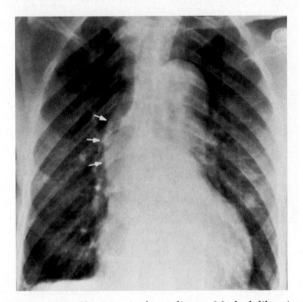

FIGURE 8-22   Hypertensive heart disease. Marked dilatation (*arrows*) of the ascending aorta caused by increased aortic pressure. There is increased left ventricle size. (Eisenberg RL. *Clinical Imaging: An Atlas of Differential Diagnosis.* 5th ed. Philadelphia, PA: Lippincott Williams & Wilkins; 2010.)

be attributed to right atrial enlargement. Although isolated right atrial enlargement is uncommon, it can be caused by subacute bacterial endocarditis or ASD.

Right ventricular enlargement is recognized radiographically by encroachment of the cardiac shadow into the retrosternal space on the lateral projection. This is an imprecise indicator, however, owing to the variability of the size of this space. The right ventricle works harder and enlarges in the presence of defects of the pulmonary vascular bed, as with pulmonary hypertension. The alterations in the pulmonary circulation

lead to pulmonary arterial hypertension, which imposes a mechanical load on right ventricular emptying. Right ventricular enlargement is usually associated with right atrial enlargement (Fig. 8-23).

Enlargement of the left atrium is seen radiographically as a rounded opacity in the retrocardiac region projecting to the left and right of the spine on the posteroanterior projection of the chest. The left atrium enlarges in rheumatic heart disease with mitral stenosis or mitral insufficiency.

Finally, **left ventricle enlargement** is demonstrated by the cardiac shadow to the left of the spine, often with a rounded lateral contour projecting below the diaphragm. The left ventricle works harder and longer with each beat when it meets increased resistance to the emptying of blood into the systemic circulation, as occurs with aortic stenosis, volume overload, and systemic hypertension. The ventricle hypertrophies because of the extra exercise, and sometimes it becomes displaced laterally.

Pericardial effusion is fluid in the pericardial sac. Causes of this condition are tuberculosis and viral infection. When there is a rapid increase in heart size seen on the chest images without other signs of heart failure,

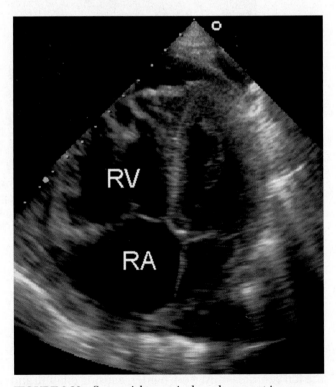

FIGURE 8-23   Severe right ventricular enlargement is demonstrated in this four-chamber view. Note the size of the right ventricle (RV) and right atrium (RA) relative to their left-sided counterparts. In both cases, the septum is shifted leftward. In addition, the RV free wall is thickened and heavily trabeculated.

pericardial effusion should be suspected. An excellent method of demonstrating pericardial effusion is echocardiography (Fig. 8-24). As little as 50 mL of fluid can be detected by this modality, whereas at least 200 mL of fluid must be present before a pericardial effusion can be detected on a radiographic image (Fig. 8-25).

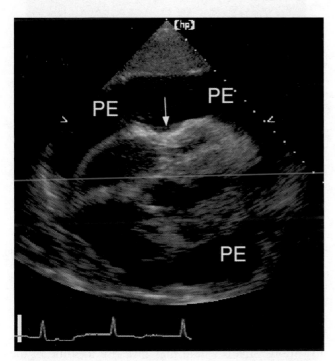

FIGURE 8-24 A subcostal four-chamber view from a patient with a large pericardial effusion (PE) is provided. From this window, diastolic right ventricular free wall collapse (*arrow*) can be demonstrated.

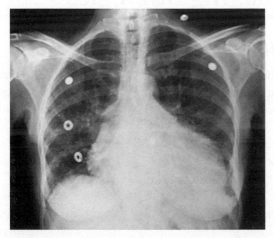

FIGURE 8-25 Chest radiograph demonstrates a large pericardial effusion, blunting of the left costophrenic angle, and patchy pulmonary infiltrates in a patient with systemic lupus erythematosus. (Crapo JD, Glassroth J, Karlinsky JB, et al. *Baum's Textbook of Pulmonary Diseases.* 7th ed. Philadelphia, PA: Lippincott Williams & Wilkins; 2004.)

TECH TIP

Patient positioning is critical so as not to give the illusion of an increased heart size. By learning the different types of hypertrophy of the chambers of the heart and about pericardial effusion, it can be seen that any deviation from proper positioning may cause a resemblance to any of these pathologies. Do not allow the patient to turn his/her head, make sure the shoulders are square against the wall unit, and ensure that the patient understands the importance of a deep inspiration. It is the technologist's duty to present the absolute best image possible and avoid any misreading due to positioning negligence.

The cause of rheumatic fever is unknown, but the attacks are preceded by Streptococcal infection. Even though the occurrence of rheumatic fever has dropped dramatically because of the antibodies used to fight Streptococcal infection, it is still the most common cause of severe valvular dysfunction. Episodes of rheumatic fever cause inflammation of the heart valves rather than the myocardium and leads to scarring deformity of the valves known as **rheumatic heart disease**. Stenosis of the mitral valve is the most common valve deformity associated with rheumatic heart disease.

At variable times following acute illness, chronic damage to heart valves may become evident. Known as **valvular disease**, the functional valve damage is produced by stenosis of the valve opening or valvular insufficiency or both. Fibrosis of the mitral valve, the valve most commonly involved, usually leads to left heart failure (Fig. 8-26). The left heart failure results either from backup of blood into the lungs caused by stenosis or from regurgitation of blood back through the insufficient valve. Stenosis and insufficiency of the aortic valve, the other commonly affected valve, cause left ventricular hypertrophy and eventually heart failure.

In addition to heart failure, the valves may become infected, producing infective endocarditis. Calcification of the mitral valve seen on the chest image is one indication of rheumatic heart disease (Fig. 8-27). Kerley B lines are often present (see Fig. 8-20). These lines eventually become permanent.

Subacute bacterial endocarditis is caused by organisms that live on the heart valves and produce

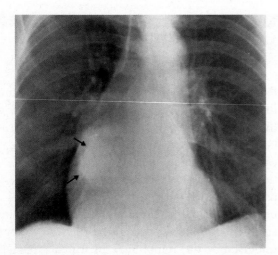

FIGURE 8-26   Mitral stenosis. Posteroanterior chest radiograph demonstrates a double contour (*arrows*) representing the increased density of the enlarged left atrium. This patient was confirmed to have rheumatic heart disease. (Eisenberg RL. *Clinical Imaging: An Atlas of Differential Diagnosis.* 5th ed. Philadelphia, PA: Lippincott Williams & Wilkins; 2010.)

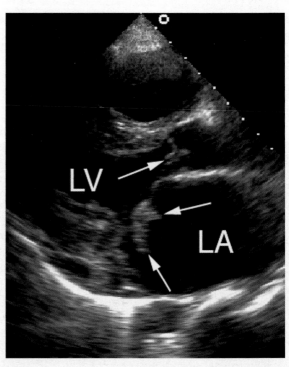

FIGURE 8-28   An example of vegetations involving the mitral and aortic valves is shown. The vegetations are indicated by the *arrows*. LA, left atrium; LV, left ventricle.

an inflammatory reaction (Fig. 8-28). Bacteria are the most common cause, hence the name bacterial endocarditis. Rheumatic valvulitis is the most common predisposing factor to the development of subacute bacterial endocarditis. Early diagnosis results in treatment that reduces the amount of damage, but the severity of this pathologic process should not be overlooked. The most striking feature of this disease is the formation of large number of emboli because of the breaking off of fragments of the vegetations.

These fragments travel in the blood stream and stick to various organs where they give rise to some of the characteristic symptoms of the disease.

Imaging Strategies

Ultrasonography

Echocardiography is used to visualize the chambers of the heart as well as the contracting and relaxation phases of the heart (see Fig. 8-24). Echocardiography is used to study the valves of the heart for motion or prolapse. It is also used to determine any septal defects, patent ductus arteriosus, and to evaluate pericardial effusion and atrial myxoma.

Carotid duplex is an ultrasound procedure performed to assess blood flow through the carotid artery to the brain. High-frequency sound waves are directed from a hand-held transducer probe to the area. These waves "echo" off the arterial structures and produce a two-dimensional image on a monitor, which will make obstructions or narrowing of the arteries visible.

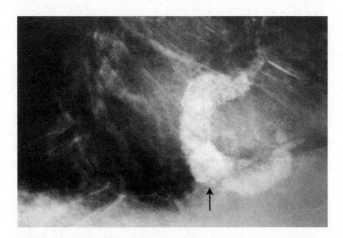

FIGURE 8-27   Mitral valve calcification, lateral chest. Note the circular calcification (*arrow*) in the typical location for mitral valve annulus. (Yochum TR, Rowe LJ. *Yochum and Rowe's Essentials of Skeletal Radiology.* 3rd ed. Philadelphia, PA: Lippincott Williams & Wilkins; 2004.)

Computed Tomography/Magnetic Resonance Imaging

A CT image may be performed if the doctor suspects a thoracic or abdominal aortic aneurysm. Contrast is injected to outline the aorta or other arteries. CT will determine the size and shape of abdominal aneurysms more accurately than ultrasonography. In cases of lymphedema, CT is an excellent method to show the obstruction of the lymph system, causing the edema.

MRI is another excellent modality to demonstrate an aneurysm and in determining their size and exact location. Magnetic resonance angiography (MRA) is a type of MRI. In this study, the patient is injected with contrast media and then undergoes a regular magnetic resonance exam. An MRA is meant to study the blood vessels and walls of the vessels. It is excellent to demonstrate an aneurysm and in determining their size and exact location, and to examine arteriosclerosis and atherosclerosis.

Nuclear Medicine

Advances in radionuclide techniques in the form of instrumentation, radiopharmaceuticals, and computer applications have revolutionized the noninvasive evaluation of cardiovascular physiology and function. Examinations by nuclear medicine now permit the detection and diagnosis of many abnormalities as well as the functional consequences of these diseases.

Nuclear medicine is a complement study that can be in the form of a gated heart scan, which is done to watch motion of the wall of the heart. Incoming information is "gated" into specific intervals from systole to diastole using an echocardiogram. Radionuclide thallium perfusion scanning is the major noninvasive study for assessing regional blood flow to the myocardium. Radionuclide scanning using technetium pyrophosphate or other compounds that are taken up by acutely infracted myocardium is a noninvasive technique for detecting, localizing, and classifying myocardial necrosis. Other nuclear medicine scans are done to demonstrate myocardial infarction, myocardial ischemia, pericardial effusion, and intracardiac shunts.

Interventional Radiology

Angiography is a general term used to describe the radiographic procedure of the vessels of the body. *Arteriography* is the study of the arterial system, *venog-*

raphy is the study of the venous system, *aortography* is the study of the thoracic or abdominal aorta, and *angiocardiography* (cardiography) is the examination of the chambers of the heart. Under sterile conditions, a catheter is fed into the femoral or brachial artery of the patient with fluoroscopic guidance. Once the radiologist is able to place the tip of the catheter into or near the area that is to be studied, a contrast medium is injected under pressure. Radiographic images are taken in a timed sequence with a rapid film changer, or more commonly, with cinefluororadiography. This allows the imaging of the body part from the moment the contrast material is visualized in the arterial phase through the venous phase and dilution and excretion. The patient is constantly monitored throughout the entire procedure for any abnormal reactions or physiologic changes.

An arteriogram is the injection of contrast material into one or more arteries to make them visible on the radiographic image. The blood flow through the area can be evaluated with fluoroscopy.

TECH TIP

Specialization into these areas varies between locations and parts of the United States and other countries. Currently, angiography can be learned on the job or there are special certificate programs that are available in some schools. Anyone who decides to do interventional radiography must be well versed in medical procedures and in performing examinations using sterile techniques. Equipment in these areas is also specialized and a good understanding of its working is essential for running the equipment during a stressful procedure.

Percutaneous transluminal angioplasty with the use of a balloon catheter is now a recognized procedure for the alleviation of symptoms in patients with arteriosclerosis. It is of special value in patients who are extremely ill and in those who would not benefit from arterial surgery. Similar to the stent graft repair described below, a catheter is threaded into the artery to the site of the plaque. At this point, a balloon is inflated, "cracking" the plaque off the arterial wall.

An **endovascular stent repair** is not a diagnostic procedure; however, it is performed with the aid of fluoroscopy. In use since 1999, a stent is threaded over a catheter and placed in the aorta where the aneurysm is found. The graft (stent) is expanded and fastened in place to form a stable channel for blood flow. The catheter is then pulled out, leaving the stent in place. This allows the blood to flow through the opening created by the stent. The graft also reinforces the weakened section of the aorta to prevent the aneurysm from rupturing.

RECAP

Anatomy

- Circulatory system
  - Heart has two atria (base) and two ventricles (apex)
  - Four valves that are important
    - Mitral valve is the left arterioventricular, also called bicuspid
    - Tricuspid valve is the right arterioventricular
    - Aortic semilunar valve is between the aorta and left ventricle
    - Pulmonary valve is between the pulmonary trunk and right ventricle
  - Vessels
    - Aorta is the major artery
    - Inferior vena cava is the major vein
    - Arteries become arterioles, then capillaries, then venules, and finally veins
- Lymphatic system
  - The major organs are the spleen, thymus, and tonsils and adenoids
  - Lymph vessels begin as lymph capillaries and are known as lymphatics
  - Lymphatics are the collecting vessels
  - Lymph nodes are found in the path of the lymphatics and are the filters

Physiology and Function

- Circulatory system
  - Pulmonary circulation
    - Blood flow is from inferior vena cava and superior vena cava into right atrium through tricuspid valve into the right ventricle
    - From right ventricle through the pulmonary valve into lungs

- Blood picks up oxygen from capillaries around alveoli and returns to the left atrium via the pulmonary veins
  - Systemic circulation
    - Blood flow is from left atrium through the mitral valve into the left ventricle
    - From left ventricle through the aortic valve and into the aorta to the body
    - Three branches off of the aortic arch send blood to upper body, while the rest goes to lower body
    - Blood gives off oxygen when in the capillaries of the tissues
  - Portal circulation
    - Blood of the abdominal digestive organs go through the portal circulation to be detoxified
    - After portal circulation, the blood goes to the right atrium for pulmonary circulation
- Lymphatic system
  - Plays a major role in immunity by
    - Producing lymphocytes and antibodies
    - Initiating phagocytosis
    - Producing blood when other ways are compromised

Congenital Pathologies

- Coarctation of the aorta
  - Narrowing of the aorta causing left ventricle enlargement
  - Two types are adult (most common) and juvenile
    - Adult has hypertension, dilated aortic arch, and rib-notching

- Shunts are from high (systemic) to low (pulmonary) and allow unoxygenated and oxygenated blood to mix
  - ASD is a hole in septum between the atria
    - They are the most common
    - Pulmonary blood flow is increased
    - Right ventricle enlargement
  - VSD is a hole in the septum between the ventricles
    - More serious than ASD because pressure is greater in ventricles than in atria
    - Shows left-sided heart enlargement
    - Heart murmur if opening is small; breathing difficulties if opening is large
    - Large openings must be surgically closed to prevent future problems
  - Patent arterial duct
    - Common in premature infants; uncommon in full-term births
    - Blood is shunted from aorta to pulmonary arteries and back to lungs
    - Lungs become overloaded with blood, and heart is overworked to balance oxygen supply and demand
    - Chest images show enlarged left ventricle and left atrium and pulmonary vascular congestion
    - Patent arterial duct must be closed off if it does not heal within a few weeks of birth
- Tetralogy of Fallot
  - Four conditions must exist: pulmonary stenosis; VSD; right ventricle enlargement; aortic displacement
  - Most common cause of "blue baby," because it causes cyanosis
  - This is a right-to-left shunt (others are left-to-right)
  - Not enough blood goes to the lungs to receive oxygen, so heart pumps harder
  - Temporary repair until child is old enough for complete repair
  - Classic sign is "Coeur en sabot" or "wooden shoe"

Other Pathologies

- Aneurysms affects the aorta
  - Aneurysm in the abdominal aorta is most likely caused by atherosclerosis
  - False aneurysm is a pulsating hematoma
  - Saccular (usually cerebral arteries)
  - Fusiform (usually distal abdominal aorta)
  - Dissecting (usually in the aortic arch)
  - Rupture is a danger and can be fatal if occurs
  - Seen by angiography or ultrasonography
  - Treated by surgery if greater than 4.5 cm
- Arteriosclerotic heart disease
  - Also known as cardiovascular disease
  - Coronary artery bypass grafting is done when disease affects heart vessels
  - Hypertension accelerates plaque
  - Continual plaque buildup results in myocardial infarction
- Congestive heart failure (CHF)
  - May affect either the right or left side of the heart
  - If one side fails, the other tries to compensate
  - Often accompanied by pleural effusion
  - Diffuse cardiomegaly and cephalization in the lower lung zones are the classic signs
- Hypertensive heart disease
  - Most common cause of CHF
  - Caused by hypertension, which causes narrowing of the systemic blood vessels
- Hypertrophy
  - Enlargement of any of the chambers of the heart
- Pericardial effusion
  - Fluid in the pericardial sac
  - Caused by tuberculosis or viral infection
  - Best demonstrated by ultrasonography
- Rheumatic heart disease
  - Scarring deformity of the heart valves
  - Caused by multiple episodes of rheumatic fever
  - Mitral valve calcification is the most common sign
- Valvular disease
  - Refers to valve that will not operate normally
  - Usually caused by acute illness
  - Valve is either incompetent or insufficient
- Subacute bacterial endocarditis
  - Caused by bacterial organisms living on the heart valves
  - Produces an inflammatory reaction

Imaging Strategies

- Ultrasonography
  - Echocardiography visualizes the chambers of the heart and the valves; determines septal defects and pericardial effusion
  - Carotid duplex scanning is performed to assess blood flow of the carotid artery

- Good method for assessing obstructions in the lymph system causing edema
- CT/MRI
  - Both are excellent to visualize thoracic or abdominal aneurysms and also any obstructions in the lymph system
  - MRA is a form of MRI done for aneurysms
  - MRI allows evaluation of the aortic root better than CT
- Nuclear medicine
  - Gated heart studies are done to watch the heart wall motion
  - Blood flow to areas of infarct, ischemia, and shunts are seen
- Interventional radiography
  - Angiography: general term for the study of blood vessels
    - Different types are arteriography, aortography, venography, and angiocardiography; these depend on what area is being studied
  - Percutaneous transluminal angioplasty
    - Uses a balloon catheter on patients who suffer from arteriosclerosis
  - Endovascular stent graft
    - This is a repair of an aneurysm
    - Catheter with a stent is inserted into the area of the aneurysm and inflated and left in place for blood to drain through the opening

CLINICAL AND RADIOGRAPHIC CHARACTERISTICS OF COMMON PATHOLOGIES

Pathologic Condition	Causal Factors to Include Age, if Relevant	Manifestations	Radiographic Appearance
Atherosclerosis	As early as the 20s High cholesterol	Narrowing of vessel	A slight increase in opacity but not due to calcium
Arteriosclerosis	Elderly Latter stages of atherosclerosis	Hardening of vessel wall	Calcification of the vessel wall
Coarctation of aorta	Congenital Narrowing of aorta	Hypertension or hypotension	Rib-notching
Atrial septal defect	Congenital	Frequent pulmonary infections	Enlarged right atrium and ventricle
Ventricular septal defect	Congenital	Heart murmur	Enlarged left atrium and ventricle
Patent arterial duct	Congenital	Asymptomatic	Enlarged left atrium and ventricle
Tetralogy of Fallot	Congenital	Cyanosis	Coeur en sabot
Aneurysms Saccular Fusiform Dissecting	Any age Weakened vessel wall Tear in vessel wall	Usually asymptomatic	Localized ballooning Uniform dilation Diffuse enlargement
Arteriosclerotic heart disease	Hypertension	Dyspnea	Calcification, cardiomegaly
Congestive heart failure (CHF)	Any age (elderly) Hypertension	Easy fatigue	Cephalization, cardiomegaly
Pericardial effusion	Any age Tuberculosis Virus infection	Usually asymptomatic	Rapid increase in heart size
Rheumatic heart disease	Unknown	Endocarditis	Calcified mitral valve, Kerley B lines

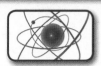 # CRITICAL THINKING DISCUSSION QUESTIONS

1. Describe blood flow in the pulmonary circulation. Describe blood flow in the systemic circulation.

2. Explain "rib-notching." What causes it and when does it occur?

3. What are left-to-right shunts? How do the lungs become overloaded with blood in a shunt? What is the shunt flow from left to right? Explain fully the three major types of left-to-right shunts. Be sure to include their names, where they occur, where the blood flows, what the shunt causes, and what the radiographic appearance is.

4. Describe tetralogy of Fallot. What must exist for this condition to occur? What does this combination of defects cause? What type of shunt is produced with this condition? This condition is the most common cause of "blue baby." Why?

5. List and describe the appearance of the three types of aneurysms. What is the danger of an aneurysm?

6. What is congestive heart failure (CHF)? What causes it? What happens to the heart in left-sided heart failure? What happens to the heart in right-sided heart failure? What is the radiographic appearance of each?

7. What is pericardial effusion? What causes it? When should this condition be suspected? What modality is best suited for pericardial effusion? Why is it the best?

8. How is hypertension related to atherosclerosis?

9. What are the complications of one or more episodes of rheumatic fever?

10. What causes subacute bacterial endocarditis? What is a predisposing factor?

9

The Nervous System

● Goals

1. To review the basic anatomy and function of the central nervous system

   OBJECTIVE: Identify the ventricles and meninges from images

2. To learn the congenital disorders of the brain and spinal cord

   OBJECTIVE: Identify the characteristics of hydrocephalus and spina bifida

3. To understand how pathologies from other systems are related to the central nervous system

   OBJECTIVE: Identify the factors that precipitate stroke and hemorrhage

   OBJECTIVE: Relate and explain how trauma of systems already studied can be related to the central nervous system

● Key Terms

Acoustic neuromas
Anencephaly
Aphasia
Arnold-Chiari
Astrocytoma
Cauda equina
Cerebral hemorrhage
Cerebrovascular accidents
Chordoma
Concussion
Contusion
Craniopharyngioma
Encephalitis
Epidural abscess
Epidural hemorrhage
External hydrocephaly
Extradural hematoma

● Goals *continued*

4. To determine how pathology of the central nervous system can be visualized for diagnostic purposes

   OBJECTIVE: Explain how the central nervous system can be imaged

● Key Terms *continued*

Germinomas
Glioblastoma multiforme
Glioma
Hematoma
Hydrocephaly
Internal hydrocephaly
Intracerebral hemorrhage
   (intraparenchymal hemorrhage)
Medulloblastoma
Meningioma
Meningitis
Microcephaly
Neurofibroma
Neurons
Stroke
Subarachnoid hemorrhage
Subdural empyema
Subdural hematoma
Transient ischemic attacks (TIAs)

The nervous system can be compared with a telegraph system. The brain acts as the main office and relays messages by way of the spinal cord through nerve fibers of the peripheral nervous system that radiate to every structure in the body. Sensory nerves bring information, or impulses, from the various organ systems, while motor nerves carry impulses from the central coordinating point to the muscles or glands, which need to respond so that the body can adjust for its own safety and welfare.

Anatomy

The nervous system is divided into central, peripheral, and autonomic systems. The central nervous system includes the brain and the spinal cord; the peripheral nervous system is composed of the cranial and spinal nerves; and the autonomic nervous system is divided into the sympathetic and parasympathetic systems. The autonomic nervous system is really a subsystem of the peripheral nervous system and is often discussed independently as it controls and harmonizes the work of the vital organs. The nervous tissue is composed of cells and fibers of many types collected together into one central axis and many peripheral strands.

Central Nervous System

The most highly organized system of the body, the central nervous system is comprised of the brain and the spinal cord together with the nerve trunks and fibers connected to them. This system is also referred to as the cerebrospinal system. The brain and spinal cord are both protected from injury by the bony components of the skull and the arched vertebrae of the dorsal body cavity.

The brain is the greatly enlarged and modified part of the central nervous system. It accounts for about 98% of the entire central nervous system. There are about 11 billion **neurons** in the brain. These carry out its functions by transmitting a message from one cell to the next through a series of axons and dendrites.

Divisions of the brain are the cerebrum and diencephalon; the brain stem and the cerebellum. The term brain stem refers to the midbrain, pons, and medulla.

Cerebrum

Also known as the forebrain, the cerebrum occupies most of the brain cavity, covering all the other parts. It is divided into two hemispheres held together by a massive bundle of white matter called the corpus callosum. The two hemispheres are arbitrarily divided into four lobes, each named after the cranial bone to which it is related: frontal, occipital, parietal, and temporal. The entire cerebrum is covered with the cerebral cortex where the highest level of neural processing takes place including language, memory, and cognitive functions.

Located below the cerebrum is the diencephalon, which is the part of the brain between the cerebellum and the cerebrum. It contains the structures called the thalamus and the hypothalamus. About the size of a walnut, the thalamus is an important relay station, distributing sensory information from the periphery to different regions of the cortex. Underneath the thalamus, is the small hypothalamus. The cavity of this part of the brain contains the third ventricle.

Brain Stem

Continuous with the spinal cord below it, the brain stem consists of the midbrain, pons, and medulla. The brain stem also contains the nuclei of the 12 cranial nerves. There are many important reflex centers which control vital functions such as heartbeat and respiration. It is also important in regulating levels of consciousness as injury to the brain stem can result in prolonged loss of consciousness or death.

The medulla oblongata is the most posterior part of the brain. It is here that the central canal of the spinal cord enlarges to form the fourth ventricle. This large cavity secretes some of the cerebrospinal fluid (CSF) and contains openings (foramina) that connect the cavity with the subarachnoid space with the lateral ventricles in the cerebral hemispheres. Connecting the cerebellum, the cerebrum, and the medulla oblongata is the pons.

Cerebellum

The second largest division of the brain is the cerebellum, which is Latin for the "little brain." It is situated just above the medulla, which it overhangs, and beneath the rear portion of the cerebrum. The pons lies anterior to the cerebellum and between the midbrain and medulla. Like the cerebrum, its surface is formed by a highly folded cortex.

Ventricles

The ventricles of the brain are located within the brain hemispheres and are a series of intercommunicating cavities. They contain CSF and communicate with the subarachnoid space surrounding the brain and spinal cord and with the central canal of the spinal cord. The ventricular system consists of four cerebral ventricles: two lateral ventricles and two others called the third and the fourth ventricles. The two lateral ventricles are located within the right and left cerebral hemispheres, while the third and fourth are midline structures.

Each lateral ventricle projects an anterior horn into the frontal lobe of the cerebrum, a posterior horn into the occipital lobe, and an inferior horn into the temporal lobe. The production of CSF is mainly by the choroid plexuses of the lateral, third, and fourth ventricles. The plexuses in the lateral ventricles are the largest and most important. The main site of absorption of CSF into the venous system is through the arachnoid granulations projecting into the dural venous sinuses (see Fig. 9-1). Each lateral ventricle connects on the medial side with the third ventricle by a narrow channel known as the interventricular foramina (foramina of Monro).

The third ventricle is a slit-like cavity located in the midline of the skull. It lies just below the level of the bodies of the two lateral ventricles. The cavity of the third ventricle extends downward to where it widens posteriorly and laterally to form the fourth ventricle. The connection between the third and fourth ventricles is known as the aqueduct of Sylvius. The lateral openings from the fourth ventricle into the subarachnoid cistern are known as the foramina of Luschka. The fourth ventricle also connects with the subarachnoid of the cerebellomedullary cistern medially through an opening called the foramen of Magendie. Through these medial and lateral recesses, the fourth ventricle communicates with the subarachnoid spaces of the brain and spinal cord. The relationship of the ventricles to

each other and to the foramina can best be understood if first visualized in the lateral aspect, as depicted in Figure 9-2. Figure 9-3 is a computed tomography (CT) scan that shows the ventricles in an axial projection. Figure 9-4 demonstrates the ventricular system from a coronal perspective in a magnetic resonance imaging (MRI) study. Figure 9-5A–E is a group of pneumoencephalograms. Although this study is no longer performed, these images demonstrate the actual ventricles filled with air and provide a historical retrospect as to the advances in radiology.

Spinal Cord

Lodged within the vertebral canal, the spinal cord is directly continuous superiorly with the medulla oblongata. It begins at the foramen magnum and terminates at the junction of the first and second lumbar vertebrae. The end of the spinal canal, called the **cauda equina**, is located from the second lumbar vertebra to the firth vertebra.

It is through the spinal cord that the brain maintains intimate association with all the peripheral organs. This is accomplished by the attachment of 31 pairs of spinal nerves along its lateral aspects. This will be discussed further in the Peripheral Nervous System section.

Like the brain, the spinal cord has three coverings known as the meninges. They are composed predominantly of white fibrous connective tissue. The dura mater is the outermost layer and is the hardest, toughest, and the most fibrous of the three. The middle membrane is called the arachnoid; it is much less dense and is web-like in appearance. The pia mater is the thin, compact membrane that is closely adapted to the surface of the central nervous system. The pia mater is very vascular and supplies the blood for the central nervous system. Frequently, the pia mater and the arachnoid are considered as one membrane called the pia-arachnoid or leptomeninges. The space between the pia mater and the arachnoid is referred to as the subarachnoid space and that space between the arachnoid and the dura mater is the subdural cavity. The area between the dura mater and the vertebral canal is the epidural space.

Peripheral Nervous System

The peripheral nervous system is made up of nerves outside of the brain and the spinal cord. There are 31 pairs of spinal nerves and 12 pairs of cranial nerves.

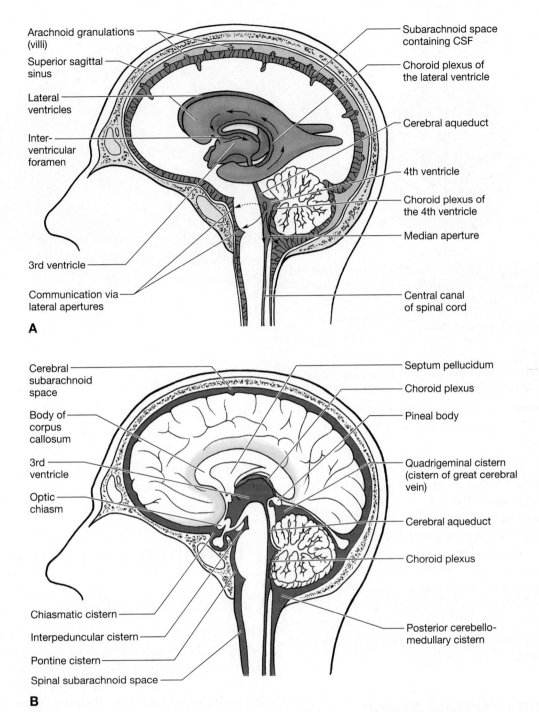

FIGURE 9-1 Subarachnoid (leptomeningeal) spaces, ventricles, and subarachnoid cisterns. **(A)** Ventricular system and circulation of cerebrospinal fluid (CSF). **(B)** Note the subarachnoid cisterns—expanded regions of the subarachnoid space—that contain more substantial amounts of CSF. (Moore KL, Dalley AF. *Clinically Oriented Anatomy.* 4th ed. Baltimore, MD: Lippincott Williams & Wilkins; 1999.)

Both voluntary and involuntary impulses are conveyed through these nerves.

The 12 pairs of cranial nerves are attached to the brain. Each leaves the skull through a foramen. In general, the cranial nerves are voluntary, except those going to the heart, lungs, salivary glands, stomach, and eyes. The spinal nerves send involuntary muscle fibers to the smooth muscles of the gastrointestinal tract,

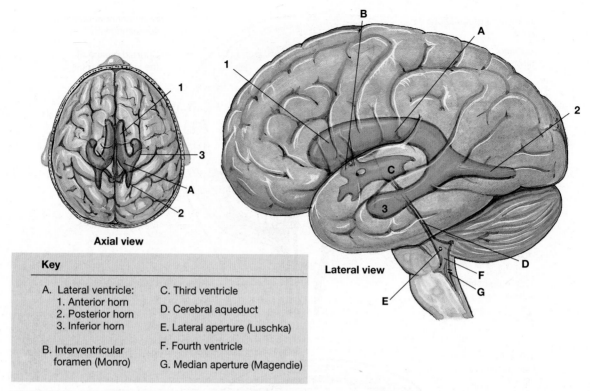

Axial view

Lateral view

Key	

A. Lateral ventricle:
    1. Anterior horn
    2. Posterior horn
    3. Inferior horn
 	
B. Interventricular
    foramen (Monro)
	C. Third ventricle
	
	D. Cerebral aqueduct
	
	E. Lateral aperture (Luschka)
	
	F. Fourth ventricle
	
	G. Median aperture (Magendie)

FIGURE 9-2   **An axial and lateral views of the brain showing the ventricles.** (Asset provided by Anatomical Chart Co.)

genitourinary tract, and the cardiovascular system. The spinal nerves that go to the muscles of the trunk and extremities are voluntary.

The spinal nerves are attached to the spinal cord. After leaving the spinal cord, the nerves are named after their corresponding vertebra. The first 8 are cervical; the next 12 are thoracic, and there are 5 lumbar, 5 sacral, and 1 coccygeal. The lower spinal nerves supply the lower extremities and extend below the level of the spinal cord in parallel strands, resembling a horse's tail; therefore, their group is called the cauda equina.

Autonomic Nervous System

As its name implies the autonomic nervous system functions automatically. It is divided into the sympathetic and parasympathetic systems. The sympathetic portion arises from all the thoracic and the first three lumbar segments of the spinal cord. The parasympathetic portion arises from the third, seventh, ninth, and tenth cranial nerves and from the second, third, and fourth sacral segments of the spinal cord. The parasympathetic system is more

advanced structurally and functionally than the sympathetic system.

Physiology and Function

Central Nervous System

The cerebrum's functions are concerned with sensation, thought, memory, judgment, reason, and the initiation or management of the functions that are under voluntary control. Optic reflex centers are located in the midbrain and serves to correlate optic and tactile impulses. Auditory reflexes are located in the midbrain which is the center for regulation of muscle tone, body posture, and equilibrium. Chief among all of its functions is bringing balance, harmony, and coordination to the motions of the body initiated by the cerebrum. To carry out its functions, it acts as an organ of integration and correlation of nerve impulses. It has connections with the motor neurons of the brain and spinal cord, and through these connections the muscles receive impulses to react.

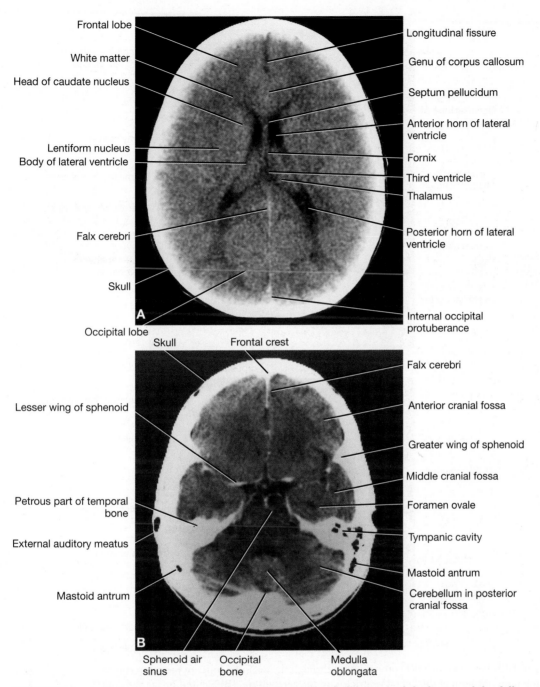

FIGURE 9-3   **Axial (horizontal) CT scans of the skull. (A) The skull bones and the brain and the different parts of the lateral ventricles. (B) A scan made at a lower level showing the three cranial fossae.** (Snell MD. *Clinical Anatomy.* 7th ed. Philadelphia, PA: Lippincott, Williams & Wilkins; 2003.)

Even though it is small in size, the hypothalamus has important functions. It has importance as the control center for body functions such as eating, drinking, and reproduction. It also plays a role in behavior, particularly in the expression of emotions, such as fear and anger.

The medulla contains three vital reflex centers: the cardiac center regulates the heartbeat; the medullary rhythmic area controls the rate and rhythm of breathing; and the vasoconstrictor center regulates the diameter of blood vessels. The function of the pons is concerned with the control of facial muscles,

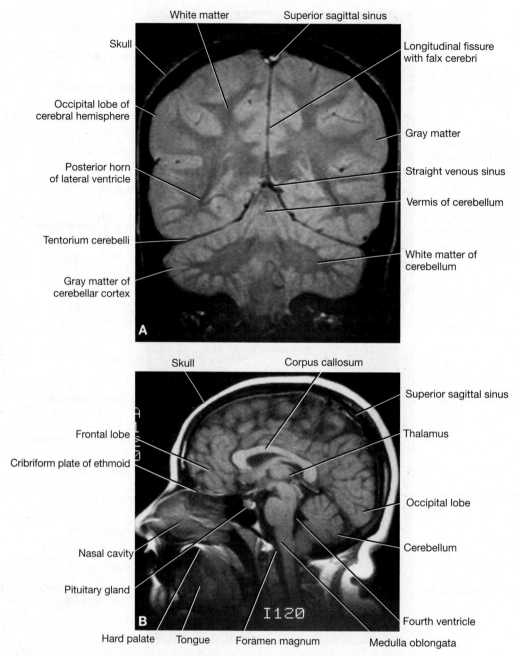

FIGURE 9-4 **(A) An MRI coronal image through the occipital lobes of the brain showing the posterior horn of the lateral ventricle and the cerebellum. (B) Sagittal image showing the different parts of the brain and the nasal and mouth cavities.** (Snell MD. *Clinical Anatomy.* 7th ed. Philadelphia, PA: Lippincott, Williams & Wilkins; 2003.)

including the muscles of mastication and the first stages of breathing.

The cerebellum plays an important role in the control of movement, particularly in the coordination of voluntary muscle activity and in the maintenance of balance and equilibrium. It is particularly sensitive to

the effects of severe drunkenness. To carry out its functions, it acts as an organ of integration and correlation of nerve impulses. It has connections with the motor neurons of the brain and spinal cord, and through these connections the muscles receive impulses to react. An extremely important area for the maintenance of

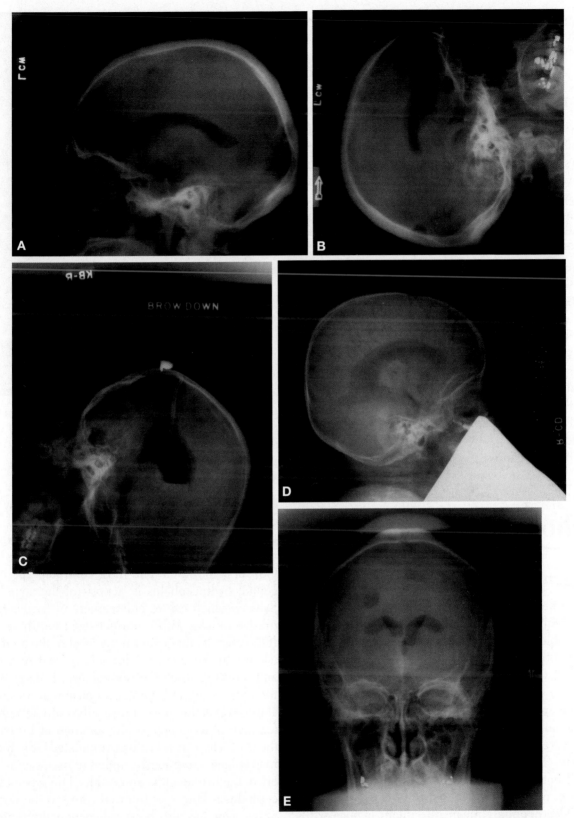

FIGURE 9-5   Pneumoencephalography demonstrating the ventricles. (A) Anterior horns and body of the lateral ventricles. The third ventricle is somewhat evident as well. (B) The anterior horn and a portion of the body of the lateral ventricles. (C) Clear image of the posterior horn and inferior horns of the lateral ventricles. (D) Lateral view demonstrating all portions of the lateral ventricles. (E) Anterior horns and portions of the bodies of both lateral ventricles. The third ventricle is seen in the midline.

homeostasis is the spinal cord, as it conducts impulses in directions between the brain and the periphery. It also serves to coordinate reflexes.

Autonomic Nervous System

This system serves to activate the involuntary smooth and cardiac muscles and glands. It also serves the vital systems that function automatically, such as the digestive, circulatory, respiratory, urinary, and endocrine systems. The two divisions—sympathetic and parasympathetic—oppose each other in function and thus maintain balanced activity in the body. For example, the sympathetic system dilates the pupils, and the parasympathetic system contracts them. The sympathetic system causes the blood vessels of the skin and viscera to contract so that more blood goes to the muscles where it is needed for fight or flight under stress. The parasympathetic system dilates the blood vessels when the need has passed. The sympathetic system causes contractions of the sphincters to prevent the emptying of bowels or bladder; the parasympathetic system relaxes these sphincters so that waste can be removed. Similarly, they regulate the body temperature, salivary digestive secretions, and the endocrine glands.

Pathology

Congenital Abnormalities

Developmental abnormalities are more important in the brain than in any other single organ, with the possible exception of the heart. Developmental abnormalities of the central nervous system are usually divided into malformations and destructive brain lesions.

Anencephaly is a severe malformation in which the cranial vault is absent and the cerebral hemispheres are either missing or markedly reduced in size (Fig. 9-6). Almost all infants with anencephaly are still born or die soon after birth. There are limited cases of infants surviving until the age of 2 or 3 years. **Microcephaly** means the infant is born with an exceedingly small head (Fig. 9-7). This occurs when there is failure of the cerebrum to develop properly.

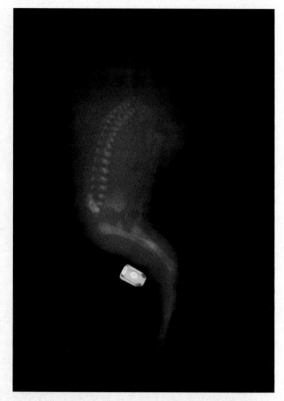

FIGURE 9-6   Anencephaly. This radiographic image of a stillborn fetus is missing the entire cranium.

Hydrocephaly literally means "water brain"; however, this occurs within the ventricles. It may occur congenitally or arise from a variety of causes at any time after birth. In hydrocephalic individuals, the ventricles enlarge as a result of a blockage in the flow of CSF at some level. The most common type of congenital hydrocephalus is stenosis of the aqueduct of Sylvius, which causes enlargement of the lateral and third ventricles with a normal sized fourth ventricle. If the obstruction occurs at the level of the foramen of Monro, the lateral ventricles enlarge, leaving the third and fourth ventricles at normal size. Enlargement of the entire ventricular system indicates an obstruction at the level of the roof of the fourth ventricle, either the foramen of Magendie or the foramen of Luschka. As the ventricles expand with accumulated CSF, the head may enlarge enormously, so that normal vaginal delivery of the live infant is impossible. This type of **hydrocephalus** is known as **internal** (fluid in the ventricles only). This has also been called noncommunicating hydrocephalus, as an obstruction in the ventricles does not allow the CSF to flow through the ventricles into the subarachnoid space and into the spinal canal.

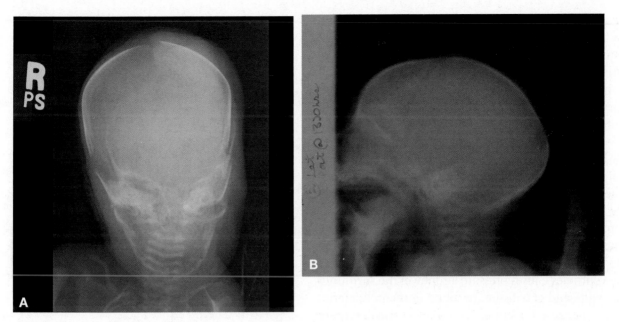

FIGURE 9-7   Microcephaly. Anteroposterior (A) and lateral (B) views.

Case Study

The axial sonogram seen in (A) is of the brain at 29 weeks of gestation which demonstrates unilateral dilatation of the left lateral ventricle (*cursers*). In image (B), a follow-up CT scan at birth confirms the finding of left hemispheric porencephaly (*arrow*). Image (C) is a transverse sonographic scan of a normal fetus at the level of the lateral ventricles. By comparing (C) with (A), the enlargement of the ventricles can be seen.

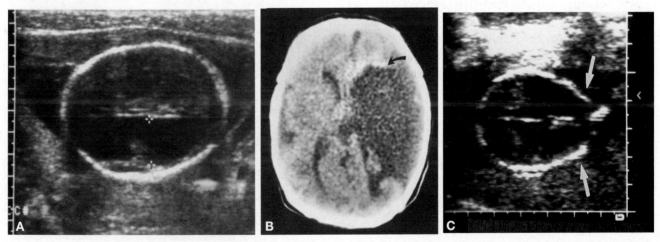

(A and B: MacDonald MG, Seshia MMK, Mullett MD. *Avery's Neonatology Pathophysiology & Management of the Newborn.* 6th ed. Philadelphia, PA: Lippincott Williams & Wilkins; 2005. C: McClatchey KD. *Clinical Laboratory Medicine.* 2nd ed. Philadelphia, PA: Lippincott Williams & Wilkins; 2002.)

In older children and adults, the cause of hydrocephalus is more often the tumors that block the flow of CSF or meningeal scarring secondary to meningitis or hemorrhage. This type of hydrocephalus is not congenital. As the tumors grow, they may press on the aqueduct, force the brain stem against the openings, or interfere with the reabsorption of CSF by the arachnoid. Usually more than one of these processes is at work. When the blockage is below the ventricular level, so that there is free flow of CSF between the ventricles and the subarachnoid space, or the cause is faulty reabsorption of the fluid, the **hydrocephalus** is known as **external**, or communicating. In this case, the head does not usually enlarge because the skull is well formed; rather, the increased pressure from the accumulated fluid in the ventricles causes pressure atrophy of the surrounding white and gray tissue, resulting in mental deterioration. Because the cranium cannot get smaller, there is a compensatory increase in fluid within the spinal canal and the spaces that the atrophy of the brain creates. This is referred to as a compensatory hydrocephalus. If the increased pressure is not relieved, the brain may herniate toward the foramen magnum. The most effective treatment is a shunt, which is placed either between the lateral ventricles and the cardiac atrium (ventriculoatrial shunt) or between the lateral ventricles and the peritoneum (ventriculoperitoneal shunt) (Fig. 9-8). The shunt is longer than necessary so that as the child grows the shunt will be extended and not need to be replaced for several years. Occasionally, the shunt can become disconnected in the area of the neck. If this happens, the lower portion of the shunt will become coiled in the pelvis (Fig. 9-9).

CT (see Image (B) in the Case Study) and MRI (Fig. 9-10) provide excellent visualization of this disorder and have replaced the use of antiquated studies such as pneumoencephalography and ventriculography. Ultrasonography may be used to diagnose hydrocephaly in utero (see Case Study) and in the newborn; however, once the fontanelles close, ultrasonography is of no use in the diagnosis of hydrocephaly.

Approximately 2,500 newborns a year in the United States are diagnosed with spina bifida. This is 1 in every 1,000 live births. More children in the United States have spina bifida than muscular dystrophy, multiple sclerosis, and cystic fibrosis combined. Since this disorder is characterized by an opening in the spine, it was discussed in Chapter 2 (see Fig. 2-13). However, a quick review of this condition is warranted since the spinal cord and the meninges can be affected depending on

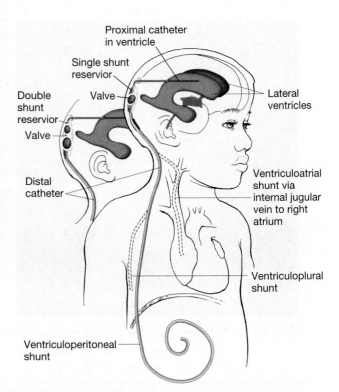

FIGURE 9-8   Diagram of a typical ventriculoperitoneal shunt.

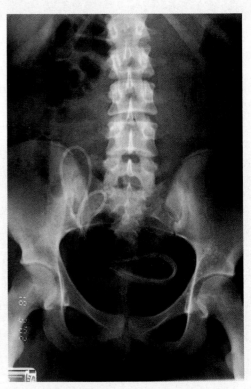

FIGURE 9-9   This radiograph shows a discontinuity in the shunt, with the distal end coiled in the pelvis. (Fleisher GR, Ludwig W, Baskin MN. *Atlas of Pediatric Emergency Medicine.* Philadelphia, PA: Lippincott Williams & Wilkins; 2004.)

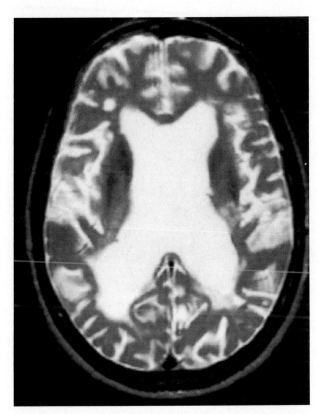

FIGURE 9-10   Normal pressure hydrocephalus. This T2-weighted axial MRI scan shows dilated lateral ventricles. (Moore KL, Dalley AF. *Clinically Oriented Anatomy.* 4th ed. Baltimore, MD: Lippincott Williams & Wilkins; 1999.)

the severity of the defect. Large defects in the lumbar or cervical spine may be accompanied by protrusion of the meninges, known as *meningocele.* As a rule, neurologic complications with meningoceles are slight or even absent, since no nerve elements are involved in the sac. If only the cord protrudes through a defect in the meninges as well as the spine, the result is a *myelocele.* In this type of spina bifida the neural tube has not closed. Myeloceles may not be compatible with life. Unfortunately, most babies with spina bifida are born with a *myelomeningocele,* in which both the meninges and the spinal cord herniate through the spinal defect. This is the most severe form for the surviving infant, as neurologic deficiencies in the control of the lower limbs, bladder, and rectum result. All three of these types of complications of spina bifida can be reviewed in Figure 2-12A & B. The severity of damage is determined by the location of the lesion. The higher up the spine, the more damage is manifested because spinal nerves are disrupted from the point of injury. As the central nervous system is freely exposed to the outside, there

is risk of infection of the meninges. Some patients with myelomeningocele demonstrate **Arnold-Chiari** syndrome, which is a cause of congenital hydrocephalus. Arnold-Chiari syndrome is a defect of the hindbrain, with bony fusion of the occiput and the upper cervical vertebrae leading to a small posterior cranial fossa. The medulla is forced through the foramen magnum into the upper cervical canal, leading to obstruction of the flow of CSF. Surgeons surgically implant a shunt to allow fluid to drain.

Most spina bifida patients have normal intelligence. Only about 3% to 5% are severely mentally disabled. Approximately 95% of children have bowel and bladder problems, since nerves that control these functions are located in the tail of the spinal cord. The bladder may be flaccid and constantly leak urine or may be spastic, causing urine to back up into the kidneys. With proper medical treatment 90% of the victims can live a normal life span.

Inflammatory Processes

Abscesses may either occur within the brain or be associated with the meninges. When the collection of pus is between the skull and the underlying dura mater, the abscess is known as an **epidural abscess.** All other are known simply as brain abscesses.

The microorganisms that cause abscesses of the brain may come from a focus of infection in the skull, the most common being from the middle ear or the mastoid region. The infection spreads inward and causes abscess formation in the adjacent part of the brain. Another source of abscess is an infection in the frontal or other sinuses that communicate with the nasal cavity. These abscesses are likely to be in the frontal part of the brain. An infecting organism can come from a systemic infection or septic process in the lung also.

The symptoms of brain abscess are not easily manifested, as many parts of the brain where an abscess is likely to occur are "silent areas." That is, a lesion in this area of the brain does not produce any characteristic symptom. The clinical sign is gradually increasing intracranial pressure, which however, may also suggest a tumor. Increased pressure coupled with an existing middle ear, mastoid, or sinus infection should be highly indicative of abscess.

CT is the best imaging modality for the demonstration of abscesses (Fig. 9-11). It can also show the underlying mastoiditis or sinusitis, thus eliminating the need

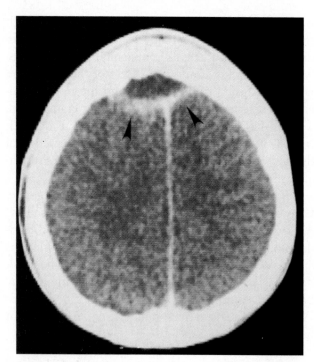

FIGURE 9-11   Epidural abscess. Biconvex hypodense lesion with contrast-enhanced dural margin (*arrowheads*) that crosses the falx and displaces the falx away from the inner table of the skull. (Eisenberg RL. *Clinical Imaging: An Atlas of Differential Diagnosis.* 5th ed. Philadelphia, PA: Lippincott Williams & Wilkins; 2010.)

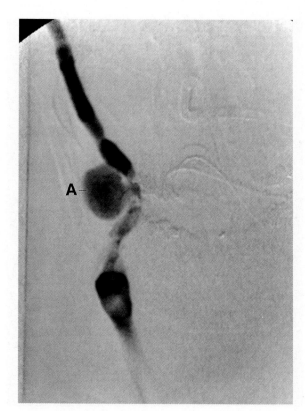

FIGURE 9-12   Giant cavernous carotid aneurysm (A).

for plain skull radiography. An untreated brain abscess eventually will rupture into the subarachnoid space or into the ventricular system. This often fatal rupture, as well as the increased intracranial pressure, is well documented on CT.

Small saccular aneurysms may occur on the intracranial vessels. Congenital "berry" aneurysms may result in intraparenchymal hemorrhages. Many aneurysms appear in middle life as a result of atheroma and hypertension. They are symptomless until they rupture and cause a subarachnoid hemorrhage. Blood is spilled into the subarachnoid space and can be detected in the CSF. Most aneurysms involve the circle of Willis, in particular the anterior communicating artery and the major subdivisions of the middle cerebral artery. In most patients, the ruptured aneurysm is characterized by sudden onset of pain, which may be around the orbit. Headaches are also a common symptom.

Not all aneurysms of the brain are the small, berry type. Figure 9-12 shows a subtraction image of a large cavernous carotid aneurysm. Noncontrast CT and MRI are now the modalities used to diagnose this condition.

Strokes were once referred to as **cerebrovascular accidents**. Strokes are the third leading cause of deaths in the United States. Thrombosis, embolism, and hemorrhage are all possible causes of a stroke. A thrombosis affects the extra cerebral arteries of the elderly more often than young to middle-aged adults. Strokes caused by thrombi have a higher risk of occurring when other factors such as smoking, obesity, and the use of oral contraceptives are involved. A middle-aged woman with all three of these factors runs a much higher risk of suffering from a cerebrovascular accident than an elderly man who is a nonsmoker and within normal weight range.

The majority of cerebrovascular accidents are caused by emboli, which occur by separating from a thrombus in a large vessel such as the carotid artery. The embolus then travels until it lodges in a smaller brain vessel and results in an infarct. This accounts for 60% of all strokes. Most thrombi initially form because the vessel in which they occur has been damaged by atherosclerosis. This is why cerebrovascular accidents become increasingly prevalent in the elderly.

Whether from emboli or thrombi, vascular occlusions result in the sudden impairment of circulation in the cerebral blood vessels. This is known as ischemic stroke and accounts for about 80% of all strokes.

This results in decreased oxygen in the brain tissue supplied by the affected vessel. The damaged brain tissue loses function within minutes and becomes soft and necrotic within a few days. This area of ischemic necrosis is known as an infarct.

Strokes are also caused by rupture of vessels and bleeding into the brain. The ruptured vessel has usually been weakened by arteriosclerosis in a patient with hypertension. Although the signs and symptoms of a brain hemorrhage depend on its location and size, almost half of the patients with large brain hemorrhages die within hours because the accumulation of blood displaces adjacent tissue, rapidly elevating the intracranial pressure.

In many cases of stroke, there is no need for imaging studies because the history of sudden onset of neurologic problems is indicative of a vascular process. However, CT can be utilized to demonstrate an acute hemorrhagic infarct, edema, and necrosis.

Immediately following a cerebral infarct, the CT shows no abnormality, as does a static radionuclide brain scan. This information is not necessarily negative, since it rules out other causes of the patient's symptoms. After 36 to 48 hours following the stroke, the involved areas become lucent on the CT scan.

Transient ischemic attacks (TIAs) often precede a stroke. These "mini" strokes are a temporary interruption of circulation usually caused by arteriosclerotic plaque. TIAs are characterized by fleeting attacks of faintness, localized paralysis, and **aphasia**. Manifestations of TIAs completely resolve within a few hours and not longer than 24 hours. The patient who presents with an obvious TIA may undergo a duplex sonographic examination of the carotid arteries to determine the extent of any further arteriosclerotic disease. If warranted, the patient may undergo angiography to study the carotid arteries. These TIAs should be considered as a "warning" sign that a major stroke may be imminent; as many as 5% of people who have a TIA suffer a stroke within 1 month and 33% go on to have major stroke within 5 years.

A suppurative process in the space between the dura mater and the arachnoid is known as a **subdural empyema**. It is most commonly caused by spread of infection from the frontal or ethmoid sinuses. Other causes may be from middle ear infection or mastoiditis, although this is less common than sinusitis. Subdural empyema is usually bilateral over the upper cerebral area. CT is best for demonstrating the involvement of the parenchyma. A skull radiograph may show diffuse areas of osteolytic destruction if the empyema has led to osteomyelitis. Even with proper treatment, a subdural empyema is associated with a high mortality rate.

Encephalitis is inflammation of the brain. This uncommon infection is almost always caused by a virus. Many of the viruses that cause encephalitis are spread by mosquitoes. Patients with encephalitis present with symptoms of irritability, drowsiness, and headache. Herpes simplex 1 can also cause encephalitis. Although it is rare, the virus can invade the brain in a susceptible person and result in severe destruction of large areas of the temporal or frontal lobes of the brain. CT is important in the clinical diagnosis of encephalitis by ruling out abscess or tumor. CT will also show the best area of biopsy in herpetic encephalitis.

Bleeding from a ruptured artery or vein into the brain tissue can be caused by disease as well as obvious head trauma that cause injury. Cerebrovascular diseases such as a hemorrhagic neoplasm, hemorrhagic infarct, or a ruptured aneurysm can cause hemorrhage. **Cerebral hemorrhage**, also known as **hematoma**, is the escape of blood from the vessels into the cerebrum. Those hemorrhages not commonly related to injury are discussed below. Two other types are discussed in Head Injuries section.

A **subarachnoid hemorrhage** is caused most commonly by rupture of a berry aneurysm in the circle of Willis. The hemorrhage is into the subarachnoid space between the arachnoid and the pia mater. As the CSF is contained in this space, blood will be found in the fluid upon lumbar puncture. Clinically, the subarachnoid hemorrhage is characterized by a history of sudden headache, clouding of vision, and blood in the CSF. The imaging procedure that most readily displays blood in the subarachnoid space is CT.

Hypertensive vascular disease is the main cause of an **intracerebral**, or **intraparenchymal**, hemorrhage. However, if the patient is young, rupture from an arteriovenous malformation is usually the cause. Hypertensive intracerebral hematoma can cause a stroke, as the hemorrhage results in blood collections within the tissue that displaces the surrounding brain. Intracerebral hematomas may occur anywhere within the brain; however, they are more often found in the basal ganglia, cerebellar hemispheres, or pons. MRI or an unenhanced CT scan will best define the area of accumulated blood (Fig. 9-13).

Meningitis means inflammation of the leptomeninges. It most often occurs by itself but may be associated with other infections such as pneumonia. This

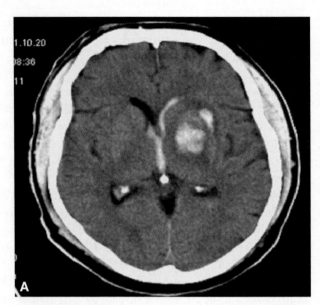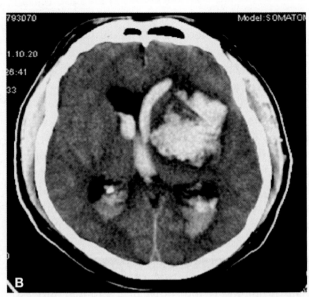

FIGURE 9-13   Computed tomography (CT) scan of hypertensive striatal intracerebral hemorrhage with intraventricular extension expanding over 6 hours. A) Image was taken when the patient was first scanned. B) This image was taken 6 hours later. (Topol EJ, Califf RM, Prystowsky EN, et al. *Textbook of Cardiovascular Medicine.* 3rd ed. Philadelphia, PA: Lippincott Williams & Wilkins; 2006.)

bacteria-caused infection has an abrupt onset, with the patient experiencing fever, headache, and muscle pain. The patient often complains of a stiff neck. The types of meningitis are named after the types of bacteria that cause them. The *Streptococcus* and *Pneumococcus* bacteria reach the meninges from the middle ear or the frontal sinus. The blood may carry the bacteria from the lung. The meningococcus comes from the nose or throat. These three organisms are pyogenic so that the meningitis they produce, *streptococcal meningitis*, *pneumococcal meningitis*, and *meningococcal meningitis*, are acute and violent. Treatment by antibiotic therapy must be immediate to avoid alterations in the blood–brain barrier, which leads to edema, increasing cranial pressure, and subsequent death of the patient.

The *tubercle bacillus-induced meningitis* is a class by itself. It has none of the acuteness of the other forms of meningitis. This is a chronic form of meningitis. The infection is carried by the blood stream from some other tuberculous lesion. The disease often sits at the base of the brain for an extended period of time as it gradually affects more and more cranial nerves. If the patient survives meningitis, there is the danger of developing hydrocephalus. Since the inflammation is in the subarachnoid space, fibrous adhesions may develop that block the flow of CSF.

Although bacterial infection is the most common cause of meningitis, there is a viral form that may be caused by mumps, polio, or herpes simplex. *Chemical meningitis* can be caused by the introduction of a foreign substance into the subarachnoid space, such as a contrast medium for myelography.

Meningitis is diagnosed clinically by evaluation of the CSF. Radiography plays a small role in this inflammatory process; however, bacterial and viral meningitis are best demonstrated on CT. Plain-film radiography shows the underlying cause of the meningitis, such as sinusitis, mastoiditis, or pneumonia.

Osteomyelitis of the skull is most often caused by pyogenic bacteria from the sinuses or mastoid air cells. Osteomyelitis is a common complication of an empyema. Skull radiographs demonstrate many small, poorly defined areas of lucency. As the weeks progress, the lucencies enlarge and unite in a central area of the skull. Osteomyelitis of the skull must not be confused with multiple myeloma, which presents a similar radiographic pattern.

Head Injuries

Normally, the brain is well protected by the skull. However, when sufficient force is applied to the head, the brain can be damaged. The major cause of head injuries today is traffic accidents. The more common among the injuries are concussion, contusion, hemorrhage, and fracture. Over one-fourth of all people who suffer fatal head wounds demonstrate no skull fracture. Trauma to the brain and brain stem is of primary concern to the emergency medical team. Because injury to the brain can occur without skull fracture, CT has replaced radiographic images of the skull in major trauma cases so that the brain tissue and brain stem can be visualized. An indication of severe trauma to the brain is the "halo sign." This occurs when there is a tear in the dura mater, which is common in fracture of the cranial base. As a patient lies supine, the fluid will drip from the ear. On a white sheet, there will be a pink center with a light yellow ring around the center.

TECH TIP

If skull radiographs are taken, a cross-table lateral projection should be done to visualize any air within the brain or fluid levels within the sphenoid sinuses.

The most common head injury is a **concussion**. A concussion occurs when there has been a violent blow or jar to the head. This causes the brain to strike the opposite side of the cranium, resulting in momentary loss of consciousness. There may be transient amnesia, vertigo, nausea, weak pulse, and slow respiration. The patient may experience a headache, but normally recovery occurs within 24 to 48 hours with no structural damage detected in the brain.

A **contusion** is more serious than a concussion. Contusions are bruises on the surface of the brain and are the result of the brain shifting inside the skull during acceleration and rapid deceleration such as a "whiplash" reaction received from a rear-end type of automobile accident. When the bruise occurs on the same side of the brain as the trauma, it is known as a coup lesion. Contrecoup lesions are contusions that occur on the opposite side of the head. Contusions result in hemorrhages from small blood vessels, which cause further vessel occlusion and edema. All of these may lead to increased intracranial pressure, which must be closely watched for.

When sufficient force is applied to the skull, fractures of various types occur. Three of the common type of skull fractures include linear, comminuted, and depressed. Fractures of the cranium are classified according to their location. Sutures and vascular grooves of the skull can appear as fractures; therefore, a thorough knowledge of the anatomy of the skull is required. Fractures are often difficult to differentiate from suture lines or vascular grooves, but if the technologist bears in mind the location of the serrated sutures and the fact that vascular markings are smooth, faint lines as seen on a radiographic image, fractures should be more readily identifiable.

A *linear* fracture appears on an image as an irregular or jagged radiolucent line (Fig. 9-14). The location of a linear fracture is important, as complications may occur. Pneumocephalus and epidural hematoma are two complications that can occur if the fracture is in the mastoid air cell area or if a vessel is lacerated.

In more severe trauma, the skull may break into three or more fragments, thus becoming a *comminuted fracture*. If any single fragment is depressed into the cranial cavity, the fracture is now known as a depressed fracture (Fig. 9-15), and the dura mater is often torn, causing hemorrhage (Fig. 9-16). If the force is sufficient to cause penetration by the fragment into the cranial vault, air and foreign material may enter the cranial cavity and even possibly the brain.

Basilar skull fractures are often difficult to diagnose on skull radiography, as the fracture may be hidden by the dense, complex anatomic structures of the temporal and mastoid areas. The cross-table lateral image may identify air-fluid in the sphenoid sinus and this is an indication of this type of skull fracture. The "halo sign", described above, is another clinical sign, in addition to the air-fluid level seen in the sphenoid sinus. CT is a better modality to determine the presence of blood in the basilar cisterns as well as demonstrate any basilar skull fractures that may not be visible on a radiographic image (Fig. 9-17).

As stated in the previous section, hematoma (hemorrhages) can be caused by injury. Collections of blood in the brain manifest in exactly the same manner as those caused by a nontraumatic rupture of a vessel. An **epidural hemorrhage**, also known as an **extradural hematoma**, is caused by a tear in the middle meningeal vessels, which causes bleeding between the bone and the dura mater. This type of hemorrhage is associated with severe trauma in which the skull has usually been fractured at the temporal area. Because of the location of the tear and bleed, the blood accumulates very rapidly. The outcome is fatal within several hours,

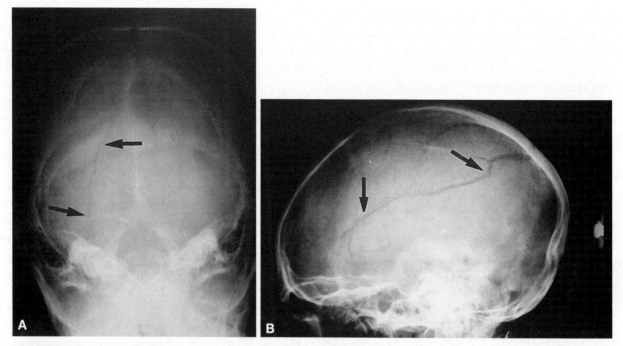

FIGURE 9-14   Linear skull fractures. (A) AP Townes view of occipital bone. Note that a linear fracture line extends through the occipital bone (*arrows*). (B) Lateral skull, parietal bone. Observe the linear fracture extending from the posterior aspect of the cranial vault anteriorly (*arrows*). (Yochum TR, Rowe LJ. *Yochum and Rowe's Essentials of Skeletal Radiology.* 3rd ed. Philadelphia, PA: Lippincott Williams & Wilkins; 2004.)

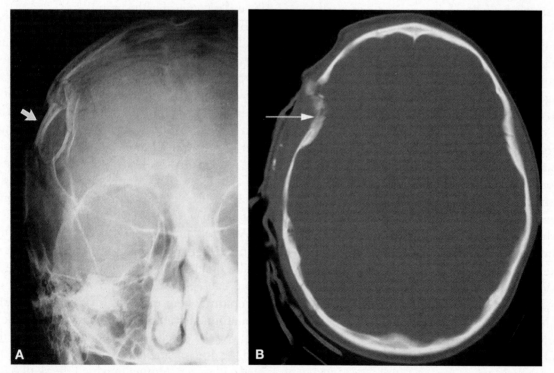

FIGURE 9-15   (A) Radiographic image of a depressed skull fracture. (B) CT image of a 6-year-old male child involved in a high-speed automobile accident. He suffered a depressed skull fracture seen at the *arrow*. (A: Yochum TR, Rowe LJ. *Yochum and Rowe's Essentials of Skeletal Radiology.* 3rd ed. Philadelphia, PA: Lippincott Williams & Wilkins; 2004.)

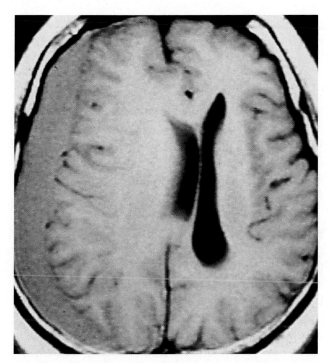

FIGURE 9-16   Subdural hematoma. This T1-weighted magnetic resonance imaging the classic appearance of a large acute subdural hematoma, with a crescent-shaped extraaxial hematoma that covers the entire right cerebral convexity. There is significant midline shift with compression of the right lateral ventricle and enlargement of the contralateral ventricle, which probably represents obstruction to CSF outflow. An emergency operative procedure was performed.

if the condition is not diagnosed and the hematoma removed surgically. Because of the rapid deterioration of the patient, radiography often plays a minor role in the diagnosis of this condition, as the patient will go straight to CT for unenhanced scans of the head (Fig. 9-18). CT will demonstrate any skull fractures, thus eliminating the need for radiographic images and saving the patient's valuable time for treatment.

A **subdural hematoma**, a common complication of injury, is the result of a tear of the veins between the dura mater and the arachnoid. Because it is venous in origin, bleeding is slow, taking hours or even days for the accumulation of blood to become large enough to cause compression of the underlying brain. Although a subdural hematoma is not as life-threatening as an epidural hematoma, surgery must still be performed to remove the blood to prevent the compression of brain tissue. Subdural hematomas (Fig. 9-19) are often found in patients who have a history of trauma to the frontal or occipital lobes caused by falling. However, these patients usually have no fractures.

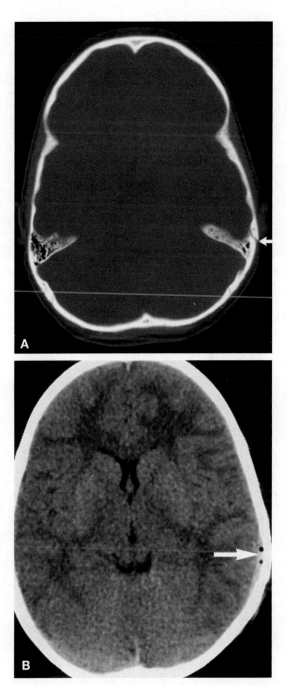

FIGURE 9-17   Basilar skull fracture. This 5-year-old girl was a pedestrian struck by a bicycle. Hemotympanum was noted on examination. (A) The *arrow* indicates a fracture of the left temporal bone. The adjacent mastoid air cells are somewhat opacified. (B) A small extraaxial hematoma with associated pneumocephaly is seen (*arrow*).

Neoplasms

Neoplasms of the brain and spinal cord are not as neatly separated into benign and malignant categories as tumors found elsewhere in the body. Although the tumor itself

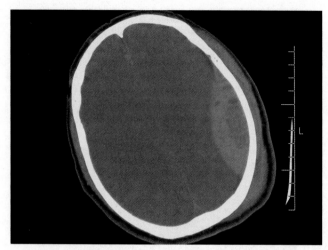

FIGURE 9-18 Left epidural hematoma in a teenager after a skateboard accident. Note the lentiform shape of the lesion. Epidural blood dissects the dura from the skull and causes this lenticular appearance, which spans the dural attachments between suture lines.

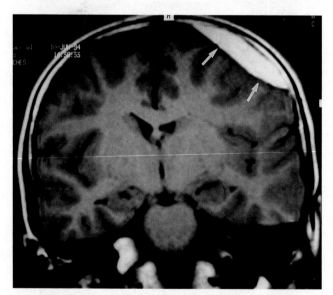

FIGURE 9-19 This coronal T1-weighted MRI scan shows the subdural hematoma (*arrows*) to greater advantage than does the CT image. Notice the compression of the brain and distortion of the left lateral ventricle. (Daffner RH. *Clinical Radiology: The Essentials.* 3rd ed. Philadelphia, PA: Lippincott Williams & Wilkins; 2007.)

may be benign, it may disrupt vital functions such as it might be found in the brain stem, killing the patient.

Neoplasms of the brain are the second most common tumors occurring in children. Leukemia occurs more often than neoplasms. Patients most often present with increased pressure and accompanying edema. Because

of the increased cranial pressure, patients may experience headaches, vomiting, blurred vision, and seizure. Surgery is almost always necessary for treatment.

Radiographic diagnosis of neoplasms is made by CT, MRI, and, in some cases, angiography. MRI is excellent for evaluating the brain stem, while CT is better for detecting calcifications within the tumor. Because the pathology of neoplasms is beyond the scope of this textbook, the definitions and manifestations of the tumors will be presented in the order from most common to least common.

The most common primary brain tumor is the **glioma** (Fig. 9-20). This tumor has a neurologic origin and occurs in the cerebral hemispheres and the posterior fossa benign forms of gliomas are known as **astrocytoma** (Fig. 9-21). The malignant variety is the fast-growing **glioblastoma multiforme**. It is the most common malignant brain tumor in adults, comprising 50% to 60% of all gliomas. Prognosis is very poor. Death usually results within 1 to 2 years of early diagnosis, less time if the diagnosis is made in the late stages of the neoplasm. Another highly malignant tumor with a very poor prognosis is the **medulloblastoma** (Fig. 9-22). This neoplasm occurs in the roof of the fourth ventricle in the midline of the cerebellum. Its victims are usually children between the ages of 9 and 12 years, but they may be as young as 5 years or as old as 15 years. Males are twice as likely to be affected. These fast-growing tumors rapidly cause death.

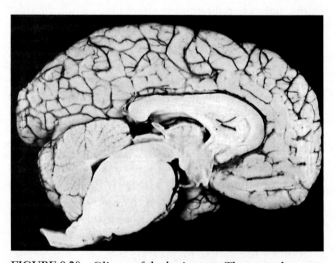

FIGURE 9-20 Glioma of the brain stem. The tumor has diffusely infiltrated the brainstem, producing hypertrophy. Note the relative lack of dilatation of lateral ventricles. (Dr. P. Cancilla, Department of Pathology, UCLA School of Medicine, University of California, Los Angeles, CA.)

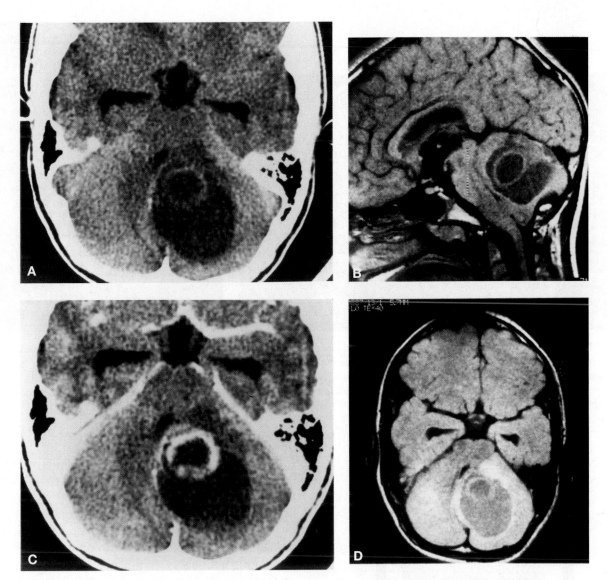

FIGURE 9-21   Computed tomographic scans revealing cerebellar cystic astrocytoma in a 13-year-old boy. Computed tomographic scans before (A) and after (B) injection of iodinated contrast material show a large lesion predominantly involving the left cerebellar hemisphere but extending to the vermis. T1-weighted magnetic resonance images in the sagittal (C) and axial (D) planes also are shown. These noncontrast magnetic resonance studies were done before gadolinium-diethylenetriaminepentaacetic acid was approved for use in children. The magnetic resonance findings are concordant with the computed tomographic scan changes. (Drs. Hervey D. Segall, Marvin D. Nelson, Jr., and Corey Raffel, Children's Hospital, Los Angeles, CA.)

Meningiomas are the next most common brain tumor, accounting for about 20% of all brain tumors (Fig. 9-23). This is a slow-growing benign neoplasm that occurs in the meninges, in particular the arachnoid and dura mater. Since the tumor does grow out of the meninges, it may also occur in the covering of the spinal cord. Although this is a benign tumor, it can eventually kill the patient as it exerts pressure on the brain. The tumor is a round, well-circumscribed lesion that usually does not invade the surrounding brain tissue, thus making excision easier and a good prognosis. Calcifications within the meningioma may be seen on regular skull radiography, but it is identified best by CT. Angiography is used to demonstrate the vascularity of the tumor, which is essential before surgical removal is attempted.

Pituitary adenomas are also common (about 15% of all tumors). The tumor grows within the sella turcica

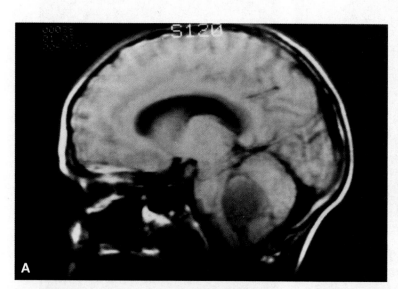

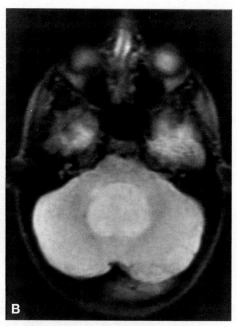

FIGURE 9-22 Primitive neuroectodermal tumor/medulloblastoma containing astrocytic elements. Sagittal (A) and axial (B) magnetic resonance images in this boy show a tumor within the fourth ventricle. It is of low signal intensity (darker than brain, but less dark than CSF) on the T1-weighted imaging (A). The lesion appeared to arise from the roof of the fourth ventricle. Although the neoplasm compressed the posterior aspect of the pons and medulla, it seemed separable from the brain stem. This was confirmed at surgery. (Drs. Hervey D. Segall and J. Gordon McComb, Departments of Radiology and Neurosurgery, Children's Hospital, Los Angeles, CA.)

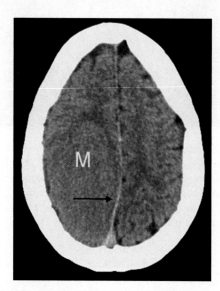

FIGURE 9-23 Meningioma. Cranial CT shows a mass (M) in the right occipital region. Notice the bowing of the septum (*arrow*). (Daffner RH. *Clinical Radiology: The Essentials.* 3rd ed. Philadelphia, PA: Lippincott Williams & Wilkins; 2007.)

where the pituitary gland is located. As it increases in size, the sella turcica become eroded and pressure is exerted on the optic chiasm, creating problems with vision. A lateral skull radiograph will demonstrate the deformity of the sella and erosion of the posterior clinoid processes (Fig. 9-24A, B). Some types of pituitary adenomas secrete growth hormones, causing acromegaly in adults or gigantism in children. Other hormones that may be secreted in excess are adrenocorticotropic hormone, causing symptoms of Cushing disease; thyroid-stimulating hormone, resulting in hyperthyroidism; and prolactin, leading to amenorrhea. A full discussion of these hormones is given in Chapter 10.

Another benign tumor that originates above the sella turcica is the **craniopharyngioma**. This tumor is more commonly found in children between the ages of 5 and 18 years, whereas the pituitary adenoma is more likely found in the adults. Because this tumor is above the sella, as it enlarges, it depresses the optic chiasm, creating vision problems. Craniopharyngiomas contain both cystic and solid components and most have calcifications that can be seen on the skull radiograph and CT scan.

Tumors that are more common in children are those that occur in the pineal gland. **Teratomas** and **germinomas** are two types of pineal tumors that occur more often in males under the age of 25 years. These tumors may compress the ventricular system causing hydrocephalus and an enlarged ventricular system. Calcification within

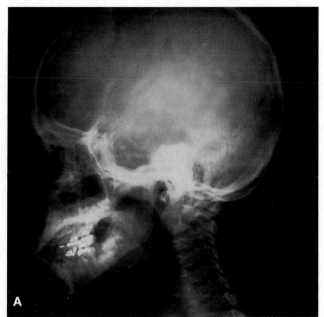

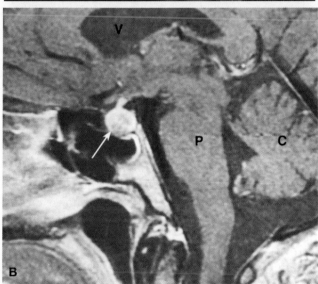

FIGURE 9-24 Pituitary adenoma. A) Erosion of the sella turcica can be seen, which is caused by a pituitary adenoma. B) An MRI scan sagittal view of the brain shows a distinct pituitary tumor (*arrow*). C, cerebellum; P, pons; V, lateral ventricle. (Rubin R, Strayer DS. *Rubin's Pathology: Clinicopathologic Foundations of Medicine.* 5th ed. Philadelphia, PA: Lippincott Williams & Wilkins; 2008.)

the adult pineal gland is common and a normal finding (Fig. 9-25). However, calcification seen within the pineal region of a child should be suspect for teratomas, as these tumors often contain teeth.

Metastatic tumors of the brain are common, accounting for another 10% of all intracranial neoplasms. Metastases are usually multiple neoplasms, whereas primary brain neoplasms are usually a solitary tumor. Usually,

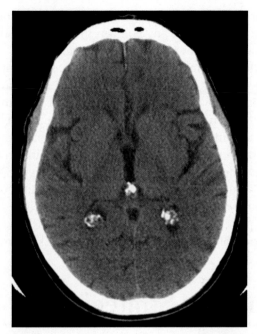

FIGURE 9-25 The calcification of the pineal gland increases with age and was, thereby, quite useful as a radiographic midline marker prior to the advent of contemporary high-resolution neuroimaging modalities. (Mills SE. *Histology for Pathologists.* 3rd ed. Philadelphia, PA: Lippincott Williams & Wilkins; 2007.)

the primary carcinoma is located in the lung or the breast, and is spread to the brain by the blood stream. Less commonly, the metastasis comes from the kidney and the gastrointestinal tract. Single metastatic tumors may be difficult to distinguish from primary tumors on the CT scan, however, since single tumors in the adult are rare, metastasis should be considered.

A tumor that is usually found at the clivus of the skull is a **chordoma**. This locally invasive tumor does not usually metastasize. On radiographic images, the destruction of the dorsum sellae and clivus, along with cloudlike calcifications, can be seen. CT can demonstrate the mass, calcifications, and bony destruction.

Acoustic neuromas are uncommon benign tumors with a very slow rate of growth. These neoplasms are more common in adults and are associated with tinnitus and deafness. The origin at the eighth cranial nerve causes the tumor to destroy the internal auditory meatus. These tumors do not invade other parts of the body.

Spinal Cord Disease

Although intracranial neoplasms are more common than spinal cord tumors, the latter cannot be overlooked. Primary spinal neoplasms include meningiomas (previous discussed) and neurofibromas. **Neurofibromas** occur with equal frequency among men and women. They may occur at any point in the spinal canal and are hallmarked by foraminal widening.

A frequent lesion of the spinal canal is herniation of the pulpy nucleus into the body of a vertebra, usually caused by degeneration or tearing of the cartilage plate that separates the nucleus from the vertebral body. An intervertebral disk may be protruded or herniated into the vertebral canal and press on the spinal cord or stretch the nerves. This is the condition known popularly as slipped disk. The most common cause of the protrusion is trauma, and manifestations include lower back pain, weakness, and sciatica. CT or MRI is used to demonstrate the location of the slipped disk or tumor.

Imaging Strategies

A skull series may be requested along with a cervical spine series in trauma cases. It is very important that radiographer knows how to obtain excellent radiographic images and NOT rely on the digital computer to post-process the image. Most trauma patients will not be able to move in a desired position and the technologist must be able to utilize acquired knowledge of the anatomy of the skull and petrous pyramids along with tube angulation to obtain images that will demonstrate the anatomy that is critical to determining any underlying pathology.

TECH TIP

Correct patient position and tube angulation is essential to avoid superimposition of anatomic features. Air-fluid levels must be demonstrated on certain images. If the patient's condition does not warrant an erect position, the technologist must be prepared to obtain cross-table lateral images with a horizontal beam.

Since skull images display the calvarium but not the brain itself, pathologic processes in the brain are made apparent by their effects of the calvarium, by the presence of abnormal calcifications or fat within the brain, or by displacement of the normally calcified pineal gland or choroid plexus. A thorough knowledge

of normal anatomy that is visualized in each projection is required in order to determine abnormalities.

TECH TIP

Blood vessel fissures can often look like a fracture. A calcified pineal gland is normal in 60% of the adult population. The sella turcica may be of various shapes, but it should by symmetrical.

Computed Tomography

Routine brain scans normally begin at the base of the skull and work superiorly. Scans may be done without the use of contrast enhancement if clinical indication warrants it. The enhanced contrast resolution of computed tomography (CT) allows visualization of fresh blood as an opaque substance. The localization of blood may be within the brain itself, in the subdural space, within the subarachnoid cisterns, or in the epidural space. CT scans allow evaluation of the ventricular size or an infarct as well as the presence of blood. The helical CT mode is used to create three-dimensional reformations or to reduce motion-related artifacts.

CT of the spine offers a noninvasive technique to evaluate the vertebrae, spinal canal, and paravertebral soft tissues. A herniated disk is often shown clearly, since its density is greater than the normal contents of the spinal canal.

CT myelography is a procedure that uses a water soluble positive contrast medium to check for herniated discs, ankylosing spondylitis, arthritis, bone spurs, cysts, injury of the spinal nerve roots, tumors and other problems. The contrast, such as Isovue or Omnipaque, is injected into the subarachoid space at the level of L-3/L-4. This is so that there is less chance of hitting nerve endings with the needle tip at the cauda equina which is at the level of L-1/L-2. The contrast will now spread throughout the spinal column outlining any defect or obstruction. The radiologist is now able to visualize the spinal cord and the nerve roots.

Magnetic Resonance Imaging

Magnetic resonance imaging is often the first imaging exam done to evaluate the spinal cord and nerve roots. This modality provides detailed spinal cord anatomy

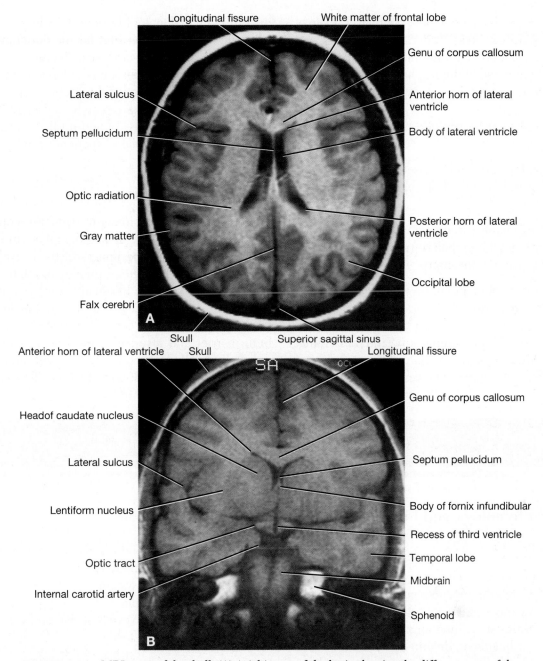

FIGURE 9-26 MRI scans of the skull. **(A)** Axial image of the brain showing the different parts of the lateral ventricle and the lateral sulcus of the cerebral hemisphere. **(B)** Coronal image through the frontal lobe of the brain showing the anterior horn of the lateral ventricle. (Snell MD. *Clinical Anatomy.* 7th ed. Philadelphia, PA: Lippincott, Williams & Wilkins; 2003.)

without the use of contrast media (Fig. 9-26). In addition, it is "blind" to bone, allowing a clear demonstration of various cranial structures. Although CT is excellent for spinal cord defects, MRI is better for soft tissue. CT can miss a soft tissue lesion that MRI will pick up.

However, there are patients for whom an MRI is not feasible. Those patients with medical devices such as a pacemaker will need to undergo CT.

Sonography

Doppler ultrasound to view intracranial basal artery blood flow has been in use since the mid-1980s. Subsequent advances in ultrasound technology have seen the use of combination Doppler blood flow imaging transcranial color-coded duplex. This more precisely identifies vessels and, if required, the direction of flow. Doppler beam angle correction gives a more accurate estimate of blood flow velocity in areas of arterial tortuosity.

Transcranial Doppler ultrasound, and more recently transcranial color-coded duplex, have been used for a variety of clinical purposes:

Screening for vasospasm following subarachnoid hemorrhage

Screening for intracranial vessel stenosis and occlusions in ischemic stroke or transient cerebral ischemia

Monitoring changes in intracranial hemodynamic and monitoring for emboli during excision of the diseased portion of the artery

Monitoring cerebral perfusion in the neurological intensive care setting

Both transcranial Doppler ultrasound and transcranial color-coded duplex provide a relatively limited view of the basal cerebral arteries. The vessels that are visible on transcranial Doppler ultrasound do, however, comprise the more common sites for the development of intracranial large artery occlusive disease.

The accuracy of transcranial Doppler ultrasound and transcranial color-coded duplex in the detection of intracranial occlusive disease can be considered acceptable when performed as "opportunistic" screening by sonographers and clinicians experienced in its use.

Nuclear Medicine

Radionuclide cerebral imaging generally consists of two phases: a dynamic or angiographic study composed of rapid sequence images of the arrival of the nuclide in the cerebral hemispheres; and static images obtained approximately 1 hour after the dynamic study to provide a record of the distribution of the nuclide in the brain. Pathologic processes often affect the blood–brain barrier and result in a focal area of increased radioactivity. Radionuclide studies will indicate an abnormality but will not point to a specific cause.

RECAP

Anatomy, Physiology, and Function

- Central nervous system
  - Brain
    - Divisions are cerebrum, brain stem, cerebellum
      - Cerebrum functions are sensation, thought memory, judgment, reason
      - Brain stem functions are cardiac center for heartbeat, rhythm of breathing
      - Cerebellum functions are control of movement, balance, and equilibrium
  - Spinal cord
- Peripheral nervous system
  - 12 pairs of cranial nerves
    - Attached to the brain
  - 13 pairs of spinal nerves
    - Attached to the spinal cord
    - Nerves end at the cauda equina
  - Voluntary and involuntary impulses conveyed through these nerves
- Autonomic nervous system

- Sympathetic system
  - Dilates pupils
  - Constricts blood vessels of skin and viscera
  - Constricts sphincters
- Parasympathetic system
  - Constricts pupils
  - Dilates blood vessels of skin and viscera
  - Dilates sphincters

Pathology

- Congenital
  - More important in brain than in any other single organ
  - Anencephaly: cranial fossa is missing in part or completely so the brain is also missing
  - Microcephaly: small head due to cerebrum failing to develop properly
  - Hydrocephaly can be either congenital or acquired
    - Congenital caused by block of flow of CSF

- Aka internal hydrocephalus and noncommunicating
  ○ Spina bifida
    - Failure of neural arch in vertebrae to form properly
    - May be associated with meningocele, myelocele, myelomeningocele, Arnold-Chiari syndrome
- Acquired
  ○ Hydrocephalus
    - Older children or adults
    - Aka external hydrocephalus and communicating
    - Tumors block flow of CSF
    - Faulty reabsorption of CSF
    - Brain may herniate to the foramen magnum
- Inflammatory
  ○ Abscesses
  ○ Strokes
  ○ Empyema

  ○ Encephalitis/meningitis
  ○ Hemorrhage/hematoma
  ○ Injuries/fractures
- Neoplasms
  ○ Benign
    - Glioma
    - Astrocytoma
    - Craniopharyngioma
    - Acoustic neuromas
    - Neurofibroma
  ○ Malignant
    - Glioblastoma multiforme
    - Medulloblastoma

Imaging Strategies

- Computed tomography
- Magnetic resonance imaging
- Sonography
- Nuclear medicine

CLINICAL AND RADIOGRAPHIC CHARACTERISTICS OF COMMON PATHOLOGIES

Pathologic Condition	Causal Factors to Include Age, if Relevant	Manifestations	Radiographic Appearance
Anencephaly	Congenital disorders Severe malformation of cranial vault	Most are still born or die within hours	Only portion of the calvarium is seen
Microcephaly	Failure of cerebrum to develop properly	Exceedingly small head	Calvarium is smaller than normal
Hydrocephaly	Congenital—stenosis of aqueduct of Sylvius Acquired—children and adults—tumors or reabsorption problems	Enlarged ventricles and enlarged head Pressure atrophy of the brain	CT and MRI show enlarged ventricles CT and MRI show smaller brain due to atrophy and increased fluid
Spina bifida	Newborn Congenital due to genetic or environmental issues	Meningocele Myelocele Myelomeningocele Arnold-Chiari syndrome Bladder and bowel problems	Defect of posterior arches of the spine
Abscesses	Infection in sinuses, middle ear, or mastoids	Intracranial pressure	CT with contrast shows a radiodense area
Aneurysm	Middle life Hypertension and atheroma	Symptomless, unless rupture	CT and MRI are now modalities of choice

(continued)

CLINICAL AND RADIOGRAPHIC CHARACTERISTICS OF COMMON PATHOLOGIES (continued)

Pathologic Condition	Causal Factors to Include Age, if Relevant	Manifestations	Radiographic Appearance
Stroke	Thrombus, embolism, or hemorrhage	Sudden onset of neurologic problems	CT shows lucencies in 36–48 h
Subdural empyema	Infection from frontal or ethmoid sinuses	Headache and pressure that is attributed to sinus problem	CT is best Skull radiograph shows diffuse area of osteolytic destruction from osteomyelitis
Encephalitis	Virus spread by mosquitoes Herpes simplex 1	Irritability, drowsiness, headache	CT rules out abscess or tumor
Hemorrhage			
Cerebral Subarachnoid Intracerebral Epidural Subdural	Injury Rupture of aneurysm Hypertensive disease; rupture of AVM Tear in middle meningeal vessel Injury	Sudden headache, cloudy vision	CT and MRI are the best modalities to show and define the area of accumulated blood
Meningitis	Bacteria or viral infection	Fever, headache, muscle pain (stiff neck): all with abrupt onset	Radiography plays a small role but CT can show bacterial or viral infection of meninges
Osteomyelitis	Pyogenic bacteria from sinuses/mastoid air cells Complication of empyema		Can be confused with multiple myeloma
Pituitary adenoma		Vision problems May secrete growth hormones	Eroded sella turcica seen on lateral skull

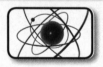

CRITICAL THINKING DISCUSSION QUESTIONS

1. Describe how the sympathetic and parasympathetic systems of the autonomic nervous system work together to maintain balanced activity in the body.

2. Describe a TIA and discuss its importance in the future occurrences of strokes.

3. Discuss the difference between congenital hydrocephalus and acquired hydrocephalus in terms of pathogenesis and clinical expression.

4. What are the causes of increased intracranial pressure? Why is increased intracranial pressure dangerous?

5. Explain the relationship between cerebrovascular accidents and atherosclerosis.

6. Explain the difference between internal and external hydrocephalus.

7. Explain the difference between concussion and contusion.

The Endocrine System

● Goals

1. To review the basic anatomy and physiology of the endocrine system

   OBJECTIVE: List the different endocrine glands and the hormones they secrete

   OBJECTIVE: Describe the physiology of the endocrine system

2. To become familiar with all of the common pathologic conditions of the endocrine system

   OBJECTIVE: Describe the various pathologic conditions affecting the endocrine system

3. To understand which imaging modalities will demonstrate the pathologies of the endocrine system

   OBJECTIVE: List the imaging modalities utilized to demonstrate the various pathologic conditions

● Key Terms

Acromegaly
Addison disease (adrenocortical insufficiency)
Cushing syndrome
Diabetes insipidus
Diabetes mellitus
Exophthalmos
Goiter
Graves disease
Hyperthyroidism
Hypoparathyroidism
Hypopituitarism
Hypothyroidism
Myxedema
Neuroblastoma
Pheochromocytoma
Primary hyperparathyroidism
Progeria
Secondary hyperparathyroidism
Simmonds syndrome
Thyroid adenoma

The complex activities of the body are carried out jointly by the endocrine system and the central nervous system. Through nerve impulses, the central nervous system is keyed to act instantaneously. The action of the endocrine system, however, is subtler. The endocrine glands slowly discharge their secretions into the bloodstream, controlling organs from a distance.

The endocrine system is made up of the ductless glands of internal secretion. They are called ductless because they have no ducts to carry away their secretions and must depend on the capillaries and, to a certain extent, the lymph vessels for this function. The substances secreted by these glands are called hormones. Although most hormones are excitatory in function, some are inhibitory.

The secretion of hormones is controlled by a feedback mechanism. The presence and amount of the hormone, or the substances released by the tissue that is excited by the hormone, regulate further secretion of the hormone by the gland. This ensures that the right amount, no more and no less, of the hormone will maintain proper balance of bodily functions.

The endocrine glands that secrete hormones are the pituitary, thyroid, parathyroid, adrenals, ovaries, testes, pineal body, and pancreas. The ovaries and testes were discussed in Chapter 7 and the pancreas was discussed in Chapter 5. Therefore, here these areas will only be reviewed briefly.

Anatomy, Physiology, and Function

Pituitary Gland

The pituitary gland, or hypophysis, is called the "orchestra leader" and "master gland" because it exerts control over all other glands. Despite its important function, it is no larger than a garden pea. Even though the pituitary is the most important gland of the endocrine system, it is controlled by the hypothalamus. The hypothalamus is the important autonomic nervous system and endocrine control center of the brain located inferior to the thalamus.

The pituitary gland lies protected within the sphenoid bone in the sella turcica. It is further protected by an extension of the dura mater called the pituitary diaphragm. A stem-like portion of the pituitary, the pituitary stalk, extends through the diaphragm and provides a connection to the hypothalamus on the underside of the brain.

The anterior lobe plays the master role, with its numerous anterior pituitary hormones influencing the actions of other endocrine organs. This internal regulation is further coordinated by action of the hypothalamus on the anterior lobe, which actually controls the release of the anterior pituitary hormones, which are of six major types.

Somatropin (a growth hormone) promotes bodily growth of both bone and soft tissues. By increasing the rate at which amino acids enter cells and their ability to convert molecules into proteins, somatropin stimulates the growth and multiplication of body cells, especially those of the bones and skeletal muscles. This hormone also resists protein breakdown during periods of food deprivation and favors fat breakdown.

A **thyrotropic (thyroid stimulating)** hormone of the anterior pituitary lobe influences the thyroid and causes secretion of the thyroid hormone. Two **gonadotropic** hormones influence the ovaries and testes and are necessary for the proper development and function of the reproductive system. A **follicle-stimulating** hormone stimulates the growth of Graafian follicles and the secretion of estrogen in the female and the development of the seminiferous tubules and sperm cells in the male. A **luteinizing** hormone stimulates the formation of the corpus luteum, and secretion of estrogen and progesterone in the female, while in the male it stimulates development and secretion of testosterone in the interstitial cells of the testes.

Prolactin, a lactogenic hormone, is responsible for breast development during pregnancy and, as its name implies, for production of milk.

Growth of the adrenal glands is under the influence of **adrenocorticotropic** hormone (ACTH), which also stimulates the adrenal cortex to synthesize and release corticosteroids. ACTH also appears to have a function in relation to pigmentation of the skin; which is primarily a function of the last of the anterior pituitary hormones, **melanocyte-stimulating** hormone.

The posterior lobe secretes two hormones, which are actually made in the hypothalamus and pass through the pituitary stalk into the posterior lobe where they are secreted into the blood stream. The first of these, an antidiuretic hormone called **vasopressin**, limits the development of large volumes of urine by stimulating water reabsorption by the distal and collecting tubules of the kidneys. The second hormone, **oxytocin**, stimulates both the ejection of breast milk and the uterine contractions in pregnancy.

Thyroid Gland

The thyroid gland is composed of two pear-shaped lobes separated by a middle strip of tissue called the isthmus, which crosses in front of the second and third tracheal cartilages. The thyroid gland perches like a butterfly with wings extended on the front part of the neck below the larynx. The lobes are molded to the trachea and esophagus down as far as the sixth tracheal cartilage, and they extend upward to the sides of the cricoid and thyroid cartilages. The thyroid may be felt slightly and may even be visible as a swelling in some diseases of the gland.

The thyroid consists of tiny sacs, or follicles, that are filled with a gelatinous yellow fluid called colloid. The colloid contains the hormone secreted by the thyroid.

The main function of the thyroid is the secretion of two iodine-laden hormones; **thyroxin** and **triiodothyronin**, which together are referred to as **thyroid hormone**. This hormone is high in iodine and vital for growth and metabolism. Thyroid hormone maintains the metabolism at a higher rate than would be maintained otherwise, and through variations in the gland activities, it alters the metabolic rate in accordance with changing physiologic demands. This hormone also helps regulate growth and differentiation of tissue during fetal development.

A secondary function of the thyroid gland is the secretion of **calcitonin**, which produces a decrease in the concentration of calcium in blood serum. It helps to maintain the balance of calcium in the blood that is necessary for a variety of bodily processes. The balance is achieved in conjunction with the functioning of the parathyroid glands.

Parathyroid Glands

The parathyroid glands are small, round glands, usually two on each side, that lie behind the thyroid gland and are usually embedded in its surface. The superior pair is located approximately at the middle lobe of the thyroid gland; the inferior pair is at the lower end of the thyroid lobe. They are not always found at these locations, and they may vary in number. They have been found implanted within the thyroid gland itself, behind the pharynx, and even in the thorax, embedded with the thymus.

Parathyroid hormone regulates the calcium and phosphorus content of the blood and bones. The regulation of calcium content is very important in certain tissue activities such as blood formation, coagulation of blood, milk production in pregnant women, and maintenance of normal and neuromuscular excitability.

Parathyroid hormone promotes calcium absorption in the blood, increasing its calcium concentration. It suppresses the concentration of calcium in the bones. This mechanism is opposite that of the hormone calcitonin from the thyroid gland. These two hormones together maintain calcium balance.

Adrenal Glands

The adrenal glands, also known as the suprarenal glands, resemble small caps perched on the top of each kidney. They are composed of two distinct parts, the cortex and the medulla, each with a different function. The cortex is indispensible to life.

All of the known adrenal hormones of the cortex are steroids, many of which can be manufactured synthetically. They are classified as **glucocorticoids**, secreted mainly by the middle zone of the cortex; **mineralocorticoids**, secreted by the outer zone of the cortex; and sex hormones secreted by the inner zone of the cortex. The glucocorticoids include cortisol (hydrocortisone), cortisone, and corticosterone and affect literally all cells in the body. Their general effect, however, is in the metabolism of carbohydrates, fats, and proteins; resistance to stress; antibody function; lymphatic function; and recovery from injury and inflammation. The mineralocorticoids are concerned with the regulation of sodium and potassium and their excretion. The principal one is **aldosterone**, which acts on the kidneys to maintain the homeostasis of potassium and sodium ions, conserve water, and decrease urine output.

The adrenal cortex in both sexes secretes large amounts of male hormone androgen and small amounts of female hormone estrogen. These hormones are produced not only by the adrenals but also by the testes in the male and the ovaries in the female, and are responsible for secondary sex characteristics, such as hair growth of muscles and bones, accounting in part for observed sexual differences. The presence of ACTH in the blood supply is necessary for the anatomic integrity of the adrenal cortex and its functions in secreting androgens and cortisol.

The adrenal medulla secretes **epinephrine** (adrenaline) and **norepinephrine** (noradrenaline). Epinephrine makes approximately 80% of the total secretions of the adrenal medulla and is considered more potent than norepinephrine. It aids the body in meeting stressful situations, such as the defense flight, attack, or pursuit. By stimulating or boosting the sympathetic nervous system, epinephrine aids in coping with stress. The effects of these hormones are increased heart rate, blood pressure, blood glucose level, respiratory rate, and airway size.

Pancreas

The pancreas was described as a part of the hepatobiliary system in Chapter 5. In brief, the specialized cells, called the islets of Langerhans, secrete **insulin** and **glucagon** into the bloodstream. Insulin is necessary for the use and storage of carbohydrates and plays a role in reducing the amount of glucose in the blood by accelerating its transport into body cells. Insulin decreases blood glucose levels, and glucagon acts to increase them. Glucagon causes the liver to convert glycogen to glucose. Blood glucose levels are also dependent on the action of many of the other endocrine secretions, such as the pituitary growth hormone, epinephrine, ACTH, and the glucocorticoids, which increase it, and the thyroid hormone, which decreases it.

Gonads

The male and female sex glands were discussed in Chapter 7. The female ovaries and the male testes produce hormones important to the functioning of the reproductive system. These glands become active at puberty under the influence of the anterior pituitary gland and produce the secondary sex characteristics of pubic and axillary hair in both of the sexes, deep voice and beard in the male, and breast development and onset of menses in the female. The hormones secreted are **estrogen** and **progesterone** in the female and **testosterone** in the male.

Pineal Gland

The pineal gland is a small, firm, oval body located near the base of the brain. Although exact functions have not been established, it is postulated that it secretes melatonin (skin-lightening agent), which inhibits secretion of the luteinizing hormone of the pituitary.

Figure 10-1 shows the location of endocrine glands in our body.

The overall effects of the endocrine system are contrasted with the nervous system. It is one of two

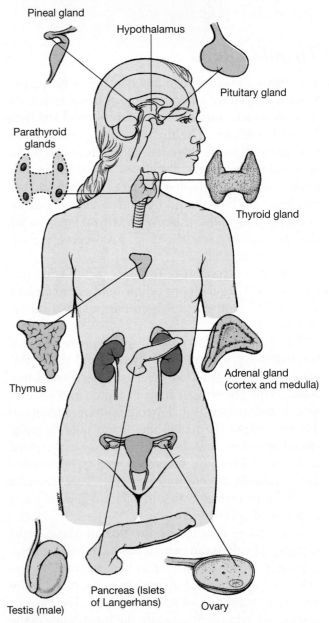

FIGURE 10-1   The major endocrine organs. (Stedman's Medical Dictionary, 27th ed. Baltimore: Lippincott Willimas & Wilkins 2000.)

major systems responsible for regulating homeostasis. Along with the nervous system, the endocrine system regulates and coordinates the activity of nearly all other body structures; failure can result in disease. Display 10-1 summarizes the endocrine glands, the hormones that they secrete, and the functions of those hormones.

Pathology

Pituitary Gland

Hyperpituitarism results from an excessive secretion of the growth hormone. The causative factor is usually a

DISPLAY 10-1 THE ENDOCRINE GLANDS AND HORMONES

Gland	Hormone	Function

Pituitary
  Anterior lobe
	Growth (somatropin)
	Thyrotropic
	Gonadotropic hormones
	  Follicle-stimulating hormone
	
	  Luteinizing
	
	Lactogenic (prolactin)
	Adrenocorticotropin
		Bone and soft tissue growth
		Causes production of thyroid hormone
		Stimulates Graafian follicle growth
		Secretion of estrogen in ovaries
		Development of seminiferous tubules
		Production of sperm cells
		Ovulation
		Secretion of estrogen and progesterone
		Development of testicle interstitial cells
		Secretion of testosterone
		Causes breasts to develop and produce milk
		Causes adrenals to release corticosteroids

Posterior lobe	Melanocyte-stimulating hormone Antidiuretic (vasopressin) Oxytocin	Forms melanin pigment in skin Causes kidney to reabsorb water Causes uterine contractions and breast milk ejection
Thyroid	Thyroxine, Triiodothyronine Calcitonin	Regulates growth, development, and metabolism Promotes calcium absorption in bones Reduces calcium content in blood
Parathyroid	Parathyroid hormone	Controls phosphorus content in blood and bone Promotes calcium content in blood Reduces calcium absorption in bones

Adrenal
  Cortex
	Glucocorticoids (hydrocortisone,
	cortisone, corticosterone)
	
	Mineralocorticoids
	Androgen and estrogen
		Causes metabolism of carbohydrates, fats, and proteins
		Causes lymphatic functions:
		  Antibody formation
		  Recovery of injury and inflammation
		Regulates sodium and potassium
		Secondary sex characteristics

Medulla	Epinephrine (adrenaline) Norepinephrine (noradrenaline)	Stimulate sympathetic nervous system responses

Gonads
  Ovaries
  Testes
	Estrogenic (estradiol, estrone)
	Testosterone
		Promote secondary sex development after puberty

Pineal	Melatonin	Skin-lightening agent Inhibits secretion of luteinizing hormone
Pancreas Islets of Langerhans	Insulin Glucagon	Regulates use of carbohydrates Reduces glucose in blood Promotes glucose in blood

tumor (Fig. 10-2) or hyperplasia of the anterior lobe of the pituitary gland. When too much growth hormone is secreted before the bone growth has ceased, a condition known as **gigantism** results. People with this condition may reach a stature of 7 or 8 feet and have long limbs. The patients may have normal or retarded mental development. Sexual development and muscular strength are below normal. The epiphyseal plate of the long bones is delayed by several years, thereby increasing the length of the long bones. The vertebral bodies show wedging. Acromegalic characteristics may develop in these patients if hypersecretion of the growth hormone continues after the epiphyseal plates close.

If the adenoma develops after growth is completed and over activity of the hormone occurs, it may produce a condition called **acromegaly**. Once the epiphyseal lines are closed at puberty, no further longitudinal growth can take place. Thus, if excessive amounts of growth hormone are secreted, appositional enlargement occurs in the bones, but all the tissues share in the overgrowth. Acromegalics are unable to increase in stature by having large hands (Fig. 10-3A), and prominent course facial features. The lips and nose are particularly large, as are the mandible, hand, and

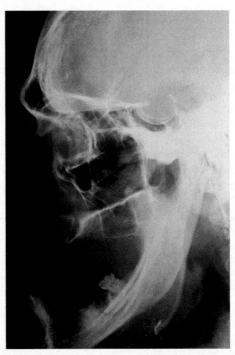

FIGURE 10-2   In this lateral facial bones image, the enlargement of the sella turcica can be seen. This is a manifestation of a pituitary adenoma. (Yochum TR, Rowe LJ. *Yochum and Rowe's Essentials of Skeletal Radiology.* 3rd ed. Philadelphia, PA: Lippincott Williams & Wilkins; 2004.)

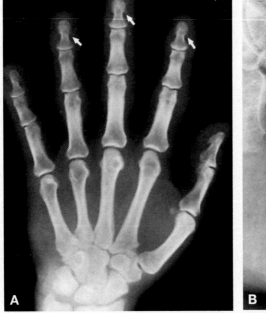
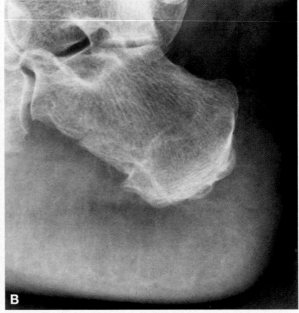

FIGURE 10-3   (A) Acromegaly can be seen on this hand image through the widening of the metacarpophalangeal joints, thickening of the soft tissues of the fingers, and overgrowth of the tufts of the distal phalanges as seen at the arrows. (B) Acromegaly can be seen on this lateral heel image. The actual measurement of the soft tissue heel pad was 32 mm. (Eisenberg RL. *Clinical Imaging: An Atlas of Differential Diagnosis.* 5th ed. Philadelphia, PA: Lippincott Williams & Wilkins; 2010.)

feet (Fig. 10-3B). Overgrowth of bones causes a curvature of the spine and the joints are more susceptible to degenerative lesions.

The pituitary gland controls the level of secretion of gonadal and thyroid hormones as well as the production of growth hormone. When there is decreased function of the pituitary gland, disturbances in bone growth and maturation are widely manifested. **Hypopituitarism** is insufficient production and secretion of the growth hormone of the pituitary gland. The most common cause of hypopituitarism is an adenoma of the pituitary gland.

In children, hypopituitarism causes dwarfism. Dwarfism caused by pituitary insufficiency is rare and may result from tumors of the anterior lobe. Because there is insufficient growth hormone to stimulate the growth of the bones in length or in width, the result is a person who is small in stature. The skeleton is small and delicately formed. This may be accompanied by thyroid, adrenocortical, and gonadal insufficiency. In true pituitary dwarfism, the children fail to develop sexually as well, but they are not mentally deficient.

Simmonds syndrome is a result of chronic pituitary insufficiency and is an example of **progeria**, or premature aging. The syndrome can occur both in children and in adolescents. Growth ceases and the patient presents as an aged person. The extremities become thin, the facial features are birdlike, and the skin becomes wrinkled. The patient will suffer complications of the elderly while still a chronologically a young person.

Diabetes insipidus is a rare type of diabetes caused by infiltrative processes such as neoplasms, head injury, or in some cases, a change in sugar levels . A patient with this type of diabetes presents with an abnormal increase in the amount of urine output. It contains no sugar and is therefore insipid, or tasteless. The excessive urination is due to failure of water reabsorption in the kidney, resulting from deficiency of antidiuretic hormone. This polyuria leads to excessive thirst.

Thyroid Gland

Iodine is the essential element of thyroid hormone. Most disorders of the thyroid gland are caused by either overproduction or underproduction of the thyroid hormone and its iodine-containing substance. The iodine in the thyroid hormone is combined with a protein in the blood, which is then referred to as protein-bound iodine. However, when the hormone enters the tissue, the separate components become unbound from the protein.

In the condition called **hyperthyroidism**, there is overdevelopment, or enlargement of the thyroid gland with excessive secretion of the thyroid hormone. This is called **Graves** disease. Graves disease most often develops in the third and fourth decades of life and affects females more often than males. In Graves disease, the thyroid gland undergoes hyperplasia and there is an associated lymphocytic infiltration. **Exophthalmos**, a protrusion of eyes, is a prominent symptom of this condition. The major clinical symptoms include nervousness, rapid pulse rate, palpitations, excessive sweating, and heat intolerance. Weight loss is frequent, despite an increased appetite. Muscular wasting is most apparent in the muscles of the shoulder girdle. Patients with hyperthyroidism have a variety of cardiac symptoms and signs. Enlargement of the heart, however, is unusual. Goiters, as described below, are another sign of Graves disease.

In **hypothyroidism** there is underdevelopment of the thyroid gland and a deficiency of thyroid hormone. During the early growth and development years, undersecretion of thyroid hormone produces dwarfism, with significant physical malformations and often mental retardation. This condition is known as **infantile hypothyroidism**. An obsolete term for this condition is cretinism. While obsolete, it is still heard occasionally. Infantile hypothyroidism is characterized by retarded mental, physical, and sexual development. Children typically have a short, stocky build, with short legs and muscular incoordination. Development of the head is abnormal, with a short forehead, broad nose, wide set eyes, and a short, thick neck. The eyelids are puffy and wrinkled. The mouth is open, with thick lips and a protruding tongue. The major radiographic abnormalities include a delay in the appearance and subsequent growth of ossification centers and retarded bone age. Skull changes are common and include an increase in the thickness of the cranial vault, under pneumatization of the air cells of the sinuses and mastoids, and widened sutures with delayed closure.

In older individuals, thyroid deficiency produces **myxedema**, with low metabolic functioning. Childhood or juvenile myxedema occurs because of thyroid dysfunction after birth. These children are usually spared the serious mental retardation of the infantile hypothyroidism patient. Adult myxedema is a form of hypothyroidism that occurs most frequently in adults between the ages of 30 and 60 years. It is four times more common in females. There is characteristic reduced intellectual and motor functioning and weight gain. The face and eyelids are edematous. The edema is quite viscous and adds firmness to the skin, which does not pit when pressed as in other types of edema. Patients with this condition will have bags under the eyes. The speech is slow or slurred. The skin is coarse, dry, scaling, and cold. On radiographs, the heart will be noted to be enlarged, which is usually caused by pericardial effusion. Because of the edema, soft-tissue swelling on the images of the extremities may be seen. In addition, there may be pleural effusion and pulmonary edema that may be caused by the lower metabolic function (Fig. 10-4).

Generalized enlargement of the thyroid with normal or low thyroid function is termed **nontoxic goiter**. It results when one or more factors occur that inhibit the ability of the thyroid gland to secrete the quantities of active thyroid hormone necessary to meet the needs of the body. Among these causes are iodine deficiency, enzymatic defects, and antithyroid compounds. By far, the most common type of goiter is caused by iodine deficiency. Goiters were once common in endemic form in inland geographic areas such as the Great Lakes region and in mountainous regions, where the iodine content of the soil and water is very low. The addition of iodine to table salt has now eliminated this cause.

Thyroid adenoma is a benign neoplasm. It is a solitary nodule of thyroid cells surrounded by a fibrous tissue capsule. These tumors are rarely symptomatic. They usually first present as a palpable mass in the thyroid gland. However, they cannot be felt unless they are over 1 cm in size. Usually located within the neck, these tumors will be surrounded by a thin zone of compressed thyroid tissue.

Thyroid carcinoma is twice as common in females as in males and can occur at any age. There are three major classifications for thyroid carcinoma: papillary adenocarcinoma, follicular adenocarcinoma, and medullary adenocarcinoma. Thyroid carcinoma differs from most other carcinomas in that it is well differentiated, with a papillary growth pattern. The most common type of carcinoma is the papillary type. This slow-growing tumor metastasizes through the lymph nodes. Follicular carcinoma is more difficult to determine as its appearance is close to that of normal thyroid tissue. A rare type of thyroid carcinoma, medullary carcinoma, is so called because the cells occur in solid masses rather than producing glands. Medullary carcinoma arises from the calcitonin-secreting cells of the thyroid.

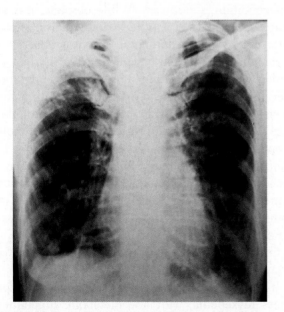

FIGURE 10-4   Right-sided pleural effusion and pulmonary edema in a patient with severe myxedema. These resolved with thyroid replacement therapy. (Crapo JD, Glassroth J, Karlinsky JB, et al. *Baum's Textbook of Pulmonary Diseases*. 7th ed. Philadelphia, PA: Lippincott Williams & Wilkins; 2004.)

Parathyroid Glands

Hyperparathyroidism is relatively common and an important disease that may be mild and go undetected for a long time. **Primary hyperparathyroidism** occurs when the cause of increased parathyroid hormone production lies in the parathyroid glands and production is not controlled by normal feedback mechanism. The causes are adenoma, hyperplasia, and carcinoma. **Secondary hyperparathyroidism** occurs with conditions associated with low serum calcium, most often chronic renal failure or vitamin D deficiency. The metabolic changes in secondary hyperparathyroidism are quite complex and will not be discussed further.

In primary hyperparathyroidism, the excess parathyroid hormone causes increased breakdown of bone, creating a lacy pattern particularly seen in the digits (Fig. 10-5), increased absorption of calcium by the intestine, and increased reabsorption of calcium by the kidney. Urine calcium is also increased because the increase in glomerular filtration of calcium is greater than the increase in reabsorption by the renal tubules.

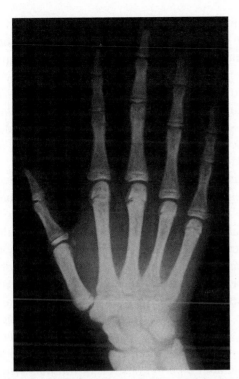

FIGURE 10-5 Secondary *hyperparathyroidism* in a 12-year-old girl with chronic pyelonephritis. There is moderate subperiosteal erosion on the radial side of the middle phalanges; note a lacy appearance of the periosteum and small-tuft erosion. Subperiosteal bone resorption is the most significant radiographic finding in hyperparathyroidism; subperiosteal bone resorption and tuft erosion are seen in both primary and secondary hyperparathyroidism. (Fleisher GR, Ludwig S, Baskin MN. *Atlas of Pediatric Emergency Medicine.* Philadelphia, PA: Lippincott Williams & Wilkins; 2004.)

Bone destruction with pathologic fracture is a less common presentation and is associated with more advanced stages of the disease. As osteoblasts attempt to repair the bone destruction, increased amounts of the enzyme alkaline phosphatase are released into the serum. When the cause of hyperparathyroidism is renal failure, there is often an associated increase in bone density known as osteosclerosis. When osteosclerosis occurs along the superior and inferior margins of the vertebral bodies, it produces the classic appearance of "rugger jersey" spine (Fig. 10-6A, B).

The bone lesions are characterized by the presence of giant multinucleated osteoclasts and fibrosis, sometimes with cyst formation (giant cell tumors). The bone resorption is commonly detected by X-rays of the hands and teeth. A ground-glass appearance is present when there has been an overall loss of bone density. Patients with hyperparathyroidism are also prone to repeat bouts of acute pancreatitis.

In **hypoparathyroidism**, functioning of the parathyroid glands is decreased. Most cases of hypoparathyroidism result from surgical removal of all four parathyroid glands, an uncommon complication of the treatment of hyperparathyroidism or of surgical removal of the thyroid gland. In rare instances it occurs idiopathically, with replacement of the parathyroids by fat. Hypoparathyroidism leads to decreased serum calcium and increased serum phosphorus, which in turn

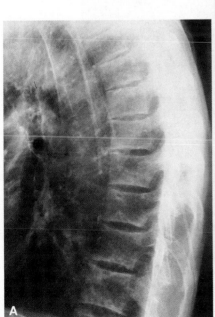

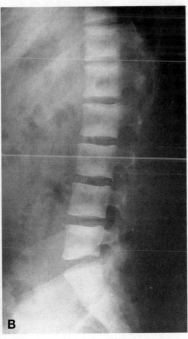

FIGURE 10-6 (A) Lateral thoracic spine. Note that the bone density is decreased, the trabecular patterns accentuated, and the endplates slightly increased in concavity. (B) Lateral lumbar spine. Note the prominent linear subendplate densities at multiple contiguous levels that produce this alternating dense–lucent–dense appearance, simulating the transverse bands of a rugby sweater (rugger jersey spine). This pattern is distinctive for hyperparathyroidism, though there is similarity to some cases of osteopetrosis. (Yochum TR, Rowe LJ. *Yochum and Rowe's Essentials of Skeletal Radiology.* 3rd ed. Philadelphia, PA: Lippincott Williams & Wilkins; 2004.)

is manifested by increased irritability of muscles and convulsions. Little or no calcium is excreted by the kidneys in the urine.

Adrenal Glands

Cushing syndrome is produced by excessive production of glucocorticoids. The most common cause is iatrogenic from the use of corticosteroids in the treatment of other diseases. Noniatrogenic Cushing syndrome may be caused by adrenal hyperplasia resulting from production of ACTH by pituitary hyperplasia or, less commonly, by corticosteroid-secreting adenomas or carcinomas of the adrenal cortex or by ACTH secreting carcinomas such as bronchogenic carcinoma.

The most obvious effect of Cushing syndrome is a peculiar obesity limited to the face and trunk. The patient has a protuberant abdomen, a "moon" face, and thin extremities. Other common findings include sexual impotence, purple striae on the skin, easy bruising, hypertension, hirsutism, muscle weakness, and

hyperglycemia. Cushing syndrome produces radiographic changes in multiple systems. Osteoporosis can be found throughout the body in a diffuse form. The demineralization of the vertebral bodies may cause them to suffer compression fracture (Fig. 10-7A, B). The femur and the humerus are common places to find a spontaneous fracture. Elevated steroid levels increase the levels of calcium in the urine, which may lead to renal calculi or nephrocalcinosis.

Addison disease, also known as adrenocortical insufficiency, is an uncommon condition characterized by insufficient production of adrenocortical hormones. In about 70% of the cases, it is the result of an autoimmune process that slowly destroys the cortex of the adrenal glands. In the remaining cases, destruction may be caused by tuberculosis, tumor growth, or inflammatory necrosis. Another cause of adrenal insufficiency is the excessive administration of steroids.

Addison disease may strike at any age, affects men and women equally, and frequently is noticed for the first time after a period of stress or trauma. Symptoms

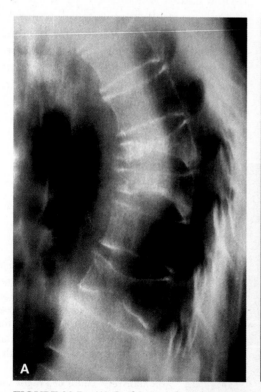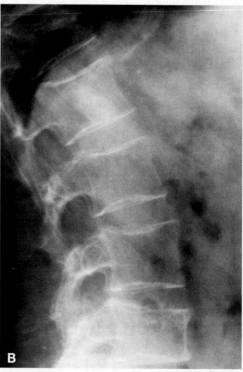

FIGURE 10-7   (A) Cushing syndrome causes demineralization of the vertebral bodies leading to compression fractures. (B) Cushing syndrome due to adrenal hyperplasia. Marked demineralization and an almost complete loss of trabecula in the lumbar spine. The vertebral end plates are mildly concave, and the intervertebral disk spaces are slightly widened. Note the compression of the superior end plate of L4. (A: Yochum TR, Rowe LJ. *Yochum and Rowe's Essentials of Skeletal Radiology.* 3rd ed. Philadelphia, PA: Lippincott Williams & Wilkins; 2004. B: Eisenberg RL. *An Atlas of Differential Diagnosis.* 4th ed. Philadelphia, PA: Lippincott Williams & Wilkins; 2003.)

include anemia, fatigue, anorexia, nausea, weight loss, and fainting due to hypotension or hypoglycemia, loss of body hair, and depression. The deficient production of corticosteroids leads to increased release of the hormone ACTH. ACTH causes a melatonin-stimulating hormone-like effect, which accounts for the increased skin pigmentation characteristic of Addison disease.

The diagnosis is made by a number of laboratory tests that search for the levels of circulating hormones in the blood or the lack of response of the adrenal gland to certain tests that normally stimulate the action of the gland. The treatment of Addison disease requires replacing the missing hormone.

A **pheochromocytoma** is a tumor that most commonly arises in the adrenal medulla. It is usually a benign neoplasm, but a small percentage of tumors may be malignant. Pheochromocytomas arise in the abdomen. The tumor may be located anywhere along the sympathetic nervous system. Even though it is a rare cause of hypertension, the removal of the pheochromocytoma will cure the hypertension. As in Addison disease, "pheos" are diagnosed mainly by laboratory tests. However, radiography, computed tomography (CT), and ultrasonography play an important role in confirming the location of the neoplasm. Masses may displace the ureter or kidney, or may appear as filling defects in the bladder on the intravenous pyelogram.

Neuroblastoma is a tumor of the adrenal medulla and is the second most common malignancy in children under the age of 5 years. Recall that nephroblastoma (Wilms) tumors are the most common malignancy found in children (Chapter 6). About 10% of neuroblastomas arise outside the adrenal gland retroperitoneally. The tumor is highly malignant and metastasizes early and fast either by permeation or embolic spread to regional lymph nodes and abdominal organs. CT is the best modality to show metastasis through the lymph nodes. Neuroblastomas tend to become quite large before detection. By that time, metastasis has occurred, and the patient has a dismal prognosis. One type of neuroblastoma (Hutchinson syndrome) is characterized by profuse osseous metastases, particularly to the skull and the orbit. Another type (Pepper syndrome) is characterized by hepatic metastases.

Features that differentiate the neuroblastoma from a Wilms tumor bear looking at. The neuroblastoma frequently has calcifications (Fig. 10-8), while this is an uncommon finding in a Wilms tumor. Since the neuroblastoma arises from the adrenal gland, which

sits superior to the kidney, this neoplasm tends to cause the entire kidney and ureter to be displaced downward (Fig. 10-9). The intravenous ureogram demonstrates

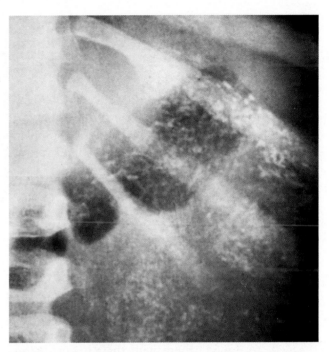

FIGURE 10-8 Diffuse granular calcification in the large left upper quadrant mass that was found to be a neuroblastoma. (Eisenberg RL. *Clinical Imaging: An Atlas of Differential Diagnosis*. 5th ed. Philadelphia, PA: Lippincott Williams & Wilkins; 2010.)

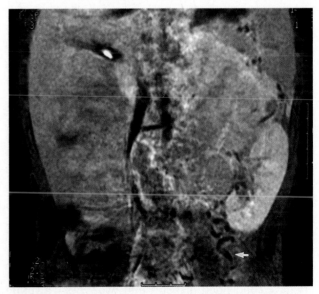

FIGURE 10-9 Neuroblastoma demonstrated on MRI scan. This coronal T1-weighted image shows a large mass on the left displacing the kidney laterally. (Daffner RH. *Clinical Radiology: The Essentials*. 3rd ed. Philadelphia, PA: Lippincott Williams & Wilkins; 2007.)

downward and lateral renal displacement. A Wilms tumor, on the other hand, has an intrarenal origin and distorts and widens the pelvocalyceal system from within.

TECH TIP

Do not confuse neuroblastoma (of the adrenal gland) with the nephroblastoma (Wilms tumor) and the hypernephroma (renal cell carcinoma). For a comparison of nephroblastoma and hypernephroma, see Chapter 6.

Pancreas

Diabetes mellitus is a generalized chronic disease resulting from a disorder of carbohydrate metabolism. It is believed to be caused by inadequate secretion of insulin by the beta cells of the islet of Langerhans in the pancreas. Without insulin, glucose cannot enter the cells to provide them with their major energy-producing nutrient.

The American Diabetes Association has recommended that the course of diabetes be divided into the four stages of prediabetes, suspected diabetes, chemical or latent diabetes, and overt diabetes. The prediabetics are offspring of diabetic parents, and it is assumed that these individuals will subsequently develop diabetes. Suspected diabetics are patients who have abnormal glucose tolerance test results of diabetic symptoms influenced by obesity, pregnancy, infections, trauma, or pharmaceutical and hormonal agents. These patients are normal in all respects and when the causative agent is removed, the metabolism returns to normal. The chemical or latent diabetics have no signs or symptoms of the disease, but have abnormal glucose tolerance test results or an elevated fasting blood glucose level independent of stress. The overt diabetics have symptoms of diabetes.

Although diabetes may develop at any time in life from a few months old to over 80 years of age, researchers have subdivided diabetes into two types—juvenile and the maturity-onset diabetes. These are based on the time of the onset of diabetes. Patients under the age of 25 years are classified as having juvenile diabetes. Patients over the age of 25 have maturity-onset diabetes.

However, maturity-onset diabetes is found more frequently in obese people over the age of 40 years.

The most common characteristics of diabetes mellitus are polyuria, increased thirst, excessive appetite, and loss of weight and strength. Increased urine output occurs because large amounts of water are taken from the body's tissue to dilute the large amounts of sugar in order to eliminate it from the body. The body is unable to utilize the carbohydrates in the sugar, and the patient becomes weak or loses strength. The loss of nutrients for energy causes the excessive appetite.

Complications of diabetes mellitus involve the vascular, endocrine, and nervous systems. Arteriosclerosis is likely to be more progressive in a diabetic patient because lipids are deposited within the walls of the blood vessels. Coronary artery disease may also develop. Gangrene is frequently the result of infection when there are circulatory disturbances of the lower extremities. Bone destruction due to osteomyelitis can be seen on the radiographs (Fig. 10-10). The retina may be damaged with impaired

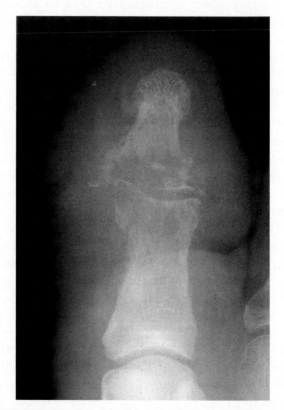

FIGURE 10-10   Osteomyelitis and joint space infection in a diabetic patient. These extensive destructive lesions involve both sides of the joint. This signifies that the process is either an arthropathy or an infection. (Daffner RH. *Clinical Radiology: The Essentials.* 3rd ed. Philadelphia, PA: Lippincott Williams & Wilkins; 2007.)

vision and sometimes blindness. Kidney symptoms are edema and hypertension. Renal failure as a complication of diabetes often causes death.

The foot is now the most common site of neuroarthropathy that occurs with diabetes mellitus. The radiographic appearance of neuropathic joint disease of the foot and ankle varies greatly as can be seen in Figure 10-11A–E. In Figure 10-11A, the patient with diabetes mellitus had only moderate discomfort with the dislocation of the navicular bone seen at the *arrow*. This was the first indication of neuropathic joint disease. In Figure 10-11B, there is massive soft tissue swelling surrounding the joint (indicated by the *arrows*). This is common in the neuropathic ankle and is frequently seen in neuroarthropathy accompanying diabetes mellitus. Figure 10-11C shows osteolysis of the metatarsals and the phalanges in this patient with chronic diabetes mellitus. The patient in Figure 10-11D exhibits destruction, fragmentation,

and displacement of the tarsometatarsal joints. Finally, Figure 10-11E shows typical soft-tissue swelling and fragmentation of the navicular bone. There is sharply defined osseous destruction at the dorsum and posterior foot and ankle.

Hypoglycemia is a condition in which the blood sugar falls below normal levels. A person who is a known diabetic must always be watchful for the signs of hypoglycemic shock, which include light-headiness, sweaty face and hands, and nervousness. Hypoglycemia occurs more often in juvenile diabetes mellitus than in the adult type.

One of the most serious complications of diabetes mellitus is diabetic acidosis or coma. It usually occurs when there is poor control of diabetes. The diabetic coma may range from drowsiness to deep unconsciousness. If the process is not reversed, the blood pressure falls and there is circulatory collapse and renal failure leading to death.

Case Study

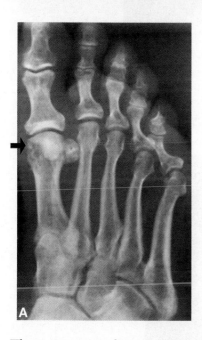
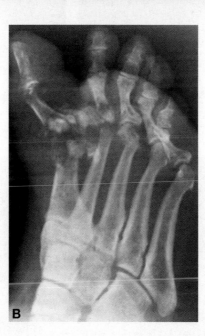

(Eisenberg RL. *Clinical Imaging: An Atlas of Differential Diagnosis.* 5th ed. Philadelphia, PA: Lippincott Williams & Wilkins; 2010.)

The two images show a patient with diabetes mellitus. In image (A), there is soft tissue involvement and minimal osteoporosis at the head of the first metatarsal with some loss of the sharp cortical outline (*arrow*). In image (B), taken 1 month later, there is severe bone destruction involving not only the head of the first metatarsal but also the rest of the big toe and the second and third metatarsophalangeal joints.

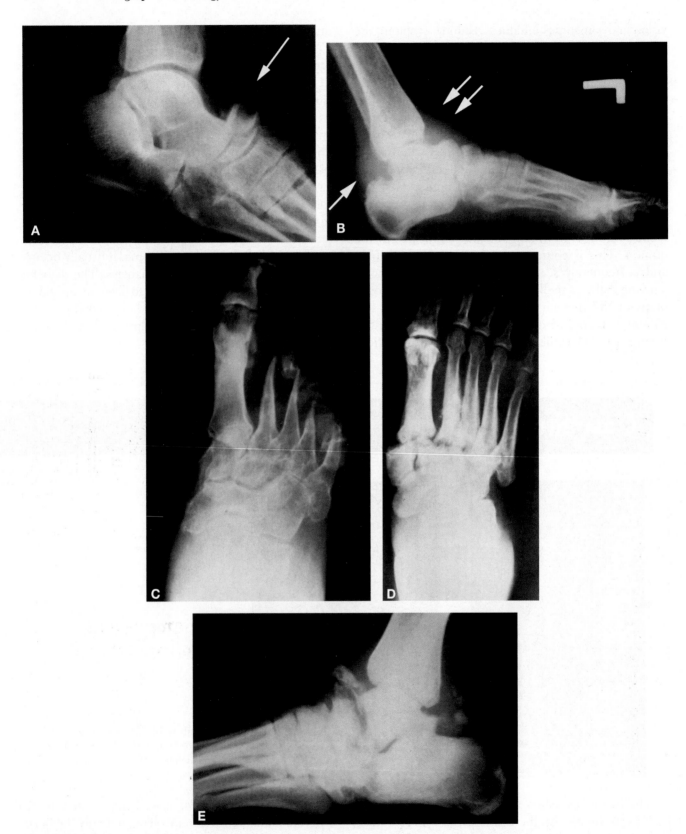

FIGURE 10-11   Various demonstrations of diabetes mellitus. A) Dislocation of the navicular bone seen at the arrow B) Massive soft tissue swelling around the joint (arrows) C) Osteolysis of the metatarsals and phalanges D) Destructive fragmentation and displacement E) Soft tissue swelling and fragmentation of the navicular. (Koopman WJ, Moreland LW. *Arthritis and Allied Conditions: A Textbook Of Rheumatology.* 15th ed. Philadelphia, PA: Lippincott Williams & Wilkins; 2005.)

DISPLAY 10-2 ENDOCRINE-RELATED DISEASES RESULTING FROM DEFICIENT OR EXCESSIVE HORMONE SECRETION

Hormone	Hormone-Deficient Diseases	Hormone-Excess Diseases
Adrenocorticotropin	Addison disease	Cushing syndrome
Growth hormone	Dwarfism, Simmonds syndrome	Gigantism, acromegaly
Antidiuretic	Diabetes insipidus	Inappropriate antidiuretic hormone secretion syndrome
Thyroid hormone	Cretinism, hypothyroidism	Hyperthyroidism, Graves
Parathyroid hormone	Hypoparathyroidism	Hyperparathyroidism
Glucocorticoids	Addison disease	Cushing syndrome
Insulin	Diabetes mellitus	Insulin shock

Display 10-2 summarizes the endocrine-related diseases that result from either deficient or excessive secretion of the various hormones.

Imaging Strategies

Imaging modalities are used to diagnose both the underlying endocrine disorders and the secondary changes that may occur in various areas of the body. Disorders of the endocrine glands themselves are usually evaluated by ultrasonography, CT, MRI, and radionuclide scanning. Secondary pathologic manifestations elsewhere in the body are generally evaluated on radiographic images. For areas that are not encased in bone, CT is often of more value because the abundance of fat may prevent an optimal sonographic examination. Ultrasonography is unable to study the glands that are embedded in bone (i.e., the pituitary and the pineal); therefore, CT and MRI are the best modalities for demonstrating abnormalities in these areas.

Ultrasound

Sonography can be helpful in imaging the thyroid gland, the adrenals, and the gonads. Testicular and ovarian ultrasound was discussed in Chapter 7.

Thyroid masses are common and can be seen in the elderly patients more often. Parathyroid masses are demonstrated by sonography to determine which of the four glands are enlarged before going to surgery (Figs. 10-12 and 10-13). If nuclear medicine demonstrates a nonfunctioning mass, ultrasound will determine if the mass is cystic or solid.

Sonography can demonstrate an adrenal tumor, but it can be a challenge for the sonographer. Thin adults and children are the best patients for ultrasound of the adrenal glands because of the prominence of the glands. A pheochromocytoma that arises off the adrenal medulla can be localized by ultrasound.

Computed Tomography and Magnetic Resonance Imaging

Adrenal glands are best demonstrated by CT. It is the method of choice to differentiate between benign adrenal masses and metastases. Abdominal spiral CT provides the best resolution to demonstrate adrenal masses as small as 1 cm in size. CT is important to detect abnormal location of parathyroid tissue.

MRI is the preferred method to study the pituitary gland. It is useful in diagnosing diabetes insipidus because of an absence of signal. MRI can accurately and quickly measure the size of the adrenal glands. Weighted T1 and T2 scans may show a difference in the intensity of the adrenal glands but are not as effective as nuclear medicine.

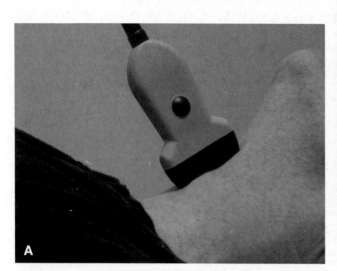

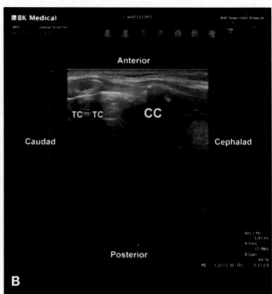

FIGURE 10-12   A) This shows the position of the transducer in order to scan the thyroid gland. B) This transverse scan of the thyroid gland is normal. (Orbaugh SL, Gigeleisen PE. *Atlas of Airway Management: Techniques and Tools.* 2nd ed. Philadelphia, PA: Lippincott Williams & Wilkins; 2012.)

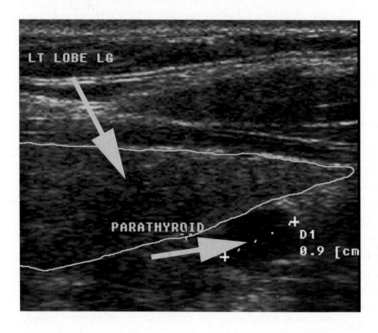

FIGURE 10-13   This sagittal image of the upper pole of the right lobe of the thyroid gland demonstrates a hypoechoic parathyroid adenoma posterior to the thyroid. (Mulholland MW, Lillemoe KD, Doherty GM, et al. *Greenfield's Surgery: Scientific Principles and Practice.* 4th ed. Philadelphia, PA: Lippincott Williams & Wilkins; 2006.)

Nuclear Medicine

A superior study for the functioning of the thyroid gland is nuclear medicine. Radioactive iodine is administered and will be diffused in the thyroid with the blood supply. If there is a hyperfunction of the gland, there will be an increased uptake of the isotope (hot spot). Hypofunction demonstrates a lack of uptake (cold spot).

Small adrenal masses can be demonstrated better by nuclear medicine than by MRI. Uptake can be seen in a mass much earlier (meaning the mass is smaller).

RECAP

Anatomy, Physiology, and Function

- Pituitary gland
  - Located in the sella turcica
  - Actually two separate glands (anterior and posterior lobes)
  - It is the master gland
- Thyroid gland
  - Two lobes; one on each side of the neck below the larynx
  - Contains colloid which holds the hormone secreted by thyroid
- Parathyroid gland
  - Two on each side of the neck (four in total)
  - Regulates calcium and phosphorus content in blood and bones
- Adrenal glands
  - Aka suprarenal glands
  - Located on top of the kidneys
  - Secretes steroids, epinephrine (adrenaline); norepinephrine (noradrenaline); androgen; estrogen
- Pancreas
  - Described in Chapter 5
  - Secretes insulin and glucagon
- Gonads
  - Described in Chapter 7
  - Female: estrogen and progesterone
  - Male: testosterone
- Pineal gland
  - Located near the base of the brain
  - Secretes melatonin

Pathology

- Pituitary gland
  - Hyperpituitarism
    - Gigantism before puberty
    - Acromegaly after puberty
  - Hypopituitarism
    - Dwarfism before puberty
    - Simmonds syndrome (progeria)
  - Diabetes insipidus
- Thyroid gland

- Hyperthyroidism
  - Graves disease
  - Exophthalmos
- Hypothyroidism
  - Cretinism
  - Myxedema
- Goiter
- Thyroid adenoma
- Parathyroid gland
  - Primary hyperparathyroidism
  - Secondary hyperparathyroidism
- Adrenal glands
  - Cushing syndrome occurs from excessive production of glucocorticoids
  - Addison disease (adrenocortical insufficiency) occurs from too little production of adrenocortical hormones
  - Pheochromocytoma is a tumor of the adrenal medulla
  - Neuroblastoma is another tumor of the adrenal medulla (malignant)
- Pancreas
  - Diabetes mellitus disorder of carbohydrate metabolism
- Gonads
- Pineal gland

Special Imaging Modalities

- Ultrasound
  - Able to see cystic versus solid in masses
  - Adrenal gland can be a challenge
  - Thyroid gland may be seen
- CT
  - Very good for adrenal gland imaging
- MRI
  - Good for the adrenal gland
  - Can show diabetes insipidus because of a lack of signal
- Nuclear medicine
  - Excellent for checking the functioning of thyroid gland

CLINICAL AND RADIOGRAPHIC CHARACTERISTICS OF COMMON PATHOLOGIES

Pathologic Condition	Age (if known) Causal Factors	Manifestations	Radiographic Appearance
Hyperpituitarism	Children Adults Excess growth hormone	Gigantism Acromegaly	Delayed epiphyseal closing Thick skull diploe, enlarged mandible and hands
Hypopituitarism	Children Young adults Deficient growth hormone	Dwarfism Simmonds syndrome	Small skeletal features Early closure of epiphyseal plates
Hyperthyroidism	30–40 y, females Excess thyroid hormone	Graves disease, exophthalmos	Atrophy of shoulder muscles
Hypothyroidism	Children Adults	Cretinism Myxedema	Thick diploe of skull, underpneumatization of sinus and mastoids Soft-tissue swelling due to edema

Hyperparathyroidism
    Primary
 	
    Secondary
	Increased hormone
	
	Chronic renal failure
		Breakdown of bone, increased absorption of calcium
		Too complex for this text
			Pathologic fractures, rugger jersey spine, ground-glass appearance

Hypoparathyroidism	Surgical removal of all parathyroid glands	Low serum calcium, high serum phosphorus	
Cushing syndrome	Use of steroids	Moon face, hypertension, hirsutism	Diffuse osteoporosis pathologic fractures, renal calculi
Addison disease	Low adrenocortical hormone	Anemia, fatigue	
Diabetes mellitus	Faulty carbohydrate metabolism	Polyuria, increased thirst, appetite	Arteriosclerosis, osteomyelitis

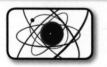

CRITICAL THINKING DISCUSSION QUESTIONS

1. Explain how exophthalmos is produced. What is it associated with?

2. Define acromegaly and how it occurs.

3. Why is it possible for spontaneous fractures to occur in persons with hyperparathyroidism?

4. Compare three manifestations that show the difference between hyperthyroidism and hypothyroidism.

5. Describe how diabetes mellitus is caused and what the early signs are that will alert a patient that something is wrong.

6. Describe the three manifestations of Graves disease.

7. Compare and contrast the conditions of infantile hypothyroidism and myxedema.

8. Describe three manifestations of Cushing syndrome.

9. Describe how "rugger jersey" spine occurs in patients with hyperparathyroidism.

10. Explain why sonography is not the modality of choice for many of the pathologic processes of the endocrine system.

Contrast Media and Their Use in Radiography

● Goals

1. To learn the types and characteristics of all contrast media

   OBJECTIVE: Differentiate between the different types of contrast media

   OBJECTIVE: List the characteristics of radiolucent and radiopaque contrast media

   OBJECTIVE: Explain the composition of positive contrast media

2. To explain the differences between ionic and nonionic contrast media

   OBJECTIVE: Describe the difference between ionic and nonionic contrast media

3. To recognize the uses and contraindications of contrast media and the treatment for reactions to the contrast

   OBJECTIVE: Explain how contrast media are chosen for a procedure

   OBJECTIVE: List the adverse reactions possible to contrast media and what treatment should be given

● Key Terms

Adverse reaction
Anaphylactic
High-osmolality contrast media (HOCM)
Hydrophilicity
Hyperosmolar
Hypertonic
Iso-osmolar
Low-osmolality contrast media (LOCM)
Miscibility
Osmolality
Persistence
Side effect
Tonicity
Toxicity
Viscosity

The basis of imaging the body's organs is the difference in density known as contrast. When two organs of the body are close in atomic number, the only way to demonstrate one is to change the density (atomic number) of one of them. Contrast media will change the difference of the densities by either adding to the atomic number of the tissue or by decreasing the atomic number and allowing the X-ray beam to pass through. When an organ is hollow, it is easy to add a contrast medium that will either attenuate or transmit the photon's energy. This will then create a density difference between the two organs, creating contrast. Regardless of the imaging modality, digital radiography or computed tomography (CT) or even nuclear medicine, these differences must exist to visualize the organs.

Classifications and Characteristics

Contrast media are classified as pharmaceuticals by the Federal Food and Drug Administration (FDA). There are three types of contrast materials: radiopaques, which have a higher density than the tissue and absorb radiation; radiolucents, which are of lower density than the surrounding tissue and therefore decrease density; and radionuclides, which emit radiation and are used in nuclear medicine.

Radiolucents are also called negative contrast media. By far, the cheapest contrast medium is air. In a number of applications such as double-contrast barium enemas and upper gastrointestinal (UGI) studies, especially through nasogastric tubes, air is the preferred medium. At times, excellent double-contrast esophageal images can be obtained when the patient swallows air together with the barium preparation. This is accomplished by having the patient drink barium through a large bore straw that has holes in the sides that help draw in air.

There were commercial preparations that had carbon dioxide added to the barium suspension. The patients were asked to drink the canned preparation as soon as it was opened so that the carbon dioxide was released in the esophagus and stomach. This was similar to drinking a bottle of soda. Effervescent granules are then used to induce air into the stomach during an UGI examination. The patient places the granules in the mouth and uses a small amount of water or barium to wash it down. The esophagus can be viewed immediately and the stomach will fill with gas shortly after. The main point is to make sure the patient does not "burp," which will release the gas.

Carbon dioxide has been used for double-contrast barium enemas because it is absorbed faster than air, and it is believed that its use results in greater patient comfort. The use of air or carbon dioxide probably does not influence the overall quality of the examination. Obviously, negative media such as air and carbon dioxide are not meant to be used for studies that involve vascular areas because of possible emboli.

Characteristics of negative contrast media are as follows:

1. Low atomic weight—therefore it will
2. Decrease the organ density—because it
3. Absorbs less radiation—which causes a
4. Greater image density
5. Radiolucent (can see through it)
6. Rapidly absorbed by the body

Radiopaques are also called positive contrast media. There are two categories of positive media: insoluble, of which barium is the only one, and soluble, which are all the others. Barium does not dissolve in water to any significant degree; it is merely suspended in solution. Mixing is necessary so that the barium crystals remain dispersed in water. If the container is allowed to stand, the barium crystals settle to the bottom. Therefore, it should be poured into individual cups for immediate use and not allowed to sit for any length of time.

Barium is termed "thick" and "thin" types. This refers to the viscosity of barium and does not infer any difference in radiodensity. "Thick" barium is a paste that is used for esophageal swallows, while the "thin" barium is the liquid form used for stomach and large and small bowel studies.

The soluble media contain iodine in some form. Iodine is used because it is readily available, has a nonmetallic atomic number, and is easily exchangeable with other ions. Water-soluble contrast media are **hypertonic**, causing water and electrolytes to be drawn into the bowel, creating dehydration. The high **tonicity** also causes dilution and reduces the degree of contrast.

Characteristics of positive contrast media are as follows:

1. High atomic weight—therefore they
2. Increase the organ density—because it
3. Absorbs more radiation—which causes
4. Decreased image density
5. Radiopaque (cannot see through it)
6. Readily excreted unchanged through the liver or kidneys (only water-soluble contrasts)
7. Relatively nontoxic

Composition

Differences in radiopaque contrast media can cause significant changes in radiodensity of tissue substance, which is related to the amount of iodine in the contrast medium. Two common iodinated substances are iothalamate and diatrizoate. Each of these contains methylglucamine (meglumine) salts or sodium salts or a combination of the two. Meglumine compounds are less toxic but are more viscous than sodium compounds. All positive contrast media are made up of a cation (a positive charge) and an anion (a negative charge). The cation is either the sodium or the meglumine compound. The anion is basically the same in all media, with the exception of one side chain, and determines the rest of the makeup of the contrast medium.

Nonionic versus Ionic Contrast Media

The chemical structures of nonionic and ionic contrast media differ significantly. A common error is made in thinking that nonionic means noniodinated, which is untrue. It must be remembered that both ionic and nonionic compounds contain iodine.

The early contrast mediums were salts of iodinated benzoic acid derivatives. These compounds became the mainstay of radiographic and CT imaging. Because they are salts, they consist of a positively charged cation and a negatively charged anion. Typically, they are organic acids with three hydrogen atoms replaced by iodine atoms and three hydrogen atoms replaced by simple side chains. These salts are strong acids and are completely dissociated (ionized) in solution. For every three iodine atoms in solution for contrast, two particles for osmolality exist—one anion and one cation. The cation most often used is sodium or a sodium and methylglucamine combination. Examples of these ionic monomers include diatrizoate sodium-meglumine (Renografin and Hypaque) and iothalamate sodium or meglumine (Conray). Figure 11-1 shows a triiodinated fully substituted benzene ring compound. Diatrizoate and iothalamate differ only in the composition of their side chains at the 3-carbon position (R). Either sodium or methylglucamine (meglumine) is attached to the carboxyl (COO⁻) group at the 1-carbon position.

The ratio between the number of iodine atoms present and the number of particles in solution are the

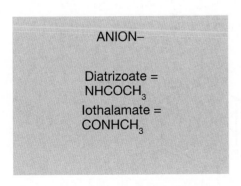

FIGURE 11-1 Diatrizoate and iothalamate differ in the composition of their side chain.

osmolality and ionicity of contrast mediums. Both of these have a bearing on the toxicity of the media. The cation was eliminated from the ionic media because cations contain no iodine and give no diagnostic information. However, it was responsible for as much as 50% of the osmotic effect of a medium, which increases the risk for adverse reactions. The ionizing carboxyl group (COO⁻) of contrasts with higher osmolality is replaced with a nondissociating group such as amide or glucose. The molecules contained in nonionic contrast media do not dissociate. When mixed with water, a nonionic compound forms a molecular (nonionizing) solution. Each dissolved molecule contains three iodine atoms and only one particle in solution, a ratio of 3:1. Figures 11-2 and 11-3 show nonionic monomeric configurations such as iopamidol or iohexol. There are five hydroxyl (OH) groups found in iopamidol and there are six in iohexol. Since the carboxyl groups have been eliminated and hydroxyl groups have been added, these are low in osmolality. Finally, in Figure 11-4, an ionic dimer, Hexabrix, is shown. This compound contains six iodine atoms but

it dissociates in solution into an anion and cation. Sodium and meglumine are attached to the carboxyl (COO⁻) group. Because Hexabrix contains six iodine atoms and two ionized particles, it still retains the 3:1 ratio of the contrasts with lower osmolality.

The development of radiopaque, iodinated intravascular contrast media of **lower osmolality (low-osmolality contrast media, LOCM)**, both ionic and nonionic nature, has made better and safer contrast media available. These contrasts have an osmolality that is closer to human plasma and thus are less likely to cause an adverse reaction. A great deal of research into the chemistry and molecular structure, toxicity, and solubility of contrast materials has resulted in the development of iodinated compounds that can be safely used in intravascular diagnostic radiology. The express purpose of these media is to provide contrast enhancement and improved diagnostic images. The molecule of contrast media are classified according to two characteristics: (1) ionic versus nonionic; and (2) monomer versus dimer. These can then be put together as ionic monomers, ionic mono-acid dimers,

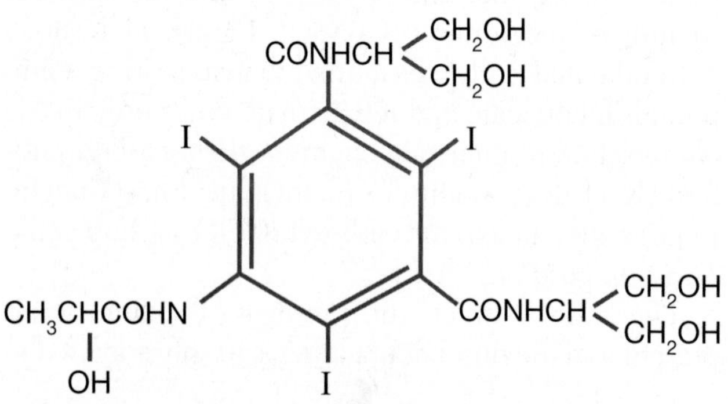

FIGURE 11-2   Iopamidol with five hydroxyl groups.

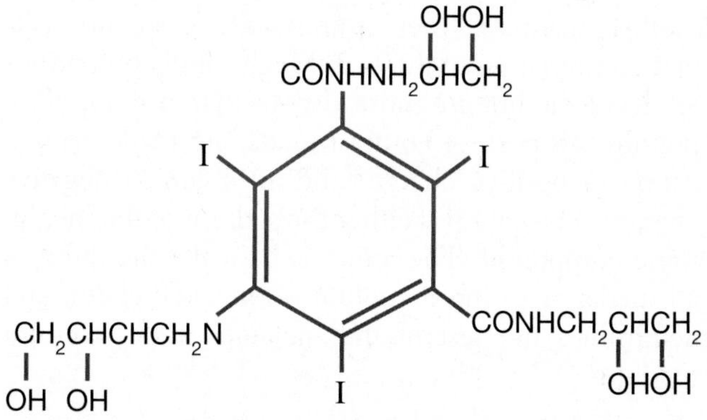

FIGURE 11-3   Iohexol contains six hydroxyl groups.

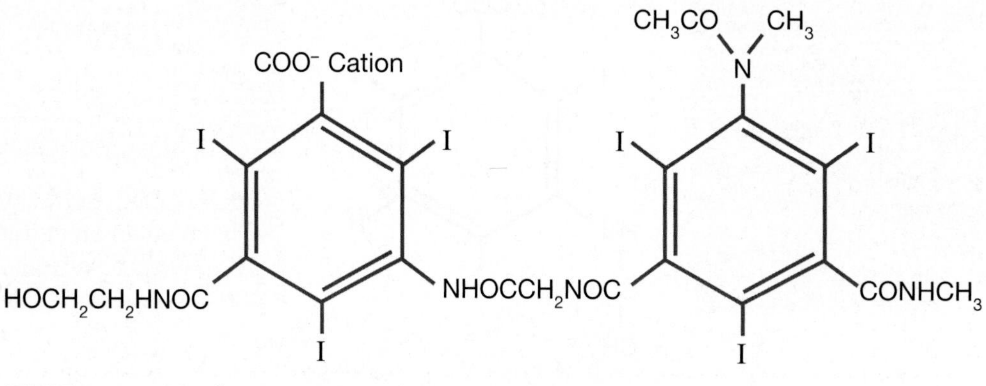

FIGURE 11-4   Hexabrix is a nonionic dimer with six iodine atoms.

nonionic monomers, and nonionic dimers. Examples of an ionic monomer include iohexol (Omnipaque), iopamidol (Isovue), and others. Ioxaglate meglumine and ioxaglate sodium (Hexabrix) are ionic dimers. These compounds provide the same ratio of atoms to ionized particles as do LOCMs. The lower **osmolality**, reduced toxicity, and high interaction with water (**hydrophilicity**) of the LOCM offer an increased safety factor for patients, especially those with known risk factors. Unfortunately, the cost of LOCM is higher, which may prevent its use on all patients.

Osmolality of a contrast medium is a significant factor to consider when adverse reactions may cause severe complications. Conventional ionic media are significantly hyperosmotic to body fluids such as blood because they dissociate into separate ions in solution. This can cause adverse effects, such as cardiac problems, vein cramping and pain, and abnormal fluid retention. Nonionic contrast media have an osmolality that is significantly closer to human plasma than a corresponding ionic medium at a similar iodine concentration because of the 3:1 ratio explained earlier. Nonionic monomeric compounds are 1 to 3 times the osmolality of human serum. Nonionic dimeric compounds can approach a hypoosmolar or iso-osmolar state with human serum and still remain viscous with high iodine concentrations. Contrast media that have less osmolality than body fluid will result in fewer and less severe side effects. Thus, nonionic contrast media are advantageous in this respect; however, there is no appreciable difference in image quality with nonionic media.

Display 11-1 compares the iodine concentration and the osmolality of the various types of contrasts media.

DISPLAY 11-1 IODINE CONCENTRATION AND OSMOLALITY FOR HOCM AND LOCM

Substance	Ionic/Nonionic	Iodine Concentration % (mg/mL)	Osmolality
Human Plasma		—	300
Intravascular Contrast Media			
Isovue	Nonionic	20% (200 mg/mL) 25% (250 mg/mL) 30% (300 mg/mL) 37% (370 mg/mL)	413 524 616 796
Omnipaque	Nonionic	14% (140 mg/mL) 18% (180 mg/mL) 24% (240 mg/mL) 30% (300 mg/mL) 35% (350 mg/mL)	322 408 520 672 844
Optiray	Nonionic	16% (160 mg/mL) 24% (240 mg/mL) 30% (300 mg/mL) 32% (320 mg/mL) 35% (350 mg/mL)	355 502 651 702 792
Oxilan	Nonionic	30% (300 mg/mL) 35% (350 mg/mL)	585 695
Ultravist	Nonionic	15% (150 mg/mL) 24% (240 mg/mL) 30% (300 mg/mL) 37% (377 mg/mL)	328 483 607 774
Visipaque	Nonionic	27% (270 mg/mL) 32% (320 mg/mL)	290 290

(continued)

DISPLAY 11-1 IODINE CONCENTRATION AND OSMOLALITY FOR HOCM AND LOCM (continued)

Substance	Ionic/Nonionic	Iodine Concentration % (mg/mL)	Osmolality
Conray	Ionic (Meglumine) Meglumine Meglumine Sodium	14.1% (141 mg/mL) 20.2% (202 mg/mL) 28.2% (282 mg/mL) 40% (400 mg/mL)	600 1,000 1,400 2,300
Hexabrix	Ionic (Meglumine sodium)	32% (320 mg/mL)	600
Hypaque	Ionic (Meglumine)	28.2% (282 mg/mL) 30% (300 mg/mL) 37% (370 mg/mL)	1,415 1,515 2,016
Reno— Renografin	Ionic (Meglumine) Meglumine Meglumine sodium Meglumine sodium	14.1% (141 mg/mL) 28.2% (282 mg/mL) 29.25% (2,925 mg/mL) 37% (370 mg/mL)	607 1,404 1,450 1,870
Gastrointestinal			
Gastrografin	Ionic	37% (370 mg/mL)	1,940
Gastroview	Ionic	37% (370 mg/mL)	2,000
Urography			
Hypaque—Cysto	Ionic (Meglumine)	14.1% (141 mg/mL)	633
Cysto—Conray	Ionic (Meglumine)	8.1% (81 mg/mL)	Instill for retrograde cystography and cystourethrography
Conray	Ionic (Meglumine)	20.2% (202 mg/mL)	1,000

Selection of Contrast Media

When choosing a contrast medium, there are certain characteristics to look for.

1. **Viscosity**: The resistance of fluid to movement (how thick it is) is known as viscosity and depends on molecular size and concentration, as well as the friction of the component molecules in solution. In general, viscosity varies proportionately with the concentration of iodine. As iodine content rises, so does viscosity. The viscosity is largely controlled by the composition of the side chain of the molecule.

Molecular structure and concentration affect the viscosity so the different compounds must be looked at to determine the usage of various contrast media. Meglumine compounds are more viscous than are sodium salt compounds. The more viscous a material is, the harder the injection is to give. There are several methods to reduce the difficulty of the injection. The contrast medium can be heated to reduce the viscosity; a needle with a larger bore or a catheter with a larger diameter can be used; the injection can be made under pressure; the injection can be delivered over a longer period of time.

2. **Type of ionic salt**: The two ionic salts most commonly used in ionic contrast media are sodium and meglumine. Each is associated with

characteristics that can influence properties of the compound. Sodium salts permit high iodine concentrations without high viscosity and are recommended for urography. Contrast media that contain a greater amount of meglumine salt deliver a smaller amount of iodine per second to the patient because of the increased weight of the meglumine ion. To illustrate this concept, compare Hypaque 50% and Conray 60%. Hypaque contains 100% sodium salt and Conray contains 100% meglumine salt, yet the iodine content of Hypaque is 300 mg/mL as compared with 282 mg/mL found in Conray. Contrast media containing meglumine salts are used in procedures such as peripheral arteriography.

3. **Iodine content**: It is the volume distribution of iodine in the contrast medium that provides the contrast enhancement for imaging. The more iodine content there is in the contrast media, the more attenuation of the radiographic beam. Contrast media may have a high, moderate, or low iodine concentration; however, 300 mg of iodine is needed to produce adequate opacity on radiographic images. For example, Reno 60% contains 292 mg of iodine and is acceptable for the renal system. However, for visualization of the blood vessels, Renographin 76%, which contains 370 mg of iodine, is needed. Higher concentrations of iodine are necessary to overcome dilution and the speed with which the contrast medium travels in blood.

4. **Miscibility**: The ability of the medium to mix with other fluids is called miscibility. Oily contrast media have either a very low or a zero miscibility factor, whereas water-soluble media have a very high factor. Media with a high miscibility factor have less of a chance of causing emboli; however, these contrasts become diluted with the fluids into which they are injected.

5. **Persistence**: Persistence refers to the amount of time the contrast medium stays in the body. This is known as the clearance rate. Once a contrast is injected, it is processed rapidly and distributed throughout the body. Positive contrast media are not metabolized and are excreted completely through the kidneys in less than 2 hours. Usually, within 45 minutes, the half-life has been reached, meaning that

one-half the dose of the contrast has been eliminated. Negative contrast media are rapidly absorbed, so the images have to be taken relatively quickly and certainly with accuracy, as a second chance to get an image may have passed.

6. **Toxicity**: An obvious consideration in the selection of a contrast medium is whether the compound is lethal when injected. Methylglucamine salt compounds are less toxic than sodium salts. The more meglumine salt, the lower the iodine content that is actually delivered to the body. Because the meglumine salt ion weighs more, the iodine delivered per second is less. However, if a contrast medium with a high iodine concentration delivery is needed, thereby causing the choice of sodium over meglumine, calcium and magnesium can be added to reduce the toxicity of the sodium salt media.

7. **Osmolality**: The osmolality is a measure of the number of dissolved particles, whether ions, molecules, or compounds, in a solution. Solutions may be **hyperosmolar** or **iso-osmolar**. The closer the osmolality of a contrast medium is to the osmolality of the body fluids, the less potential there is for adverse reactions caused by differences in osmolality. Hyperosmolar compounds cause more direct endothelial damage. The media with high osmolality may cause more abrupt or severe hemodynamic changes, such as decreased cardiac output, changes in pulmonary artery pressure, and changes in heart rate. All contrast media have a greater osmolality than body fluids, but they differ in the degree of their hyperosmolality. Contrasts today are classified as either **high-osmolality contrast media (HOCM)** or low-osmolality contrast media (LOCM). Contrasts that are classified as HOCM may be as high as seven times the osmolality of blood, whereas those contrasts that are considered to be LOCM can have lower osmolality than blood. Visipaque 270 and Visipaque 320 are two such media with an osmolality of 290.

Of course, the ultimate choice is left up to the radiologists, but the imaging technologist needs to be aware of why certain media are used to help educate patients to alleviate concerns about reactions.

Complications of Barium

Barium sulfate is poorly soluble in water and therefore is highly constipating. Patients must be educated to increase their fluid intake after undergoing any procedure that involves barium. Aspiration of small amounts of barium is of little significance as the barium clears the major bronchi and trachea within hours, leaving little or no residual findings. Aspiration of large amounts can result in pneumonia or even significant compromise of pulmonary function.

Extraperitoneal perforation allows the spill of barium into the mediastinum, causing an immediate inflammatory reaction followed by fibrosis. The barium will persist in the mediastinum for a period of time. Perforation occurs in the rectum as well, which will again lead to inflammation and fibrosis. However, if there is escape of bacteria along with the barium, peritonitis is possible. Sepsis and shock are likely within hours and death can occur if the condition is not treated immediately with antibiotic therapy and large volumes of intravenous fluids. If perforation is suspected, barium should not be used for the study. A water soluble iodinated contrast should be used instead that will be absorbed by the body without harm.

Adverse Reactions of Iodinated Contrast Media

The number of mild and moderate reactions related to the administration of contrast media has decreased dramatically in the recent years as the use of HOCM changes over to LOCM. Even though those have decreased, the numbers of severe and life-threatening reactions still occur without any predictability. Because of this, the technologist must be adequately trained and vigilant in patient care after contrast is administered. It is now within the scope of the technologist to administer drugs (contrast media); however, unless the technologist is properly schooled in pharmacology and venipuncture, it is best to allow a radiologist or radiology nurse to inject contrast media and other drugs. Many facilities provide training to technologists to prepare them to perform venipuncture. The ASRT curriculum requires radiography programs to teach pharmacology. The different states have different requirements regarding venipuncture, so all technologists need to determine the requirements in the state where they will be employed.

Contrast media are not always accepted into the body without any physical or functional changes because of the molecular structure of the compound used. When the body reacts to contrast in a manner that is of little or no consequence, the patient is experiencing a **side effect**. Side effects are common and can be expected to happen in the majority of the patients. These include a metallic taste and a feeling of warmth. Both of these effects usually last only a few moments. It is possible that these mild effects advance to nausea and vomiting, both of which again last for about 5 minutes. Patients should be told that these effects might occur so that they do not panic and will know what to expect.

The body's reactions that are more toxic are considered **adverse reactions**. Adverse reactions are also known as idiosyncratic reactions. Depending on the osmolality of the contrast, there may be a reaction or one of little consequence. There are essentially three different types of reactions to contrast media. The American College of Radiology (ACR) has classified these three categories of adverse reactions as mild, moderate, and severe.

Mild Reactions

The majority of adverse reactions are mild and non-life-threatening. These reactions include nausea and vomiting and urticaria. Dermal reactions are usually the least significant of adverse effects associated with contrast media and may not require treatment. Although most dermal reactions are self-limiting and probably do not need treatment, antihistamines are chosen if treatment is indicated. Drowsiness is a frequent side effect of the drug. If urticarial (hives) is severe, an antihistamine is probably not adequate. In that event, subcutaneous administration of epinephrine is the recommended treatment. Feelings of warmth and flushing are of short duration. These reactions increase in incidence with increasing osmolality. Mild reactions require only observation, reassurance, and support, but because they may evolve into a more severe reaction, the patient should be observed for a minimum of 20 minutes to ensure clinical stability. If the reaction is serious enough to require epinephrine, an intravenous line to manage possible further complications is advisable. As stated earlier, most minor reactions do not require treatment. Usually, reassurance by the technologist is all that is needed. It is important, however, to recognize that a minor reaction may be followed by a more severe one. Pain at the injection site is usually a function of hypertonicity. With the use of LOCM, these symptoms have been decreased and with the use of iso-osmolar contrasts, pain has virtually been eliminated.

Moderate Reactions

These reactions are not immediately life-threatening but often require treatment. Certainly, these reactions must be monitored as the reaction may progress to a more severe state. The symptoms include the symptoms of mild reactions, namely nausea, possible vomiting and urticaria. Additionally, mild bronchospasm, tachycardia, and mild hypotension will also be experienced by most patients experiencing moderate reactions. These symptoms may be treated using diphenhydramine for the hives, an inhaler for the bronchospasm, and elevation of the legs with fluid therapy for hypotension. Establishing an intravenous line for possible future medications is advisable as well as preparing to administer oxygen. Vital signs should be obtained in the first stages of moderate reactions and then be monitored throughout the patient's stay in the imaging department.

Severe Reactions

Severe adverse reactions are potentially life-threatening within a short time frame. They rarely occur but it is essential for all technologists who administer contrast media to understand how unpredictable these reactions are and that they require immediate recognition and treatment. Symptoms start with anxiety and respiratory difficulty related to bronchospasm, laryngospasm, and angioedema of the upper airway. Severe hypotension and pulmonary edema may also occur, particularly if the patient is already suffering from congestive heart failure. This will lead to sudden cardiac arrest.

Cardiac and pulmonary arrest requires cardiopulmonary resuscitation (CPR) and advanced life-support equipment. It is of utmost importance that the technologist be well versed with current CPR training and techniques for life support. Current (2011) CPR techniques require that the compressions now be done before opening the airway. Drug intervention

depends almost exclusively on whether the patient has bradycardia or tachycardia. Tachycardia represents an **anaphylactic** reaction. Peripheral vasodilation and increased capillary permeability result in diminished circulating blood volume, falling blood pressure, and rising heart rate.

Vasomotor Reaction

There is a fourth reaction to contrast administration known as vasomotor reaction. This is not a true reaction to contrast media but is rather caused by fear of the examination itself. Manifestations include pallor, cold sweats, rapid pulse, and near syncope. Bradycardia and hypotension together are true indicators of a vasomotor reaction. The patient should be placed in the Trendelenburg position, and, if warranted, an intravenous line should be started for infusion with isotonic fluids. If the treatment is inadequate, then intravenous atropine can increase the heart rate.

Risk Factors Contributing to Reactions

Before the injection of contrast material into a patient, the technologist must always question the patient about the presence of an allergic history, since it has been noted that an instance of adverse reaction is more likely to occur in a patient who has an allergic history. A negative history does not guarantee that the patient will be reaction-free. Any patient who reports an allergy to a food or a contrast should be questioned further to clarify the type and severity of the allergy or the reaction. It is important to note that patients that have an allergy to shellfish or seafood are at no greater risk for a contrast reaction than patients who have any other food allergy. In the past, a seafood allergy had raised concerns. This has since been proven to be unfounded. A history of asthma may indicate an increased likelihood of a contrast reaction. There is a reported risk of 5 to 8 times greater of a reaction as compared to patients that do not suffer with asthma. Patients with renal insufficiency or significant cardiac disease may be at increased risk and therefore, the volume and the osmolality of the contrast media must be carefully determined before any is given to such a patient. Patients that have had a previous contrast reaction may or may not experience one during the current procedure; however, repeated exposure to contrast may lead to more serious reactions.

The dose, route, and rate of delivery of the contrast media and how these are related to adverse reactions are not fully understood. Although a test dose is recommended for medicolegal purposes, studies have shown that a test dose does not decrease the incidence of severe reactions. Any intravascular injection of contrast media may cause an adverse reaction, whether mild or life-threatening.

Incidence of Adverse Reactions

The number of actual adverse reactions to intravenous contrast media is not easily determined because similar symptoms may be due to other medications that are being taken at the same time as the administration of contrast. Most adverse reactions are mild and do not require treatment, thereby not being reported. Adverse reactions have occurred in 5% to 15% of all patients who receive HOCM. Most of the patients experience warmth or heat upon introduction of the contrast. When using LOCM, the reported incidences of adverse reactions range from 0.2% to 0.7%.

Severe contrast reactions are rare and have occurred in 0.2% when HOCM is used, and with the use of LOCM the rate drops to 0.002%. The rate of fatalities is not known. There is a conservative estimate of 1 fatality per 170,000 contrast administrations. Low fatality rates are most likely a reflection of improvements in the treatment of reactions and the use of LOCM.

During any injection of a contrast medium, the patient should be monitored closely for abnormal response or reaction, and emergency drugs, equipment, and medical personnel should be immediately available. The technologist must be watchful for extravasation of the medium into the arm. If this occurs, the application of a warm wet cloth will help reduce the pain.

Delayed Reactions to Contrast Media

While most reactions will occur within 5 minutes after injection of the contrast medium, some reactions can occur much later, even after the patient has left the imaging department. The incidence of delayed adverse reactions range from 0.5% to 9% with those reactions starting from 3 hours to 7 days following the administration of a contrast medium. Delayed reactions are unusual in that there is a high rate of recurrence. Any reaction or side effect to contrast injection must be documented appropriately according to the facilities protocols. The very minimum that must be documented includes the dose and type of contrast that was injected, any signs and symptoms that the patient exhibited, any treatment and medications that were given to the patient to counteract the reaction, and the patient's response to the treatment.

RECAP

Classifications and Characteristics

- Radiolucents (negative)
  - Decrease density
  - Transmit energy of the X-ray beam
  - May cause an emboli if injected into the blood stream
- Radiopaque
  - Insoluble
    - Barium
  - Water soluble
    - Iodinated contrast
      - Ionic and nonionic
  - Composition
    - Anion (positive charge)

- Cation (salts) (negative charge)
  - Iothalamate or diatrizoate salts
    - Each of these contain methylglucamine (meglumine) or sodium salts
    - Meglumine is less toxic, more viscous

Nonionic versus Ionic Contrast

- Both contain three particles of iodine, but the nonionic had the cation removed and replaced with a hydroxyl group
- It is the iodine that causes the contrast difference. There is no difference in the image, only in the reactions that might happen to the patient

- Lower-osmolality contrast media (LOCM) offers lower osmolality, reduced toxicity, and increased safety for those patients with known risk factors to contrast
  - These contrasts have osmolality closer to the human plasma and result in fewer and less severe side effects
- High-osmolality contrast media (HOCM) contain the cations (salts) that are known to cause 50% of the adverse reactions from contrast use
  - Osmolality is much higher than human plasma

Selection of Contrast Media

- Viscosity: resistance of fluid to movement
- Type of ionic salt
  - Sodium permits higher iodine concentrations without high viscosity
  - Meglumine delivers smaller amount of iodine to patient because of the weight of the atom
- Iodine content: the more the iodine, the greater the attenuation of the beam
  - May have a high, moderate, or low iodine concentration
  - Need a minimum of 300 mg of iodine to produce adequate opacity on images
  - Higher concentrations of iodine are needed to overcome the dilution of the blood and the speed with which the contrast travels in the blood stream
- Miscibility: ability of the contrast to mix with other fluids
- Persistence: amount of time the contrast medium stays in the body
- Toxicity: how lethal is the contrast?
  - Meglumine salts are less toxic than sodium salts
  - If sodium in needed, then magnesium and calcium can be added as buffers
- Osmolality: the number of dissolved particles in solution
  - Solutions may be hyperosmolar or iso-osmolar
  - The closer to the osmolality of the body fluid, the less potential for adverse reactions

Reactions and Treatments

- Complications resulting from the use of barium
  - Aspiration
  - Constipation
  - Fibrosis
  - Peritonitis

- Three classifications accepted by the ACR for iodinated contrast
  - Mild reactions
    - The majority of reactions are mild. These are non-life-threatening
    - They include nausea, vomiting, and urticaria
    - Warmth feeling, flushing of face are normal and of short duration
    - Reassurance by the technologist may be all that is necessary
    - Usually self-limiting but may need an antihistamine
    - If urticaria is severe, subcutaneous epinephrine is recommended
    - Pain at the injection site is caused by hypertonicity of the contrast and is not usually present with the use of LOCM
  - Moderate reactions
    - Not immediately life-threatening but often require treatment
    - Symptoms include the mild one plus bronchospasm, tachycardia, and mild hypotension
    - Intravenous line is established in case further action is necessary if reaction progresses
    - Legs are elevated for hypotension, bronchodilator is given, and oxygen should be ready in case of need
  - Severe reactions
    - Rarely occur but are potentially life-threatening and occurring very quickly
    - Symptoms start with anxiety due to inability to breathe; there is laryngospasm and angioedema of the upper airway
    - Patient may suffer cardiac arrest if they already have congestive heart failure
    - CPR is usually necessary
    - Drug intervention depends on if the patient is in tachycardia or bradycardia; tachycardia represents true anaphylactic reaction
  - Vasomotor reaction
    - Not a true reaction but caused by fear
    - Symptoms include pallor, cold sweats, rapid pulse, and near syncope
    - Bradycardia and hypotension are indicators of vasovagal reaction
    - Place patient in the Trendelenburg position
    - Atropine may be needed to increase heart rate
- Risk factors
  - Allergic history must be taken, but a positive history is not a indication that another reaction will occur

- ○ History of asthma may indicate an increased likelihood of a reaction
- ○ History of renal insufficiency or cardiac disease may be an indication of an adverse reaction
- Incidence rates
  - ○ Most reactions are mild and therefore, not reported
  - ○ There may be delayed reactions that are also not reported; delayed reactions can occur from 3 hours to 7 days following administration
  - ○ There are 5% to 15% of reported reactions to HOCM
  - ○ There are 0.2% to 0.7% of reported reactions to LOCM
  - ○ Severe reactions occur in 0.2% when using HOCM, and occur in 0.002% when using LOCM
  - ○ 1 fatality per 170,000 contrast administrations

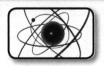 **CRITICAL THINKING DISCUSSION QUESTIONS**

1. Explain the composition difference between nonionic contrast and ionic contrast media.

2. How does the composition of nonionic contrast media affect the reactions to the medium a patient may experience?

3. Explain why water-soluble compounds would be used to examine the gastrointestinal tract. What side effects might these produce?

4. Describe the composition of positive contrast media.

5. Why is it important to watch a patient for 20 minutes after a contrast administration?

6. Why should someone who has asthma be watched more closely for an adverse reaction than someone who does not have asthma?

7. Why does contrast media affect kidney function?

8. Why is an allergy to shellfish food not a reliable indicator that the patient will have an adverse reaction to contrast media?

9. Explain the three reasons that iodine is used in soluble contrast media.

Glossary

Abscess. Localized collection of pus and necrotic tissue

Achalasia. Failure to relax such as sphincters that open into other organs (cardia, sphincter of Oddi)

Achondroplasia. Congenital abnormal conversion of cartilage into bone

Acoustic neuromas. A benign tumor arising from the cells of the auditory nerve symptoms include dizziness and unsteady gait

Acromegaly. Hypersecretion of the growth hormone after adulthood and results in abnormal enlargement of the extremities

Addison disease (adrenocortical insufficiency). Uncommon condition characterized by insufficient production of adrenocortical hormones

Adenocarcinoma. A malignant tumor that originates in glandular epithelium

Adenomyosis. Benign ingrowth of the endometrium into the uterine musculature

Adverse reaction. Undesirable reaction to contrast media that may be harmful to the patient

Aganglionic megacolon. Aka Hirschsprung disease; pertains to a colon that has a congenital absence of ganglions that cause loss of peristalsis, as a result, the colon enlarges (mega)

Alcoholic liver disease (alcoholic hepatitis; alcoholic cirrhosis). A set of diseases that are caused by the abuse of alcohol

Altered tissue growth. Also known as growth disturbance, it is a departure from normal tissue growth caused by multiplication of cells

Alveoli. Plural of alveolus; when pertaining to the pulmonary system, the alveolus is a thin-walled, saclike terminal dilation of the respiratory bronchiole

Ampiarthrodial. Cartilaginous joints that are slightly moveable

Anaphylactic. Manifesting extremely great sensitivity to foreign material

Anastomosis. A natural communication between two tubular structures created either surgically or through disease

Anencephalus. A fetus lacking all or most of the brain

Aneurysm. Dilation of an artery due to an acquired or congenital weakness of the wall

Ankylosing spondylitis. Arthritis of the spine that resembles rheumatoid arthritis; characterized by stiffness

Anoxia. Absence or almost complete absence of oxygen

Aphasia. Impaired or absent ability to communicate due to an injury in the brain

Appendicular. Classification of the skeleton relating to the limbs, shoulder girdle, and pelvic girdle

Arnold-Chiari. Deformity of the posterior cranial fossa structures, it is associated with spina bifida

Arteriosclerosis. Hardening of the arteries due to calcium deposits and plaque buildup

Arthritis. Inflammation of a joint

Ascites. Accumulation of serous fluid in the peritoneal cavity; it is a complication of cirrhosis, congestive heart failure, malignancy, or peritonitis; ascites presents problems with technical factors

Asthma. Inflammatory disease of the lungs which is usually reversible; the airway is narrowed causing difficulty in breathing

Astrocytoma. Glioma that arises from different parts of the brain depending on the age of the patient and accounts for about 3% of all intracranial neoplasms

Atelectasis. Reduction or absence of air in a part of the lung or in the entire lung

Atherosclerosis. Irregularly distributed lipid deposits in the lumen of arteries

Atresia. Congenital absence of an opening or an open lumen

Atrophy. A wasting away of tissue, organs, or the entire body

Axial. Classification of the skeleton relating to the vertebral column and head

Bacteriuria. The presence of bacteria in urine

Barrett esophagus. Chronic peptic ulceration of the lower esophagus resulting from chronic esophagitis

Benign neoplasm. Noncancerous tumor

Bezoar. A ball of matter located in the alimentary canal; it is classified by the type of material that forms the ball. phytobezoar is a food ball; trichobezoar is a hairball; trichophytobezoar is a hair and vegetable fiber mixed ball

Bifid system. Two of any part of the urinary system; it can include a double renal pelvis and/or ureter

Bile. Fluid secreted by the liver and discharged into the duodenum to aid in the emulsification of fats; increases peristalsis and retard putrefaction

Bone cyst. A wall of fibrous tissue filled with clear fluid that develops beneath the epiphyseal plate

Bronchiectasis. Chronic dilatation of the bronchi or bronchioles caused by inflammation or an obstruction

Bronchitis. Acute inflammation of the mucous membrane of the bronchial tubes

Bronchogenic carcinoma. Squamous cell or oat cell cancer that comes from the mucosa of the large bronchi; it may cause a bronchial obstruction

Bursitis. Inflammation of a bursa

Cancellous. Spongy bone located beneath the compact bone

Cardiac dilation. References to any enlargement to the ventricles or atria of the heart

Cardiac heterotaxia. The heart is a mirror image of a normal heart, with the chambers and great vessels being reversed

Cardiomegaly. Enlargement of the heart as a whole, not just a ventricle and/or atrium

Cardiovascular disease. A broad term to describe any disease process of the heart and/or the blood vessels or the circulation

Cauda equina. The bundle of spinal nerves arising from the lumbar sacral region

Cerebral hemorrhage. Hemorrhage into the substance of the cerebrum

Cerebrovascular accidents. A term that is used for cerebral stroke, however, the term is imprecise

Chocolate cysts. Cysts that are composed of old endometrial tissue that is found outside of the uterus with endometriosis

Cholangitis. Inflammation of the bile ducts or of the entire biliary tree

Cholecystitis. Inflammation of the gall bladder

Cholecystokinin (CCK). A hormone released by the upper intestinal mucosa that stimulates contraction of the gallbladder and release of pancreatic enzymes

Cholelithiasis. Presence of gall stones in the gall bladder or in the bile ducts

Chondroma. Benign neoplasm that forms cartilage

Chordoma. A rare neoplasm of the skeletal tissue in adults

Chronic obstructive pulmonary disease (COPD). Group of pathologies that obstruct the airway making it increasingly difficult to breath; usually comprised of chronic bronchitis and/or emphysema

Chyme. Semifluid, partially digested food that is passed from the stomach into the duodenum

Cirrhosis. Liver disease characterized by diffuse damage to the liver parenchyma

Coarctation. A constriction or stenosis in particular relating to the aorta

Concussion. An injury of the soft tissue of the brain as a result of violent shaking or blow with partial or complete loss of function

Congenital dislocated hip. Developmental abnormality in which a neonate's hips easily become dislocated

Congenital. Existing at birth

Congestion. Increase blood supply at the site of injury caused by vasodilation

Congestive heart failure. Failure of the heart to supply adequate amount of blood to maintain circulation

Contusion. An injury as a result of a blow that causes bleeding beneath the unbroken skin

Corpus luteum. A yellow endocrine body formed in the ovary at the site of a ruptured ovarian follicle

Cortical. Compact bone

Craniopharyngioma. Neoplasm that arises in the sella turcia area of the brain

Cretinism. Obsolete term for congenital hypothyroidism; now known as infantile hypothyroidism

Crohn disease. Aka regional enteritis

Croup. Bronchitis of the larynx and trachea in infants and toddlers that is caused by the parainfluenza virus

Cryptorchidism. Failure of one or both testes to descend into the scrotum

Cushing syndrome. Adrenal hyperplasia caused by ACTH secreting adenoma of the pituitary

Cystic fibrosis. A congenital metabolic disorder that affects the pancreas causing mucus obstruction of the bile ducts and bronchi

Degeneration. Deterioration

Delayed union. When bone fragments do not heal in the normal time frame

Dermoid. *See* teratoma

Dextrocardia (Dextroposition). Displacement of the heart to the right side of the body

Diabetes insipidus. A rare type of diabetes caused by the kidneys' failure to reabsorb water due to deficient antidiuretic hormone

Diabetes mellitus. Results from a disorder of carbohydrate metabolism; the cause is believed to be failure of the pancreas to secrete adequate insulin

Diagnosis. The determination of the nature of a disease

Diarthrodial. Freely moveable joints

Differentiation. The possession of one or more characteristics or functions different from that of the original type of tissue

Disease. Any abnormal change of the function or structure within the body

Dislocation. Displacement of any organ or body part

Displacement. Any organ or body part that is not in the normal location

Distraction. Pulling apart of bone fragments to realign proximity to each other

Diverticula. This is the plural of diverticulum; diverticula are herniation of mucosa and submucosa of the major muscle layers of the colon

Dysmenorrhea. Difficult and painful menstruation

Dyspnea. Shortness of breath; difficulty breathing and is usually associated with diseases of the heart or lungs

Dysuria. Difficulty in pain or urination

Embolus. A mass occluding a vessel usually thought of as a blood clot

Emphysema. An increase in the size of the alveoli through trapped air causing destructive changes in the walls and reduction of the number of the alveoli

Encephalitis. Inflammation of the brain parenchyma

Enchondroma. Benign cartilaginous neoplasm located in the medullary cavity

Endocarditis. Inflammation of the endocardium (lining of the heart)

Endogenous. Infection caused by an agent already present in the body

Endometriosis. Tissue that resembles the endometrial lining of the uterus that is located in abnormal locations within the pelvic cavity

Endosteum. A layer of cells on the inner surface of the medullary cavity

Enzymatic necrosis. Death of one or more cells due to the release of enzymes

Epididymitis. Inflammation of the epididymis

Epidural abscess. Abscess that occurs on or outside the dura mater

Epidural hemorrhage. A bleed located in the space above the dura mater

Etiology. The science and study of the causes of disease

Exogenous. Originating or produced outside the organism

Exophthalmos. Protrusion of the eyes caused by edema associated with hyperthyroidism

Exostosis. Cartilage-capped bone neoplasm

External hydrocephaly. Hydrocephalus that occurs from faulty reabsorption of the cerebrospinal fluid

Extracorporeal shock wave lithotripsy. Focused shock waves to disintegrate renal stones

Extradural hematoma. An accumulation of blood between the skull and the dura mater

Exudate. Thick cloudy fluid full of live and dead protein

Fatty liver. Fatty degeneration of the liver cells thus causing a yellow discoloration

Fibroadenoma. Benign neoplasm commonly found in the breast

Fibroid. Old term for leiomyoma occurring in the uterus; it is a mass composed of fibrous tissue

Fibrous dysplasia. Areas of bone undergoing lysis being replaced with abnormal fibrous tissue

Fistula. An abnormal passage from one surface of epithelium area to another; it can be either congenital or acquired

Fracture. Discontinuity of bone structure

Frequency. Rate of occurrence of a pathologic process

Functional disease. Disease that alters function of the organ

Gastritis. Inflammation of the mucosa of the stomach

Gastroesophageal reflux disease (GERD). A syndrome of chronic epigastric pain due to reflux of acid gastric juice into the lower esophageal sphincter; it may lead to Barrett esophagus

Germinoma. Neoplasm that arises from the gonads or the pineal region of the brain

Giant cell tumor. Osteolytic tumor composed of multinucleated giant cells that are sometimes malignant

Glioblastoma multiforme. A rapidly growing, invasive malignant neoplasm of the cerebrum

Glioma. Benign neoplasm derived from various types of cells that form the interstitial tissue of the brain or spinal cord

Glomerulonephritis (Bright disease). Renal disease characterized by inflammatory changes in the glomeruli, which are not the result of an infection

Goiter. Enlargement of the thyroid gland causing a swelling in the front of the neck

Grading. Classification of the degree of malignancy

Graves disease. Also known as hyperthyroidism

Growth disturbance. *See* altered tissue growth

Gynecomastia. Enlargement of the male breast

Hamartoma. An abnormal development of tissue that resembles a neoplasm but is actually not a tumor

Hemangioma. Congenital anomaly where there is a proliferation of blood vessels that creates a mass appearance

Hematoma. Localized mass of extravasated blood that is relatively or completely confined within an organ

Hepatic encephalopathy. Associated with cirrhosis of the liver, passage of toxic material from the portal system to the systemic system leading to cerebral manifestation that may include coma

Hepatitis. Inflammation of the liver, usually from a viral infection

Hepatoma. A malignant neoplasm arising from parenchymal cells of the liver

Hereditary. Transmitted by parent to offspring through germ cells

Hernia. Protrusion of a part through the tissues that would normally contain it

Hiatal hernia. Protrusion of a part of the stomach through the esophageal hiatus of the diaphragm; there are two types. sliding esophageal and paraesophageal

High-osmolality contrast media (HOCM). Contrast media that has an osmolality greater than human plasma

Hirschsprung disease. *See* aganglionic megacolon

Horseshoe kidney. Congenital anomaly where the lower poles of each kidney are fused by a band that extends across the midline of the body

Hydrocele. Collection of fluid in the testes or along the spermatic cord

Hydrocephaly. Excessive accumulation of cerebrospinal fluid causing dilation of the ventricles and increased intracranial pressure

Hydronephrosis. The result of some obstruction in the ureter or renal pelvis

Hydrophilicity. A tendency of the blood and tissues to absorb fluid

Hypernephroma (Grawitz). Malignant tumor arises from renal tubule cells, destroying the kidney and invading the blood vessels, in particular the renal vein and inferior vena cava

Hyperosmolar. A solution that has higher osmotic concentration of particles in solution as compared to blood plasma

Hyperplasia. Exaggerated response to stimuli causing an increase in number of cells

Hypertensive heart disease. Refers to heart conditions that arise from hypertension

Hyperthyroidism. Excess thyroid hormone that usually occurs in women between the ages of 30 and 40 years

Hypertonic. The same as hyperosmolar; when a fluid is hypertonic, it will create dehydration

Hypertrophy. Increase in the size of an organ

Hypoparathyroidism. Increased secretion of the parathyroid hormone

Hypopituitarism. Results from a deficiency of the growth hormone; in children it results in dwarfism and in adults it results in Simmonds disease

Hypothyroidism. Undersecretion of the thyroid hormone

Hypoxia. Decrease of oxygen to below normal levels

Iatrogenic. Unfavorable response that is induced by the treatment for another process

Idiopathic. Of unknown cause

Incidence. Number of new persons falling ill with a specific disease in a given time frame

Incompetent. Incapable of performing the required function even though the anatomy required is present

Infarct. An area of necrotic tissue

Infections. Invasion of the body with organisms that have potential to cause disease

Inflammation. Response of tissue to injury or destruction

Insufficient. Anatomical features required to perform a function are not adequate

Internal hydrocephaly. Hydrocephalus that occurs from a blockage in the foramen from the ventricles into the subarachnoid space causing the cerebrospinal fluid to stay within the ventricles

Intracerebral hemorrhage (intraparenchymal hemorrhage). Bleeding within the substance of the brain tissue

Intussusception. The telescoping of one segment of the bowel into another

Invasion. A method of metastasis to occur; direct extension of neoplastic cells into surrounding tissue

Ischemia. Deficiency of oxygen and blood in the muscle

Iso-osmolar. Having the same osmolality as another fluid; in this case, any contrast that has the same osmolality as human plasma

Jaundice. Denotes a yellowish cast to the skin and sclera; there are medical (nonobstructive) and surgical (obstructive) types

Legg-Calvé-Perth. Necrosis of the femoral head epiphyseal ossification center

Leiomyoma. A benign smooth muscle tumor

Lesions. Pathologic change in tissue

Low-osmolality contrast media (LOCM). Contrast media that has osmolality that is closer to that of human blood plasma

Malignant neoplasm. Cancerous tumor

Malunion. Bone fragments do not heal in proper relationship to each other

Manifestations. Observed changes of the patient due to disease

Mechanical small bowel obstruction. Obstruction of the bowel due to some structural cause such as adhesions, stones, tumors, etc.

Meckel diverticulum. The remains of the yolk stalk of the embryo persists on the ileum of the adult instead of being absorbed into the bowel wall after birth

Medullary. Bone marrow cavity found in the center of the shaft of long bones

Medulloblastoma. Malignant neoplasm that occurs most often in children arising from the cerebellum

Meningioma. A benign encapsulated neoplasm of arachnoid origin

Meningitis. Inflammation of the membranes of the brain and spinal cord

Menopause. Permanent cessation of the menses

Menstrual cycle. The period of time in which an egg matures, ruptures from the ovary, enters into the uterus through the fallopian tube, and endometrium of the uterus sloughs off

Metaplasia. Transformation of a differentiated tissue into an abnormal tissue

Metastasis. Spread of diseased cells from one location to another

Microcephaly. Abnormal smallness of the head

Miscibility. Capable of being mixed with some other fluid and remaining mixed

Morbidity rate. Proportion of people in a population with a given disease in a given time frame

Mortality rate. Estimate of number of population that will die from a disease during a specific period of time

Myocardial infarction. Necrosis of an area of the heart muscle, most often caused by an occluded coronary artery

Myxedema. Condition of nonpitting edema associated with hypothyroidism

Necrosis. Death of cells in an injured area

Neoplasia. Abnormal tissue growth by cellular proliferation more rapidly than normal

Nephroblastoma (Wilms tumor). This malignant tumor occurs in children under the age of 5 years; found deep within the flank

Nephron. A long convoluted tubular structure that is the functional unit of the kidney

Nephroptosis. A floating kidney, which occurs when the kidney is not fixed to the peritoneum

Nephrosis. Degeneration of the renal tubular epithelium

Neuroblastoma. A tumor of the adrenal medulla affecting children under the age of 5 years

Neurofibroma. A benign encapsulated tumor occurring in the spinal cord and characterized by foraminal widening

Neurons. Functional unit of the nervous system consisting of the cell body with dendrites and axons

Nocturia. Excessive urination at night

Nonunion. Bone fragments that do not heal

Nosocomial. New process associated with being treated in a hospital

Nulligravida. A woman who has never conceived a child

Nullipara. A woman who has never given birth to a child

Orchiectomy. Excision of one or both testes

Orchiopexy. Fixation of undescended testes in the scrotum

Osgood-Schlatter. Inflammation with partial avulsion of the tibial apophysis

Osmolality. The concentration of a solution expressed in weight of the molecule in solution

Ossification. Formation of bone

Osteitis. Inflammation of the bone

Osteitis deformans. *See* Paget disease

Osteoblast. A bone-forming cell

Osteochondritis dissecans. When a portion of joint cartilage and underlying bone separate

Osteoclast. A cell that absorbs and removes osseous tissue

Osteoclastoma. *See* giant cell tumor

Osteodystrophy. Defective formation of bone

Osteogenesis imperfecta. Abnormal fragility and plasticity of bone with recurring fractures with little or no traumatic effects

Osteomalacia. Disease characterized by a gradual softening and bending of the bones due to lack of calcium

Osteomyelitis. Inflammation of the bone marrow and adjacent bone

Osteopenia. A series of diseases that show a decreased calcification or density of bone

Osteopetrosis. Excessive formation of calcium in bones creating overly dense bones

Osteoporosis. Disease process in which the skeletal tissue is reduced and there is a lack of calcium

Ovulation. Release of mature ova from the ovarian follicle

Paget disease. Generalized skeletal disease of older persons where bone resorption and formation are both increased

Pancreatitis. Inflammation of the pancreas

Paralytic ileus. Aka adynamic ileus; obstruction of the bowel due to paralysis of the bowel wall causing failure of peristalsis

Pathogenesis. Sequence of events that renders the disease apparent

Pathology. Science concerned with all aspects of disease

Pelvis inflammatory disease (PID). Inflammation of the fallopian tubes (uterine tubes)

Perfusion. The flow of blood per unit volume of tissue

Pericardial effusion. Increased amount of fluid in the sac around the heart (pericardium); may be due to inflammation

Periosteum. Thick outer membrane that covers the entire surface of bone

Peristaltic asynchrony. Esophageal motility becomes tertiary contractions

Persistence. In terms of contrast media, it means the ability of the contrast to stay in the body

Phagocytosis. Engulfing microbiological organisms by phagocytes in order to neutralize and destroy injurious agents

Pheochromocytoma. Benign neoplasm that most commonly arises in the adrenal medulla

Pleural effusion. Fluid in the pleural cavity that is caused by inflammation

Pneumonconiosis. Inhalation of certain dusts that causes inflammation leading to fibrosis of the lungs

Pneumonia. When the lung parenchyma becomes inflamed, the alveoli are filled with exudate

Pneumothorax. Air or gas in the pleural cavity

Polycystic ovarian disease. An endocrine disorder resulting from long-term anovulation, in which the enlarged ovaries contain many follicles that fail to reach maturity and rupture

Polycystic renal disease. A progressive disease characterized by formation of multiple cysts of different sizes scattered throughout both kidneys

Prevalence. Refers to the number of people who have a given pathologic process

Primary hyperparathyroidism. Caused by the parathyroid gland secreting excess parathyroid hormone

Procedures. An act or treatment conducted to make a diagnosis

Progeria. Normal development in the first year followed by retardation of growth, and a senile appearance characterized by dry, wrinkled skin, total alopecia, and birdlike facial features

Prognosis. A forecast of the probable course or outcome of a disease

Prostatic calculi. A concentration of calcium formed in the prostate gland

Prostatic hyperplasia. Benign enlargement of the prostate gland leading to urinary dysfunction

Pseudocysts. Accumulation of fluid in a cyst-like loculus

Pulmonary edema. Fluid in the lung tissues (not in the vascular system) usually caused by mitral valve stenosis

Pulmonary emboli. Embolism in the pulmonary arteries that frequently come from the leg or pelvis following a surgery or confinement to bed

Pulsion diverticula. A diverticula that was caused by pressure from inside of the lumen

Purulent. Containing pus

Pyelonephritis. Inflammation of the kidney and renal pelvis

Pyloric stenosis. A narrowing of the pylorus that occurs either congenitally or is acquired

Pyosalpinx. Accumulation of pus in the fallopian tube

Pyuria. Presence of pus in the urine

Regional enteritis. Idiopathic chronic enteritis of the terminal ileum; there are deep ulcers and narrowing and thickening of the bowel

Renal agenesis. Total failure of a kidney to develop

Renal calculi. Stones that form anywhere in the urinary system

Renal cell carcinoma. *See* hypernephroma

Renal ectopia. Condition of a misplaced kidney, usually found in the pelvis

Renal failure. Impairment of renal function, with retention of urea, creatinine, and other waste

Respiratory distress syndrome (RDS). A condition that occurs primarily in premature infants who are born with insufficient surfactant in the lungs, causing the alveoli to collapse

Respiratory syncytial virus (RSV). A virus that can cause a minor respiratory infection in adults but a more serious infection in young children; severe bronchitis and bronchopneumonia are commonly caused by the RSV in children

Rheumatic heart disease. Disease of the heart caused by rheumatic fever; the valves of the heart are most affected

Rheumatoid spondylitis. *See* ankylosing spondylitis

Schatzki ring. A radiographic demonstration of a narrow constriction that occurs at the distal esophagus with a sliding hiatal hernia

Scoliosis. Abnormal lateral curvature of the spine

Secondary hyperparathyroidism. Excess parathyroid hormone is secreted because of some influence on the parathyroid gland rather than from something being wrong with the glands themselves

Seminomas. Malignant neoplasm of the testes

Septal defects. Defects in the septum in the heart; particularly referring to openings between the atria or the ventricles; *See* shunts

Sequestrum. Piece of dead or necrotic bone tissue

Shunts. A bypass of fluid from one area to another

Side effect. An unintended reaction to contrast media that is of little or no consequence

Signs. Abnormality indicative of disease that is discovered by the patient

Simmonds syndrome. Trauma or inflammation (including tumors) of the anterior pituitary lobe creating insufficiency of hormone secretions

Situs inversus. Reversal of position or location; referring to the organs of the body when their positions are a mirror image of normal

Spermatocele. Cystic dilation of the epididymis containing spermatozoa

Spermatogenesis. The entire process by which spermatogonial stem cells divide and differentiate in sperm

Spina bifida. Failure of one or more vertebral arches to fuse

Staging. Description of the extent of involvement of a disease process

Stenosis. A stricture or narrowing of any canal, but especially a narrowing of a cardiac valve or blood vessel

Stroke. Any clinical event that involves the circulation of the cerebral area and lasting longer than 24 hours

Structural disease. Physical and biochemical changes within the cell that alter the organ

Struvite calculi. A type of calculus in which the crystal component consists of magnesium ammonium phosphate

Subarachnoid hemorrhage. A bleed located in the space beneath the arachnoid membrane and above the pia mater

Subdural empyema. Area of pus located in the subdural space

Subdural hematoma. An accumulation of blood in the subdural space

Sub-lethal cell injury. Injury to a cell that does not cause it to die

Subluxation. An incomplete dislocation

Suppurative inflammation. An inflammation that exudes pus

Symptoms. Departure from the normal as experienced by the patient

Synarthrodial. Fibrous joints that are immovable

Teratoma. A true neoplasm, either benign or malignant, made up of different types of tissue, usually found in an ovary or testes (also called a dermoid)

Testicular torsion. The twisting of the testicle upon its cord within the scrotum

Tests. Method to determine the presence or absence of a disease in fluid, tissue, or excretions of the body

Thrombus. A clot in the cardiovascular system

Thyroid adenoma. Benign neoplasm of the thyroid gland; it is rarely symptomatic but palpable

Tonicity. The osmotic pressure of a solution relative to that of blood

Toxicity. The state of being poisonous

Traction diverticula. A diverticula that is formed from a pulling force from outside the lumen of the distal esophagus

Transient ischemic attacks. A sudden focal loss of neurologic function with complete recovery usually within 24 hours

Transitional vertebra. Appearance of vertebrae mimics the one above or below it

Transudate. Fluid that has passed through a normal membrane as a result of an imbalance of osmotic pressure

Trauma. Refers to a physical injury, but can be a mental injury

Tubal ovarian abscess. An abscess formation in the pelvic adnexa region of the ovary and the uterine tubes

Tuberculosis. Caused by *Mycobacterium tuberculosis*, this opportunistic infection affects most often the lung tissue but can affect almost any tissue

Ulcer. A lesion that penetrates a cutaneous or mucosal surface and is accompanied by inflammation

Ureterocele. Cyst-like dilatations of a ureter near its opening into the bladder

Uric. Relating to urine; uric stones contain uric acid, which are white crystals that are hard to dissolve and are found in urine

Valsalva (maneuver). A forced exhalation or strain causing the venous return to the right atrium to be impeded; this study is done to study cardiovascular effects or to determine hiatal hernias

Valvular disease. Any process that changes the structure or function of the valves of the heart, causing other pathologies to exist

Varices. The plural of varix, varices are dilated veins that become enlarged and tortuous

Vesicoureteral reflux. Backward flow of urine from the bladder into the ureter

Viscosity. The resistance to flow (the thickness of a material)

Volvulus. A twisting of the bowel that will cause an obstruction

References

Chapter 02

1. Berquist T. *Musculoskeletal Imaging Companion*. 2nd ed. Baltimore: Wolters Kluwer, Lippincott: Williams & Wilkins; 2007:532–542.
2. Brusin JH. Radiologic technology. *Osteogenesis Imperfecta*. 2008;79(6).
3. Dirckx J, ed. *Stedman's Concise Medical Dictionary for the Health Professions*. 4th ed. Baltimore; 2001.
4. Greenfield G. *Radiology of Bone Diseases*. 3rd ed. Philadelphia: Lippincott; 1980.
5. Manaster BJ. *Handbook of Skeletal Radiology*. 2nd ed. St. Louis: Mosby; 1997.
6. Resnick D. *Bone and Joint Imaging*. 2nd ed. Philadelphia: Saunders; 1996.
7. Yochum T, Rowe L. *Essentials of Skeletal Radiology*. 3rd ed. Vol. 1 and 2. Baltimore: Lippincott, Williams & Wilkins; 2005.

Chapter 03

1. Albertson D. *The Recipe to Respiratory Health*. Ebsco Publishing; 2006.
2. Dahnert W. *Radiology Review Manual*. 3rd ed. Baltimore: Williams & Wilkins; 1996.
3. Gamsu G, Patel, MD. *Diagnostic Imaging Review*. Philadelphia: Saunders; 1998.
4. Juhl JH, Crummy AB. *Essentials of Radiologic Imaging*. 5th ed. Philadelphia: Lippincott; 1987.
5. McPhee SJ, Lingappa VR, Canong WF, Lange, JD. *Pathophysiology of Disease, an Introduction to Clinical Medicine*. Stamford, CT: Appleton & Lange; 1995.
6. Mettler F. *Essentials of Radiology*. Philadelphia: Saunders; 1996.
7. Reed JC. *Chest Radiology, Plain Film Patterns and Differential Diagnoses*. 4th ed. St. Louis: Mosby; 1997.
8. *Stedman's Concise Medical Dictionary for the Health Professions*. 4th ed. Baltimore: Lippincott Williams & Wilkins; 2001.

Chapter 07

1. Dahnert W. *Radiology Review Manual*. 3rd ed. Baltimore: Williams & Wilkins; 1996.
2. Eisenberg RL. *Clinical Imaging: An Atlas of Differential Diagnosis*. 5th ed. Philadelphia, PA: Wolters Kluwer Lippincott, Williams & Wilkins; 2010.
3. Gamsu G, Patel MD. *Diagnostic Imaging Review*. Philadelphia: Saunders; 1998.

4. Juhl JH, Crummy AB. *Essentials of Radiologic Imaging*. 5th ed. Philadelphia: Lippincott; 1987.
5. McPhee SJ, Lingappa VR, Canong WF, Lange JD. *Pathophysiology of Disease, an Introduction to Clinical Medicine*. Stamford, CT: Appleton & Lange; 1995.
6. Mettler F. *Essentials of Radiology*. Philadelphia: Saunders; 1996.
7. *Stedman's Concise Medical Dictionary for the Health Professions*. 6th ed. Baltimore: Lippincott Williams & Wilkins; 2008.
8. U.S. Cancer Statistics Working Group. *United States Cancer Statistics: 1999–2007 Incidence and Mortality Web-Based Report*. Atlanta GA: Department of Health and Human Services, Center for Disease Control and Prevention and national Cancer Institute; 2010. http://www.cdc.gov/uscs
9. Weissleder R, Rieumont MJ, Wittenberg J. *Primer of Diagnostic Imaging*. 2nd ed. St. Louis, MO: Mosby; 1997.
10. *Your Daughter Could Become 1 Less Life Affected by Cervical Cancer.* "Gardasil" Pamphlet Produced by Merck & Co., Inc.; 2006.

Chapter 08

1. Eisenberg RL. *Clinical Imaging: An Atlas of Differential Diagnosis*. 5th ed. Philadelphia, PA: Wolters Kluwer Lippincott, Williams & Wilkins; 2010.
2. Dahnert W. *Radiology Review Manual*. 3rd ed. Baltimore: Williams & Wilkins; 1996.
3. Gamsu G, Patel MD. *Diagnostic Imaging Review*. Philadelphia: Saunders; 1998.
4. Higgins C, de Roos A. *MRI and CT of the Cardiovascular System*. Baltimore: Lippincott, Williams & Wilkins; 2006.
5. Juhl JH, Crummy AB. *Essentials of Radiologic Imaging*. 5th ed. Philadelphia: Lippincott; 1987.
6. McPhee SJ, Lingappa VR, Canong WF, Lange JD. *Pathophysiology of Disease, an Introduction to Clinical Medicine*. Stamford, CT: Appleton & Lange; 1995.
7. Mettler F. *Essentials of Radiology*. Philadelphia: Saunders; 1996.
8. *Pathophysiology Made Incredibly Easy*. 5th ed. Baltimore MD: Lippincott; 1997.
9. *Stedman's Concise Medical Dictionary for the Health Professions*. 6th ed. Baltimore: Lippincott Williams & Wilkins; 2008.
10. Weissleder R, Rieumont MJ, Wittenberg J. *Primer of Diagnostic Imaging*. 2nd ed. St. Louis, MO: Mosby; 1997.

Chapter 09

1. Dahnert W. *Radiology Review Manual.* 3rd ed. Baltimore: Williams & Wilkins; 1996.
2. Eisenberg R. *Clinical Imaging an Atlas of Differential Diagnosis.* 5th ed. Philadelphia: Wolters Kluwer Lippincott, Williams & Wilkins; 2010.
3. Gamsu G, Patel MD. *Diagnostic Imaging Review.* Philadelphia: Saunders; 1998.
4. Juhl JH, Crummy AB. *Essentials of Radiologic Imaging.* 5th ed. Philadelphia: Lippincott; 1987.
5. McPhee SJ, Lingappa VR, Canong WF, Lange JD. *Pathophysiology of Disease, an Introduction to Clinical Medicine.* Stamford, CT: Appleton & Lange; 1995.
6. Mettler F. *Essentials of Radiology.* Philadelphia: Saunders; 1996.
7. *Pathophysiology Made Incredibly Easy.* 5th ed. Baltimore MD: Lippincott; 1997.
8. Romans LE. *Computed Tomography for Technologists Exam Review.* Philadelphia: Wolters Kluwer Lippincott, Williams & Wilkins; 2011.
9. Scott A, Fong E. *Body Structures & Functions.* 11th ed. New York: Delmar Cengage Learning; 2009.
10. *Stedman's Concise Medical Dictionary for the Health Professions.* 6th ed. Baltimore: Lippincott Williams & Wilkins; 2008.
11. Weissleder R, Rieumont MJ, Wittenberg J. *Primer of Diagnostic Imaging.* 2nd ed. St. Louis, MO: Mosby; 1997.

Chapter 10

1. Eisenberg RL. *Clinical Imaging: An Atlas of Differential Diagnosis.* 5th ed. Philadelphia, PA: Wolters Kluwer Lippincott, Williams & Wilkins; 2010.

2. Gamsu G, Patel MD. *Diagnostic Imaging Review.* Philadelphia: Saunders; 1998.
3. Gould BE, Buttle G. *Pathophysiology for the Health Professions.* 10th ed. Philadelphia: Saunders, Elsevier; 2006.
4. *Pathophysiology Made Incredibly Easy.* 5th ed. Baltimore MD: Lippincott; 1997.
5. Romans LE. *Computed Tomography for Technologists Exam Review.* Philadelphia: Wolters Kluwer Lippincott, Williams & Wilkins; 2011.
6. Scott A, Fong E. *Body Structures & Functions.* 11th ed. New York: Delmar Cengage Learning; 2009.
7. *Stedman's Concise Medical Dictionary for the Health Professions.* 6th ed. Baltimore: Lippincott Williams & Wilkins; 2008.

Chapter 11

1. *ACR Practice Guidelines for the Use of Intravascular Contrast Media.* American College of Radiology; 2007.
2. Katzberg RW. *The Contrast Media Manual.* Baltimore: Williams & Wilkins; 1992.
3. Peppers M. Pharmacological mechanisms of radiologic contrast media. *Sem Radiol Technol.* 1995;3(3).
4. Romans LE. *Computed Tomography for Technologists Exam Review.* Philadelphia: Wolters Kluwer Lippincott, Williams & Wilkins; 2011.
5. *Stedman's Concise Medical Dictionary for the Health Professions.* 6th ed. Baltimore: Lippincott Williams & Wilkins; 2008.

Index

Page numbers followed by *f* indicate figures; those followed by *t* indicate tables.

A

abscess, 6
  lung, 62, 63*f*
achalasia, 96, 98*f*
achondroplasia, 22, 23*f*
acoustic neuromas, 255
acromegaly, 266, 266*f*
Addison disease (adrenocortical insufficiency), 270
adenocarcinoma, 110, 111*f*, 121, 145
  infiltrating (linitis plastica), 110, 111*f*
  papillary (fungating) tumors, 110, 110*f*
  ulcerating tumors, 110
adenomyosis, 192
adrenal glands, 263–4, 270–2
  anatomy, physiology, and function, 263–4
    aldosterone, 263
    epinephrine, 264, 264*f*
    glucocorticoids, 263
    mineralocorticoids, 263
    norepinephrine, 264
  pathology, 270–2
    Addison disease, 270
    Cushing syndrome, 270*f*
    neuroblastoma, 271, 271*f*
    pheochromocytoma, 271
adrenocorticotropic hormone (ACTH), 262
adult respiratory distress syndrome (ARDS), 62–3, 63*f*
adverse reaction, 286
aganglionic megacolon, *see* Hirschsprung disease
alcoholic liver disease, 133
aldosterone, 263
altered tissue growth, 7
alveoli, 58
amphiarthrodial joints, 13
ampulla of Vater, 131
anaphylactic, 287
anastomosis, 215–16
anencephaly, 242, 242*f*
aneurysm, 219–20, 227–8
ankylosing spondylitis (rheumatoid spondylitis), 45
anoxia, 5
aphasia, 247
appendicular skeleton, 13

Arnold-Chiari syndrome, 245
arterial aneurysm, 220*f*
arteriosclerosis, 214, 215*f*
arteriosclerotic heart disease, 221, 222
arthritis, 42
  osteoarthritis (degenerative joint disease (DJD)), 42–3
  rheumatoid arthritis (RA), 43, 49*f*
ascites
asthma, 63
  extrinsic, 63–4
  intrinsic, 64
astrocytoma, 252
atelectasis, 64–5, 65*f*
  adhesive, 65
  cicatrizing, 65
  compressive, 64–5, 65*f*
  obstruction, 64, 64*f*, 65*f*
  passive, 65, 65*f*
atherosclerosis, 213, 219, 221, 227
atresia, 96, 97*f*
  rectal, 115, 115*f*
atrial septal defect (ASD), 216*f*
atrophy, 5
  disuse, 5
  endocrine, 5
  pressure, 5
  senile, 5
autonomic nervous system, 238
axial skeleton, 13

B

bacteriuria, 166
Barrett esophagus, 103, 103*f*
basilar skull fracture, 251*f*
benign neoplasm, 8
bezoar, 106–7
  gastric, 107
    phytobezoar, 107, 107*f*
    trichobezoar, 107, 107*f*
bifid system, 155, 156*f*
bile, 132
bile ducts
  anatomy, 130–1